To Kathrin

Contents

Part 2: Keeping Cancer at Bay

Part 3: Menu Planning for Side Effect Management

Part 4: Recipes for Cancer Treatment and Beyond

Foreword

This book answers the basic questions you will have about your cancer. It systematically reviews the steps that patients go through during a course of cancer treatment, be it surgery, radiation, or chemotherapy, and identifies the relevant nutritional considerations.

I would like to congratulate Jean LaMantia on the completion of this book. When she first presented her vision of it to me, I was immediately interested in contributing to the project. Nutrition and diet are essential to the health of all cancer patients, helping them to feel good about their quality of life and enabling them to better cope with cancer treatments and their side effects. Until now, evidence-based information on the nutritional needs of cancer patients has been scattered, but this thoroughly researched book brings together the best evidence in one place, providing informed guidance for those who have been touched by cancer. Jean LaMantia is a practicing registered dietitian who speaks from experience in battling her own cancer and her father's cancer.

This book answers the basic questions you will have about your cancer. It systematically reviews the steps that patients go through during a course of cancer treatment, be it surgery, radiation, or chemotherapy, and identifies the relevant nutritional considerations. Jean explains the mechanisms behind many cancer-related symptoms and provides logical recommendations on strategies to minimize these symptoms. In addition, she gives practical advice on how to maintain healthy nutritional intake on assessment and treatment days and how to benefit from family members or friends who are willing to help you. She answers basic questions such as "What should I eat?"; "What shouldn't I eat?"; and, most importantly, "How can I optimize my nutrition to reduce the risk of cancer development or recurrence?"

You will also find answers to questions about complementary and alternative cancer remedies, including information on how nutraceuticals, prebiotics, and probiotics work, and how omega-3 fatty acids, antioxidants, vitamins, and other nutrients can reduce inflammation, boost the immune system, and even kill cancer cells.

Oncologists know — unfortunately, all too well — that there may come a time when a cancer has progressed too extensively for active treatments to be available. New questions arise. Perhaps a patient cannot eat well, or is not sufficiently alert to do so. What are the nutritional options? What can be done to optimize patient comfort?

Many patients with cancer have pre-existing conditions or illnesses that must also be managed. Some of these conditions — including diabetes, heart disease, and obesity — have an impact on cancer, and vice versa. In addition, certain treatments for cancer may have an impact on these conditions, so patients need a heightened awareness of what could happen.

Jean provides current, state-of-the-art information on how to favorably modify your diet and, once treatments are completed, how to optimize your body's ability to suppress or prevent cancer recurrence or development. One note of caution: when it comes to alternative remedies that do not have a high level of clinical trial evidence to prove their efficacy, we must be careful not to compromise standard cancer therapies that have been well researched. That being said, there may be roles for some of these complementary therapies in certain situations. It is always best to discuss alternative therapies with your oncologist before proceeding.

This book is also a living feast. The recipes are delicious creations designed to optimize the nutrition you require either during or after cancer treatment. Each recipe includes a "recommended for" list that makes it easy for you to choose the best recipes for your symptoms. Cancer patients, cancer survivors, family members, friends and anyone who wants to optimize their diet to reduce the risk of developing cancer will find this book their "go-to" resource.

I am delighted to have contributed to this book. I provided input on common clinical issues, validating Jean's research, and helped provide interpretations of the medical literature she cites. She has collected, analyzed, and synthesized a wealth of knowledge, not only from thorough research but also from her busy practice and, more poignantly, from personal battles with cancer — both her own and her father's. These experiences have helped her create an exceptional book that is relevant to anyone coping with cancer.

As a clinical medical oncologist and cancer researcher, I am pleased to see a book of this quality available to the public and to health-care providers, including oncologists. This book will help me provide better and more factually sound nutritional advice to my patients and their families. I will highly recommend it to the cancer patients I look after, to other cancer patients around the world, and to my oncology colleagues.

— *Neil L. Berinstein, MD, FRCP(C)*

This book is also a living feast. The recipes are delicious creations designed to optimize the nutrition you require either during or after cancer treatment.

Introduction

This book is written for cancer patients, to help you and your caregivers get through your treatment plan by maximizing your nutritional health.

This book is written for cancer patients, to help you and your caregivers get through your treatment plan by maximizing your nutritional health. Cancer and its treatment can have an immediate impact on your nutrition in many ways, making it difficult to swallow due to mouth sores or dry mouth, reducing your appetite, changing your taste for food, and disturbing your normal digestion by causing acid reflux, constipation, or diarrhea. This book contains a detailed nutrition guide for managing these symptoms and side effects, as well as concurrent conditions, such as diabetes and heart disease.

I start by helping you understand cancer basics, and follow this with clear step-by-step strategies focused on specific side effects and conditions. Chief among these strategies is preparing meals with your condition in mind. To this end, I provide nutrient-rich recipes that are not only delicious but also take into account the dietary challenges cancer creates. Keeping yourself well nourished should help you persevere with your treatment plan, get home from the hospital sooner, and experience a speedier recovery.

The Evidence

This book is uniquely trustworthy. I have worked with Dr. Neil Berinstein, a research scientist and medical oncologist at Sunnybrook Health Sciences Centre in Toronto, to interpret the latest evidence-based research dealing with cancer and nutrition so we could make this material easy for you to understand. The reference section located in the back of this book is testament to this effort. These citations are provided for professionals so they can feel confident in recommending this book and for patients and family members who may want to share this information with their health-care team. In addition, I have provided a list of resources you can use to pursue questions specific to your case.

I also bring a unique personal perspective to the subject of cancer and nutrition. I am a cancer survivor, a registered dietician specializing in cancer care, and a family member of a cancer patient. When I was 27 years old, I was diagnosed with Hodgkin's lymphoma. This cancer originates in the white blood cells (lymphocytes) and then spreads to the lymph nodes. My treatment involved 6 months of chemotherapy, followed by another month of daily radiation treatment. I experienced many of the nutrition-related side effects of treatment, including loss of appetite, weight loss, nausea, and vomiting.

In addition, I am a registered dietitian. As a professional, I have counseled many clients with cancer. My first job as a dietitian was working at a large hospital with patients who were at various stages of their cancer treatment and needed help in managing their nutrition during their stay in hospital. A few years later, and after my own fight with cancer, I worked for several years with a home-care agency, which exposed me to many cancer patients living in different households with varying levels of support.

Then my father was diagnosed with a rare form of cancer originating in his gallbladder. Although it had been 14 years since my family had dealt with my cancer, we once again came face to face with this threat. We struggled to help my father maintain his weight and strength so he could survive not only the cancer but also the treatments that were meant to extend his life. Unfortunately, just five months after his diagnosis, he succumbed to his illness. The treatment had devastated his body, but he took the risk. Many cancer patients accept the treatment in the hope that they can beat the cancer into submission and come out of this battle with a good quality of life. I have learned from his experience, and this knowledge is contained in this book.

I have also been blessed to meet a group of cancer survivors who served as my sounding board. Their wisdom and experience is presented throughout this book as "Survivor Wisdom." If you have cancer, you will likely find your concerns and fears mirrored and perhaps allayed in these stories.

Besides providing coping strategies for side effects, dietary therapy may strengthen your immune system while you are fighting cancer and help prevent a recurrence or the development of a new cancer following cure or remission. Your diet can influence whether a cancer cell will thrive and multiply or simply lie in a dormant state. The dietary information presented in this book may spur you to improve your diet, thereby taking an active and positive role in maintaining your health.

Besides providing coping strategies for side effects, dietary therapy may strengthen your immune system while you are fighting cancer and help prevent a recurrence or the development of a new cancer following cure or remission.

The Nutritional Program

My dietary approach to cancer is based on the relatively new field of nutritional immunology. Although I do not claim to have discovered "the" cancer diet, research has shown that foods that are anti-inflammatory, high in whole grains, low on the glycemic

Research has shown that foods that are anti-inflammatory, high in whole grains, low on the glycemic index, and rich in nutraceuticals, phytonutrients, antioxidants, probiotics, and prebiotics may be therapeutic for patients with cancer.

index, and rich in nutraceuticals, phytonutrients, antioxidants, probiotics, and prebiotics may be therapeutic for patients with cancer. These foods support the immune system and have been shown in laboratory studies to be able to stop cancer cells. I have provided lists of foods high in required nutrients throughout the text, as well as many risk-reduction recipes.

I will expand on this evidence, but up front, let me tell you the two key dietary recommendations to support your treatment and reduce the risk of cancer returning:

❶ Eat a plant-based diet with lots of fruits, vegetables, herbs, spices, legumes (pulses), whole grains, and cold-water fish. This will provide the nutrients you need to maintain general good health and help eliminate factors that lead to the development and spread of cancer.

❷ Limit your intake of red meat, refined grains, and alcohol and avoid processed meats and soft drinks (soda pop). This will reduce the dietary sources of inflammation and elevated insulin levels that have the potential to promote cancer, and will help enable beneficial foods and nutrients to do their therapeutic job.

The Recipes and Meal Plans

While I love to cook and try new recipes, I have only a handful of recipes that are my own creation. Thankfully, my publisher had a cast of recipe developers and cookbook writers ready to help. I sifted through their vast catalog of recipes to pick the best ones for this book. I made the selections with several criteria in mind.

First, I selected recipes that would help with symptom management, including appetite loss, weight loss and gain, nausea and vomiting, taste changes, diarrhea, constipation, and mouth sores. Look for the "Recommended for" box at the top left of each recipe and choose the ones that apply to your situation and appeal to your appetite at the moment. As an added benefit, many of the recipes contain suggestions on how to adjust the recipe to accommodate your side effects.

A second criteria was recipes that are simple to prepare, with easy-to-find ingredients — not only for your use, but also for caregivers who may be preparing your meals. These recipes should make cooking and eating easier. Some of the meals and snacks are portable so you can take good food with you to your medical appointments. Many can be prepared ahead. These benefits are highlighted in the "Bonus features" box that accompanies many of the recipes.

Third, a portion of the recipes needed to have the potential to reduce the risk of cancer cell recurrence or development. Research studies have shown that certain foods can reduce inflammation and boost your immune system, while other foods are carcinogenic, feeding the cancer by promoting uncontrolled cell division. Recipes with cancer-fighting potential specify "Risk reduction" in the "Bonus features" box.

To make it easy for you to find recipes that are suitable for your priorities, the index at the back of the book lists recipes by what symptom they help manage. For example, if your appetite is low, look under "L" for the entry "low appetite, recipes for" to see all the recipes suggested for this side effect. The bonus features of the recipes are also indexed in this way.

I have put together a few one-day sample menus. There is no single meal plan that will work for all patients with cancer, so I have devised three to accommodate the more common nutrition issues. In this section, you will find sample menus for an antidiarrhea diet, a liquid and soft foods diet, and a high-energy, high-protein diet.

In addition, to be sure you have anticancer foods on hand, I have assembled a shopping list. Not everyone will want to prepare a meal or a snack, so I have included some ready-to-eat foods you can have on hand. You'll also find information on food safety and storage — highly relevant to cancer patients, given their compromised immune systems.

Certain foods can reduce inflammation and boost your immune system, while other foods are carcinogenic, feeding the cancer by promoting uncontrolled cell division.

The Hope

I hope that this book serves you well, that there is something in these pages that relieves your symptoms, encourages you to eat better, helps you feel empowered, and benefits you in some other wonderful way.

Despite everything that happened to me during my cancer — the fear, the pain, the worry, the countless side effects — I see my cancer as a gift. I will never take my health for granted again. I live my life in a different way — a better way, I think. Even with my father's cancer and death, there was a gift there, too. I was able to communicate with my father in a way that had not been possible up until that point in our lives. I hope that you and your loved ones are able to find a gift in your experience as well. I trust there is something in these pages that makes your cancer journey a little easier.

Wishing you well on your journey,
Jean LaMantia, RD

Part 1

Cancer Therapies and Their Side Effects

1

Conventional Cancer Therapies

Cancer Basics

Most of us have been touched by cancer, as patients or as patients' relatives and acquaintances. According to World Health Organization estimates, there were 12.7 million cases of cancer diagnosed in 2008. Although survival time improved by 4.5% for all cancers combined in the 10 years between 1992–94 and 2002–04, the road between being diagnosed and being cured or progressing into remission can still be a rocky one. Statistics offer some comfort, but understanding how nutrition affects the development of cancer may ease your anxiety more and offer you the opportunity to participate in your own healing process.

Cancer Cells

Our bodies are made up of billions of cells. Throughout our lives, these cells replace themselves through a process of division. Occasionally, cell renewal goes out of control. Cells will rapidly divide in an uncontrolled way, no longer under the control of normal growth factors. Cancer by definition is a group of cells that are growing out of control.

For a normal cell to change into a cancerous cell, its deoxyribonucleic acid (DNA) must be damaged. The DNA is the genetic code of the cell. Things that damage the DNA of cells are called carcinogens. These could include radiation, smog, pollutants, cigarette smoke, or other factors in our body's environment, including chronic inflammation.

Once the DNA change takes place, this altered cell can live for a long time. If our bodies provide an environment that promotes the life of this cell, the cell will grow into a lump or tumor and will make itself known in our lifetime. If we do not make that cancerous cell feel welcome, it can remain in our bodies but won't bother us. Keeping the immune system healthy is a key factor in controlling or even eliminating cancer cells. Cancer treatments may kill cancer cells directly or create an unfavorable environment in the body, so that cancer cells cannot grow.

Survivor Wisdom

There is fear and anxiety with cancer, and friends want to help "fix it," and this takes the form of giving advice. Thank them for their interest and know it is well intended.

Diagnostic Procedures

There may be a delay from the time that cancer is first suspected until a diagnosis is confirmed and a treatment plan can be initiated. During this time, the pathology of the tumor will be examined to determine if it is benign or malignant and, if malignant, the type and stage of development. "Staging" describes the severity of the cancer at the tumor site and the spread, or metastasis, of the cancer to other parts of the body.

Diagnostic procedures include medical imaging — such as X-rays, computed tomography (CT) scans, and magnetic resonance imaging (MRI) — and biopsies. Biopsy involves using a needle to aspirate, or surgically remove, a sample of the tumor cells or conducting local surgery to scrape suspicious cells off the tumor for study. To biopsy tissue in the gastrointestinal tract, you may need to undergo an endoscopy or colonoscopy, which involves inserting a probe through your mouth or anus. The cells are then sent to the hospital laboratory. There, a lab technician will prepare the cells for analysis and a pathologist will determine the specific type of the cancer cells. For example, there are two major types of lymphoma — Hodgkin and non-Hodgkin. The cancer cells from these two types look different under the microscope. The cells behave differently and have different immune characteristics. Analyzing your cells during diagnosis is essential for your oncologist to determine the best treatment to fight the specific cancer cells that are present in your body.

Standard Treatment Procedures

Most people diagnosed with cancer receive at least one of several possible standard treatments: chemotherapy (which includes cytotoxic, hormone, and biological or immunological therapy), radiation, surgery, or stem cell transplant therapy. These therapies are collectively known as standard, mainstream, or, most commonly, conventional therapies. The word "conventional" is defined in this case as medically accepted or established. Conventional therapies are thoroughly and scientifically researched, refined, and tested on an ongoing basis.

These therapies have become part of the standard of care for cancer patients because there is scientific and clinical evidence that they are effective and safe. They have shown some clinical antitumor activity against your type of cancer. However, they are often accompanied by side effects that in some cases can be extreme.

> **Survivor Wisdom**
>
> *After each chemo session, I felt like I had been hit by a truck and totally flattened. I needed 3 weeks to get back up.*

> **Survivor Wisdom**
>
> *I had lymphoma (cancer of the lymph nodes in my neck), and whenever I drank alcohol, pain would start in my neck and shoot down my arm. I couldn't tolerate alcohol.*

Cancer Talk

Like most medical conditions, cancer has a specialized vocabulary. Here is a brief glossary of key terms to help you understand the language of cancer care.

Adenoma: benign growths that start in the gland cells that line the inner surface of some organs in the body, including the stomach, salivary glands, parotid gland (sides of the face), small and large intestines, and the pituitary, adrenal, thyroid, and prostate glands. They are benign but can progress to become malignant, at which point they are called adenocarcinomas.

Adenocarcinoma: a tumor in a gland that has become a malignant tumor. For example, 95% of stomach cancers are adenocarcinoma.

Adjuvant: treatment used in addition to the primary treatment. Chemotherapy or radiation treatment after surgery, for example, is referred to as adjuvant.

Angiogenesis: the process by which the tumor cells develop their own blood supply to survive.

Anorexia: loss of the desire to eat.

Apoptosis: the normal, preprogrammed cell death that is part of the life of a cell.

Bile acids: acids made in the liver and stored in the gallbladder. After a meal, these acids are secreted into the intestines, where their job is to help the body process dietary fat and remove cholesterol.

Benign: a noncancerous growth that does not spread to other parts of the body; it usually is not life-threatening.

Cachexia: progressive loss of both body fat and muscle, often but not always accompanied by loss of appetite.

Carcinogen: a cancer-causing substance or agent.

Chemotherapy: drugs used to treat cancer.

Colonoscopy: a procedure in which a doctor will use a thin scope (an endoscope) with a light, camera, and magnifying lens to examine the inside of the colon and rectum.

Complementary therapy: cancer treatment that enhances or supports conventional therapies.

Conventional therapies: chemotherapy, radiation therapy, and surgery.

DNA: nucleic acid (deoxyribonucleic acid) that contains genetic information.

Early satiety: feeling full soon after eating a small amount of food.

Endoscope: a thin flexible or rigid tube with a light and lens and a tool for removing tissue samples.

Endoscopy: a procedure that allows a doctor to look inside the body using an endoscope.

Gland: an organ that can secrete a substance, such as hormones or stomach acid.

Gray (Gy): a unit of measure to indicate the radiation absorbed during a treatment.

Immune system: a network of cells and barriers designed to protect the body against destructive forces from inside and outside the body.

Mantle field radiation: radiation directed at the neck, chest, and underarms.

Margin: the healthy tissue surrounding a tumor that is sent with the tumor for laboratory analysis after surgery.

Malignant: cancerous growths or lumps of cells.

Metastasis: the spread of a tumor to other parts of the body.

Mucositis: inflammation and ulceration of the mucus membranes lining the digestive tract.

Nausea: a sensation of unease in the stomach, with an urge to vomit.

Needle biopsy: procedure in which a needle is used to take a sample of tissue from a tumor for laboratory analysis.

Neoadjuvant: preliminary therapy. For example, chemotherapy or radiation given first, before surgery, would be neoadjuvant.

Oncology: the branch of medicine that deals with cancer and tumors.

Oncologist: physician who specializes in chemotherapy (medical oncologist), radiation (radiation oncologist), or surgery (surgical oncologist).

Oral mucositis: inflammation and ulceration of the mouth.

Osteoradionecrosis: injury to the jaw bone as a complication of radiation treatment.

Pathology: the medical study of cells.

Pathologist: a physician specially trained to analyze cells.

Radiation: high-energy rays or particles used to destroy cancer cells.

Recurrence: a disease that is still present after treatment but poses no problem and then "flares up" again.

Relapse: a disease that goes away but comes back.

Relative survival: a rate calculated by dividing the overall survival rate after diagnosis of a disease by the survival rate observed in a similar population that was not diagnosed with that disease. A similar population is composed of individuals with at least age and gender similarities to those diagnosed with the disease.

Remission: absence of disease in patients with chronic conditions.

Satiety: sensation of feeling full while eating.

Staging: the way of classifying a cancer based on the extent of cancer in the body, the size and location of the tumor, and its spread to other body parts.

Tumor: a solid or fluid-filled cyst that may be benign, premalignant, or malignant.

Trismus: inability to open the mouth as a result of radiation treatment.

Surgical biopsy: surgery performed to remove a tumor or part of a tumor for laboratory analysis.

Xerostomia: dry mouth caused by a reduced amount of saliva.

Guide to Preparing for Cancer Therapy

If you have not started your treatment yet, or even if you are in the midst of a treatment plan, you can prepare yourself for therapy or improve your situation by following these 11 guidelines:

1 Get organized at home. You may be surprised how time-consuming your treatment will be. There may be little time for self-care. If you can, do the shopping you need to do so that you will have necessary household items on hand. You may want to start preparing and freezing some meals. Many of the recipes in this book have freeze-thaw instructions with this purpose in mind. In addition, you can consult the suggested shopping list to get ideas for healthy foods to have in your pantry for days you won't feel like cooking. Don't forget to stock up on other items you use regularly, such as tissues, toilet paper, pet supplies, and other toiletry and household items.

2 Make contingency plans in the event that you aren't able to keep up to your normal routine. This could include finding backup drivers who may be able to take your children to school or events, or finding a dog walker or a bird cage or litter box cleaner. You may not need the backup people, but if you have the conversation beforehand, you may find it easier to ask for help when you need it.

3 Consider the logistics of getting to and from your appointments. For many of the treatments, it is not recommended that you drive yourself.

4 Keep in mind that these appointments can take a long time. In the case of chemotherapy, you will usually need to see your oncologist first and have blood work taken. It is not until your oncologist determines that you are fit to proceed that the pharmacy will start to prepare your chemotherapy. Some IV chemotherapy can take hours to infuse, so it is best to talk to your health-care team about the time commitment that will be involved. Radiation treatments are much faster, but time is required to remove your clothes and get positioned properly. Although it takes less time than chemotherapy, radiation is usually scheduled every day for a period of time, whereas chemotherapy is given weekly, biweekly, or on another schedule, depending on your particular regimen.

5 Plan how to communicate your progress with your group of support people. This is one area where you will find that technology can be a big help. Friends and family may be calling to find out how you are doing. Speaking on the phone, especially saying the same thing several times, may exhaust you. What may work for you is to designate a spokesperson. This has worked well for many people when there are a lot of concerned friends and family who would like to know the latest medical update. Your spokesperson can get regular updates from you and then send email, Facebook, or Twitter updates to the people you want to keep in the loop. You will be rewarded with lots of encouragement and support that comes back to you. It is a nice way to keep in touch but doesn't drain your energy by having to speak with people individually on the phone. If your support group is not computer-savvy, you can still have a spokesperson, but they can disseminate the information via telephone to certain people, who can then pass on the report to others. This is a more difficult way to control the accuracy of the update, however, because it relies on people's memory and their understanding of the information.

6 Begin or maintain an exercise routine. In a study looking at pretreatment exercise and quality of life, exercise prior to treatment was shown to reduce anxiety and depression and was associated with a better overall mental and physical quality of life. Walking is probably the best exercise, but find something that works for you.

7 Establish or strengthen a stress-reduction or relaxation routine. There are many community resources that can help with this (see the Resources, page 306). Practicing meditation, visualization, positive affirmations, prayer, and other mindfulness-based strategies can be a big help as you navigate the journey ahead of you.

8 Prepare for reactions from friends and family. Decide how to tell your friends, family, coworkers, and others about your progress. Who will you tell, and when? What are the questions that you need to be prepared to answer? People will react to your news in a variety of often unpredictable ways. It is best to be as informed as you can about your situation so that you can answer questions they may have. You will find that some of your friends and family will rise to the challenge and become more supportive than you could have imagined, while others may retreat and draw back from you. This is not a reflection on you or on the strength of your relationship, but rather an insight into their fear or inability to cope with the news.

9 Be specific in asking for support. When telling people about your diagnosis, it can help if you are as specific as possible about the help you are expecting from them. For example, you may ask a friend to prepare a recipe that you have selected from this book. That is a practical way for them to provide support. Another idea is to ask someone to come to appointments with you or to drop by for a visit on a day when you are feeling up to company.

10 Get your finances in order. You may need to cut down on certain expenses. If you are stopping work, your income replacement will likely not cover 100% of your previous earnings. And some drugs may not be fully covered by your health plan.

11 Improve your diet. This is a good time to start focusing on your diet. Eating healthy, nourishing food will allow you to feel that you are doing your part to help combat the cancer. Consider food to be a complementary therapy for the treatment that you are about to begin. Here are a few recommendations for improving your diet that will be discussed further in this book:
- Reduce your intake of simple sugars and refined carbohydrates.
- Choose whole grains as often as you can.
- Increase your intake of fruits, vegetables, herbs, spices, and legumes (beans, peas, lentils).
- Limit your intake of red meat.
- Avoid processed meats and alcoholic drinks.
- Eat small meals and snacks throughout the day.

Side Effects

Many side effects have a direct impact on your nutritional status and general good health. These side effects are far-ranging, and are outlined in Chapter 2.

Most likely, your cancer support team will brief you on the expected side effects and medical complications of your particular treatment before you begin. You are not alone in your fight against cancer. Your health-care team will likely include an oncologist and nurses specialized in cancer care, as well as a pharmacist, physiotherapist, psychotherapist, speech pathologist, and registered dietitian.

Chemotherapy

Chemotherapy, often simply called chemo, is the medical or drug treatment of cancer. There are three kinds of chemotherapy: cytotoxic therapy, hormone therapy, and biological or immunotherapy.

Cytotoxic Therapy

Cytotoxic therapy refers to the use of drugs designed to stop cancer cells from growing, multiplying, or spreading to other parts of the body. Specific chemotherapy drugs are selected for specific types of cancer. They are toxic to cancer cells and normal body cells, such as bone marrow cells, which have a fast rate of cell turnover.

Common Cytotoxic Medications

There are many kinds of cytotoxic drugs. In some chemotherapy treatment plans, or regimens, individual medications are used. In other regimens, the oncologist will prescribe a "cocktail" of drugs or a sequence of related drugs. Get to know your medications by discussing them with your oncologist and pharmacist. They can help you prepare for any medical and nutritional side effects.

Double-Edged Effect

One advantage of chemotherapy is that it can reach all the cells in your body. Because you either ingest the medication in pill or liquid form or receive it as an injection or intravenously (IV), it gets into the bloodstream and can travel throughout the body. On the one hand, this means it can reach small tumors or cells that may have spread from the original mass. On the other hand, side effects can be wide-ranging and sometimes unpredictable, causing, for example, tingling in your feet and hands and a dry mouth. Unfortunately, chemotherapy has not yet evolved to the point where it can target only the cancer cells and leave all the other, normal cells in the body alone.

Hormone Therapy

Hormone therapy is referred to as chemopreventive because it inhibits cancer progression but does not eliminate the cancer cells. Hormones are made naturally in our bodies by glands and organs and can be made artificially in the laboratory. They travel throughout our bodies in the bloodstream and carry important messages about metabolism, growth, and reproduction. Certain glands and organs, such as the breast, prostate, endometrium, testes, pancreas, adrenal, thyroid, and pituitary glands, are often the site of cancer tumors. Two common drugs used in chemotherapy for breast cancer, for example, are tamoxifen and raloxifene. These drugs work by blocking the effects of estrogen on the growth of malignant breast cancer cells, but they do not stop the production of estrogen.

Side Effects

Possible side effects of hormonal drugs include osteoporosis, hot flashes, decreased libido, impotence, constipation, increased appetite, weight gain, and menstrual irregularities. When glands that produce these hormones (such as the testes or the ovaries) are resected, certain common surgical side effects result. And sometimes side effects are chronic, in that hormones must be taken for a lifetime.

Immunotherapy

Immunotherapy, also known as biological response modifier therapy (BRMT), is designed to "boost" the immune system, enabling it to overcome the invading cancer.

Immune-enhancing agents and BRMT include treatments such as interferon alfa, epoetin alfa, filgrastim, angiogenesis inhibitors, cytokines, colony-stimulating growth factor, bevacizumab, rituximab, and trastuzumab. Immunotherapy also encompasses cancer vaccines and some forms of gene therapy, relatively new techniques in oncology.

These agents work by slowing the growth and spread of cancer cells, stopping some cancers from coming back after treatment, or managing side effects caused by other cancer treatments.

Side Effects

Side effects of immunotherapy include fatigue, weight loss, flu-like symptoms, low blood pressure, chills, fever, bone pain, impaired wound healing, fluid retention, rash, and peripheral neuropathy.

Did You Know?

Hormone Dependent
Some cancers, such as certain types of breast and prostate cancer, are considered hormone dependent, meaning that hormones promote the growth of the cancer. Treatment of these cancers involves adjusting hormone levels, which may involve drugs or surgically removing the hormone-producing gland, such as the thyroid, the ovaries (which produce estrogen), or the testicles (which produce testosterone).

Survivor Wisdom

The process of cancer affects people very differently; some people who were hardly in my sphere were champions for me, and some I thought I could count on were gone, never to return. I had to realize that three great new friends are better than ten associates.

Nutrition-Related Side Effects of Common Chemotherapy Medications

If you do not find the drug that has been prescribed for you on this list, ask your oncologist for information on your medications. Knowing what side effects you may encounter can help you be better prepared.

Medication (Brand)	Therapeutic Target	Administration Site	
carboplatin (Paraplatin)	Ovarian cancer	Intravenous (IV)	
cisplatin (Platinol) (Platinol-AQ)	Cancers of the bladder, ovary, testicles	Intravenous (IV)	
cyclophosphamide (Cytoxan) (Neosar) (Procytox)	Lymphoma, breast cancer, ovarian carcinoma, leukemias	Intravenous (IV) or oral	
daunorubicin (Cerubidine)	Leukemias, lymphomas	Intravenous (IV)	
docetaxel (Taxotere)	Breast cancer, lymphomas, multiple myeloma, lung cancer, prostate cancer	Intravenous (IV)	
doxorubicin (Adriamycin)	Cancers of the breast, bladder, endometrium, and uterus, as well as myelomas	Intravenous (IV)	
etoposide (Vepesid) (VP-16) (Etopophos) (Eposin)	Lung cancer, testicular cancer, leukemias, lymphomas	Intravenous (IV)	

Nutrition-Related Side Effects	Nutrition Notes
• Nausea and vomiting • Salt imbalance • Increased calcium in the blood • Constipation • Diarrhea	• A magnesium supplement may be required.
• Nausea and vomiting that usually occur for 24 hours or longer • Loss of appetite (anorexia) • Diarrhea • Metallic taste • Fluctuations in blood electrolytes	• Drink plenty of fluids (at least 8 cups/2 L per day). • Empty your bladder often.
• Nausea, vomiting, abdominal pain • Decreased appetite • Inflammation of mucus lining of mouth and esophagus • Dry mouth (xerostomia) • Abdominal pain	• No grapefruit, pomegranate, starfruit, Seville oranges, or their juices, as they may interfere with the drug or cause side effects. • Drink plenty of fluids.
• Nausea and vomiting • Poor appetite • Mouth and esophageal ulcers • Diarrhea • Dry mouth • Change in taste acuity	
• Nausea, vomiting, abdominal pain • Diarrhea • Fatigue • Decreased appetite • Numbness and tingling in hands and feet • Liver effects	• No grapefruit, pomegranate, starfruit, Seville oranges, or their juices, as they may interfere with the drug or cause side effects.
• Diarrhea • Nausea and vomiting • Mouth sores	
• Nausea and vomiting • Mouth ulcers • Low blood pressure (during administration) • Decreased appetite • Flu-like symptoms • High blood pressure	• No grapefruit, pomegranate, starfruit, Seville oranges, or their juices, as they may interfere with the drug or cause side effects.

Medication (Brand)	Therapeutic Target	Administration Site	
fluorouracil (5-FU) (Adrucil)	Cancers of the colon, breast, stomach, head, neck	Intravenous (IV)	
irinotecan (Camptosar) (Campto)	Cancers of the colon, rectum	Intravenous (IV)	
methotrexate (Folex) (Mexate) (Amethopterin) (methotrexate sodium)	Cancers of the breast, lung, blood, bone, lymph system	Intravenous (IV), intrathecal (into the spinal column), or oral	
paclitaxel (Taxol) (Abraxane)	Kaposi sarcoma and cancers of the breast, ovary, lung	Intravenous (IV)	
vincristine (Oncovin) (Vincasar PFS)	Leukemias, lymphomas, sarcomas	Intravenous (IV)	

Nutrition-Related Side Effects	Nutrition Notes
• Decrease in blood cell counts • Diarrhea • Mouth ulcers	
• Diarrhea	• No grapefruit, pomegranate, starfruit, Seville oranges, or their juices, as they may interfere with the drug or cause side effects.
• Nausea and vomiting • Mouth ulcers • Poor appetite • Diarrhea • Decreased absorption of B_{12}, folate, and D-xylose • Change in taste acuity	• Keep well hydrated — drink at least 8 glasses of fluid per day. Urinate frequently.
• Nausea and vomiting • Loss of appetite • Change in taste acuity • Mouth and esophageal ulcers • Diarrhea • Fatigue	• Talk to your doctor about grapefruit or grapefruit juice consumption.
• Nausea and vomiting (mild) • Poor appetite • Mouth and esophageal ulcers • Jaw pain • Alternating diarrhea and constipation or abdominal cramping	• No grapefruit, pomegranate, starfruit, Seville oranges, or their juices, as they may interfere with the drug or cause side effects.

Adapted from www.caring4cancer.com; McCallum PD and Grant B, *The Clinical Guide to Oncology Nutrition*, 2nd ed, New York: American Dietetic Association, 2006; Cancer Care Ontario, www.cancercare.on.ca.

Radiation Therapy

Radiation therapy uses energy from X-rays, gamma rays, and electrons to kill or injure cancer cells. Radiation can be given externally or internally. Prior to receiving radiation treatment, your radiation oncologist and the technicians who make up the team will spend time pinpointing exactly where your cancer is located. In this way, they can aim the radiation beam directly at the cancer cells. Unlike chemotherapy, which is exposed to the entire body, radiation is directed as closely as possible to the exact source of the cancer.

Side Effects

Despite efforts to aim the radiation at the cancer cells, some normal cells are caught in the radiation field. This is the source of the side effects of radiation. As well as the skin surface above and below the targeted cancer, any other cells caught in the radiation field will also experience changes. Many times these changes are temporary and the cells will return to normal after the treatment has stopped, but there are some side effects that can remain even after treatment.

The National Cancer Institute at the National Health Institutes in the United States has created a chart itemizing the side effects of radiation treatments. These side effects depend on the part of your body being treated and the form of cancer. Some people will undergo radiation therapy for a longer period than others and the side effects may be more severe. (This information is summarized in the chart on pages 31–33.)

FAQ

Q. *My friend had radiation and she was really tired. Is this common?*

A. Yes, fatigue is a common side effect of radiation, and it doesn't matter which area of your body is being treated. A generalized level of lower energy will likely last throughout the treatment and may persist for several weeks once the treatment is complete. There are several strategies for managing low energy levels, including dietary therapy. These energy-boosting strategies are discussed starting on page 67.

Surgery

Surgery is commonly used to remove a piece of tumor for a biopsy to determine the specific kind of cell in the mass. This will assist your medical team in planning an appropriate treatment, possibly including additional surgery to resect or remove the solid tumor.

Almost any solid tumor, if caught early and found to be localized, can be treated with surgery alone. For example, a common protocol now for colon cancer stage I and II is to treat with surgery without adjuvant chemotherapy. This is also true for early-stage lung cancer and localized renal cancer. A complete resection removes the entire tumor, as well as some healthy surrounding tissues. The healthy tissue surrounding the tumor is referred to as the "margin." The size of the margin depends on the type and location of the tumor.

Sometimes, the entire tumor cannot be removed because it is too large or too close to vital organs. When it is not possible to remove the entire tumor, a procedure called debulking may be used to reduce the size of the tumor. This may make you more comfortable. Debulking can also make chemotherapy and radiation more effective because there is a smaller mass left in the body for these treatments to tackle. In some regimens, surgery may be combined with radiation, chemotherapy, or both.

Adjuvant and Neoadjuvant

When surgery is performed first and followed by radiation or chemotherapy, the chemo or radiation is referred to as "adjuvant" therapy. Your treatment may be done in this order to make sure that any cancer cells that have spread to other parts of the body can be killed and to reduce the risk of your cancer returning or recurring.

In some cases, this order is reversed. Chemotherapy and radiation are given first and then surgery is performed afterwards. In this case, the chemotherapy and radiation are referred to as "neoadjuvant," meaning they are the first but not the only therapy. Performing the treatment in this order can result in the tumor shrinking before surgery. In addition, it can help doctors see the surrounding tissue that has been infiltrated by cancer cells and distinguish it from the margin that is free of cancer but inflamed.

Stem Cell Transplant Therapy

For some cancers, high-dose chemotherapy and/or radiation treatments are required to kill the cancer cells. One side effect of these treatments is that they destroy bone marrow cells, the site of stem cell production.

Stem cells mature into white blood cells (which fight infection), red blood cells (which carry oxygen), or platelets (which help the blood to clot). After high-dose chemotherapy and radiation, the patient can no longer make blood cells that will carry oxygen, fight infection, or prevent bleeding.

Did You Know?

Reconstructive Surgery may also be performed to repair or reconstruct areas of the body, as in the case of breast cancer, for example. Whatever the reason for the surgery, a surgical wound will be a side effect. The healing of the wound is an essential part of the recovery.

Hematopoietic (blood) stem cells are required to provide these cells. Blood stem cells are found chiefly in the marrow, but some, called peripheral blood stem cells, circulate in the bloodstream. Stem cells are also found in blood from the umbilical cord after birth.

Transplant Procedures

Transplanting bone marrow is a complex medical procedure that requires hospitalization with close monitoring.

Bone Marrow

Transplantation can be autologous (the patient's own marrow is removed and banked before chemo or radiation treatments), syngeneic (the marrow is donated by an identical twin), or allogenic (the marrow is donated by someone else with a compatible blood profile). After the patient is anesthetized, the stem cells are drawn using a needle injected into the hip bone. The procedure to harvest the stem cells takes about an hour. The cells can then be frozen or banked.

Peripheral Blood

If the source of the stem cells is the peripheral blood, the blood is removed through a vein and enters a machine that removes the stem cells. The harvested stem cells are then frozen for later transplantation. The procedure is called apheresis.

Cord Blood

Umbilical cord blood stem cells can be banked after birth or acquired from a cord blood bank that stores donated cord blood. Many mothers are now donating their baby's umbilical cord blood so that it can be banked and used later by those in need.

Side Effects

Following chemotherapy or radiation treatments, the banked stem cells can be transplanted intravenously. After 2 to 3 weeks, patients can again make their own healthy blood cells. During this time, the patient is immunocompromised and has a low resistance to infection. Common problems following stem cell transplant therapy include inflammation of the mouth or esophagus (mucositis), dry mouth (xerostomia), thick, ropey saliva, altered taste, poor appetite (anorexia), nausea, vomiting, diarrhea, and constipation.

Special Diet

A special diet will be recommended to help prevent infection following transplantation surgery. The risk of infection can be reduced by avoiding certain foods. Your dietitian will give you a complete list of dietary dos and don'ts during this process; the list that follows is an example.

Foods to Avoid During Recovery from Stem Transplant Therapy

- Raw or undercooked meat
- Luncheon meats
- Nonpasteurized dairy products
- Soft and blue-veined cheeses
- Raw eggs
- Unwashed fruits or vegetables
- Miso
- Moldy or out-of-date foods

> **Survivor Wisdom**
>
> *When people say, "Recovery time is X," this is not a hard-and-fast rule.*

Treatment Protocols

Some people reading this book may be recently diagnosed with cancer and quite anxious about how treatment will proceed. Others may be in the midst of their treatment regimen but are still concerned about the course of what follows. Although every case is different and demands individual care, this chart highlights the standard protocols your oncologist may follow, with the help of your health-care team, for the three major treatment groups.

Medical Oncology	Surgical Oncology	Radiation Oncology
Diagnosis by biopsy	Referral to surgeon for biopsy and/or resection	Referral to radiation oncologist, usually by medical oncologist or surgeon
Pathology review	Biopsy	Review of radiology
Staging	Pathology review	Planning clinic if proceeding with radiation Decision on field of treatment and number of treatments
Selection of treatment	Staging investigations	Discussion of potential side effects with radiation oncologist
Selection of chemotherapy regimen or appropriate hormonal or targeted immunotherapy	Assessment by medical oncologist or radiation oncologist concerning additional therapies that may be required postoperatively (occasionally, chemotherapy is recommended prior to surgery)	Outpatient treatments with daily visits to radiation delivery device

Medical Oncology	Surgical Oncology	Radiation Oncology
Discussion of potential side effects	Admission to hospital for resection Blood work Anesthetic risk assessment	Periodic assessments by radiation oncologist during treatment
Booking of chemo bed	Surgery and pathology review post-surgery	Post-treatment scans to assess response
Nursing assessment concerning intravenous access and chemo education	Repeat assessment of wound healing by surgeon	Continued care with referring physician after completion of radiation treatment
Psychosocial assessment (if required)	Additional treatments by medical or radiation oncologist as required	
Blood assessment prior to chemo visit		
Chemo visit		
Assessment by oncologist before each chemo appointment Discussion of side effects Optimization of supportive care		

Chapter 2

Managing Side Effects and Concurrent Conditions

If you are currently dealing with a cancer diagnosis, your first priority is to get through your treatment program while minimizing side effects. Adjusting your diet is one way to help you manage the nutrition-related side effects of treatment. If you are a caregiver for someone with cancer, you now have the dual role of caring for yourself and your friend or family member.

The side effects you may experience during treatment will depend on the location and size of the tumor, as well as the treatment protocol. The nature, number, and severity of side effects vary from person to person.

The following table outlines the possible effects of the cancer tumor and the corresponding treatment on factors that have an impact on your nutrition. These nutritional side effects can instigate or aggravate quite serious medical conditions, including anorexia, anemia, and diabetes.

> **Survivor Wisdom**
>
> *Your hair may be thin and more brittle during radiation. My fingernails were brittle too. I put lemon juice and olive oil on my nails, and it helped with the discoloration.*

Tumor Site	Tumor's Effect	Nutritional Side Effects		
		Chemotherapy	**Radiation**	**Surgery**
Bladder and urethra		• Nausea • Vomiting	• Inflammation of small intestines	
Breast	• Weight gain	• Weight gain (with hormonal treatment) • Inflammation	• Inflamed esophagus • Nausea	
Central nervous system	• Difficulty swallowing • Headaches • Neurologic symptoms	• Fluid retention • High blood sugar • Increased appetite • Weight gain	• Nausea • Altered taste	

Tumor Site	Tumor's Effect	Nutritional Side Effects		
		Chemotherapy	Radiation	Surgery
Colon and rectum	• Bowel obstruction • Malabsorption of nutrients	• Nausea • Inflammation • Diarrhea	• Inflammation • Narrowing of colon • Malabsorption of nutrients	• Gas • Diarrhea • Sodium imbalance • Fluid imbalance
Esophagus	• Difficulty swallowing • Regurgitation after meals	• Nausea	• Upset stomach • Inflamed esophagus • Acid reflux (heartburn) • Narrowing of esophagus • Fistula • Nausea • Swelling	• Decreased movement of food through the stomach • Decreased stomach acid • Fistula • Narrowing of esophagus • Regurgitation • Fatty diarrhea
Lung	• Difficulty swallowing • Difficulty eating • Shortness of breath • Cough • Chest pain	• Nausea • Vomiting • Inflammation • Altered taste	• Inflamed esophagus • Acid reflux (heartburn)	
Lymph nodes	• Depends on location • Difficulty swallowing • Malabsorption of nutrients	• Nausea • Vomiting • Inflammation of mouth	• Depends on location • Inflamed esophagus or small intestines • Nausea	
Neck, mouth, throat	• Difficulty chewing or swallowing	• Nausea • Vomiting • Diarrhea • Inflammation of the mouth	• Inflammation • Altered or reduced taste • Dry mouth • Difficulty chewing or swallowing • Thick saliva • Mouth and/or throat ulcers • Bone death (usually lower jaw) • Fistula • Difficulty opening jaw	• Impaired chewing or swallowing • Dry mouth

Tumor Site	Tumor's Effect	Nutritional Side Effects		
		Chemotherapy	Radiation	Surgery
Pancreas and biliary tree	• Malabsorption of nutrients • Diabetes • Altered taste • Nausea	• Nausea • Vomiting • Inflammation • Diarrhea	• Nausea • Vomiting	• Diabetes • Malabsorption of fat, protein, fat-soluble vitamins, minerals
Small intestines	• Bowel obstruction or crampy abdominal pain • Malabsorption of nutrients	• Nausea • Inflammation • Diarrhea	• Ulcers • Malabsorption of nutrients • Fistula • Narrowing • Obstruction • Bleeding	• Acidic blood • Kidney stones
Stomach	• Feeling full quickly • Vomiting after meals • Heartburn or pain associated with meals • Vomiting • Black bowel movements	• Nausea • Vomiting • Inflammation • Diarrhea	• Nausea • Vomiting	• Fat malabsorption and diarrhea • Slow emptying of stomach • Flushing of stomach contents into intestines • Low blood sugar • Protein malabsorption • Deficiencies of calcium, fat-soluble vitamins, B_{12} • Swollen esophagus
Uterus, ovaries, and cervix	• Bowel obstruction • Fluid retention • Feeling full quickly • Weight gain	• Nausea • Vomiting • Weight gain (with hormonal drugs)	• Inflammation of small intestines • Fistula • Narrowing • Gas	• Malabsorption of nutrients if there is bowel resection

Adapted with permission from Fisher S, Bowman A, Mushins T, et al., *British Columbia Dietitians' and Nutritionists' Association Manual of Nutritional Care*, Vancouver: British Columbia Dietitians' and Nutritionists' Association; 1992:151–61.

Anemia

The word "anemia" means "low blood" in ancient Greek. When you have anemia, the red blood cells cannot deliver oxygen to other cells in your body as effectively. The symptoms include fatigue, weakness, dizziness, loss of appetite, shortness of breath, loss of energy, looking pale, headaches, difficulty concentrating, and increased susceptibility to infection. If untreated, anemia may cause a delay in planned chemotherapy or radiation treatment.

Iron Deficiency Anemia

Iron deficiency anemia, also known as microcytic anemia, is the most common kind of anemia. Iron is needed to make hemoglobin, which is the main component of red blood cells. Almost two-thirds of the iron in the body is found in the hemoglobin. Hemoglobin carries oxygen to cells throughout the body.

Anemia that responds to iron therapy can occur because of blood loss, poor dietary intake, or poor absorption of iron. Cancer can also suppress red blood cell production. Anemia from chemotherapy will not be helped by iron supplements.

In most cases, anemia from iron deficiency develops gradually. The body maintains a store of iron, and this will be used up first. After iron stores are used up, hemoglobin levels will start to decline.

Recommended Dietary Allowance for Iron

The recommended dietary allowance (RDA), sometimes referred to as recommended daily allowance, is defined as the average daily dietary intake level that is sufficient to meet the nutrient requirements of nearly all (approximately 98%) healthy individuals.

Age	Nonvegetarians	Vegetarians
RDA for Women		
19–50 years	18 mg	33 mg
51+ years	8 mg	14 mg
RDA for Men		
19+ years	8 mg	14 mg

Source: National Academy of Sciences.

Foods with Heme Iron

All iron values or amounts are for cooked meat, fish, shellfish, and poultry. Please note that liver is high in cholesterol, so people with high blood cholesterol levels should not eat it often. In addition, pregnant women should not eat liver. It has a very large amount of vitamin A, which can be harmful to the baby.

Food	Serving	Iron
Liver, pork	2½ oz (75 g)	13.4 mg
Liver, chicken	2½ oz (75 g)	9.2 mg
Oysters	2½ oz (75 g)	6.4 mg
Mussels	2½ oz (75 g)	5.0 mg
Liver, beef	2½ oz (75 g)	4.8 mg
Beef	2½ oz (75 g)	2.4 mg
Shrimp	2½ oz (75 g)	2.2 mg
Clams	2½ oz (75 g)	2.0 mg
Sardines	2½ oz (75 g)	2.0 mg
Lamb	2½ oz (75 g)	1.7 mg
Turkey	2½ oz (75 g)	1.2 mg
Tuna/herring/trout/mackerel	2½ oz (75 g)	1.2 mg
Chicken	2½ oz (75 g)	0.9 mg
Pork	2½ oz (75 g)	0.8 mg
Salmon (canned/fresh)	2½ oz (75 g)	0.5 mg
Flatfish (flounder/sole/plaice)	2½ oz (75 g)	0.3 mg

Source: HealthLink BC.

Blood Loss

Iron deficiency anemia from blood loss is more likely to occur in patients who have had cancers arising in some part of the gastrointestinal system. Some chemotherapy treatments, such as oral corticosteroids, may predispose patients to blood loss. Of course, surgery also causes blood loss, which varies by surgical site. You may not necessarily notice blood loss from cancer because it can leave the body gradually in small amounts via the stool over a long period. Black tarry stools, called melena, are one sign that blood could be leaving the body via the stool.

Foods with Non-heme Iron

Items with an asterisk (*) are fortified with iron. Read the Nutrition Facts table for exact amounts. Iron amounts in some enriched foods vary; check the label for accurate information. If the iron amount is given as a percentage of the daily value (DV), the standard used is 14 milligrams. For example, if a serving of cereal has 25% of the daily value, it has 3.5 milligrams of iron (0.25 × 14 mg).

Food	Serving	Iron
Pumpkin seeds, hulled, roasted	¼ cup (60 mL)	8.6 mg
Tofu, medium-firm or firm	5 oz (150 g)	2.4–8.0 mg*
Soybeans, dried, cooked	¾ cup (175 mL)	6.5 mg
Instant enriched oatmeal	1 package (35 g)	2.8–5.6 mg*
Lentils, cooked	¾ cup (175 mL)	4.9 mg
Hummus	¾ cup (175 mL)	2.9–4.5 mg
Enriched cold cereal	1 oz (30 g)	4.0 mg*
Dark red kidney beans, cooked	¾ cup (175 mL)	3.9 mg
Molasses, blackstrap	1 tbsp (15 mL)	3.6 mg
Spinach, cooked	½ cup (125 mL)	3.4 mg
Refried beans	¾ cup (175 mL)	3.1 mg
Cream of wheat, instant, prepared	¾ cup (175 mL)	3.1 mg*
Soy beverage	1 cup (250 mL)	2.9 mg
Wheat germ, ready to eat, toasted, plain	3 tbsp (30 mL)	2.7 mg
Chickpeas, canned	¾ cup (175 mL)	2.4 mg
Soybeans, green (edamame), cooked and shelled	½ cup (125 mL)	2.4 mg
Tahini (sesame seed butter)	2 tbsp (30 mL)	2.3 mg
Lima beans, cooked	½ cup (125 mL)	2.2 mg
Swiss chard, cooked	½ cup (125 mL)	2.1 mg
Shredded wheat	1 oz (30 g)	1.8 mg*
Quinoa, cooked	½ cup (125 mL)	1.7 mg
Prune juice, canned	½ cup (125 mL)	1.6 mg
Cream of wheat, regular, prepared	¾ cup (175 mL)	1.5 mg
Green peas, cooked	½ cup (125 mL)	1.3 mg
Tomato sauce, canned	½ cup (125 mL)	1.3 mg

Food	Serving	Iron
Sunflower seeds, hulled, roasted	¼ cup (60 mL)	1.2 mg
Whole wheat bread	1 slice	1.2 mg
Eggs	2	1.2 mg
Potato, baked, with skin	1 medium	1.1 mg
Oats, prepared	¾ cup (175 mL)	1.1 mg
Molasses, light (fancy)	1 tbsp (15 mL)	1.0 mg

Source: HealthLink BC.

Poor Diet

In some cases, anemia can develop from poor diet. If your blood levels of iron are low, then it is a good idea to adjust your diet so you include more iron-rich foods. You will likely still need an iron supplement, but the form of iron added to iron-enriched and iron-fortified foods can help bring the level back to normal sooner and keep it there after you've finished the supplements.

There are two forms of dietary iron: heme and non-heme. Heme iron is found in animal foods that originally contained hemoglobin, such as red meats, fish, and poultry. Iron in plant foods is called non-heme iron. Heme iron is absorbed better than non-heme iron. Therefore, the iron requirement for vegetarians is 1.8 times higher than for nonvegetarians, as recommended by the U.S. National Academy of Sciences.

Iron Supplements

Your doctor will likely recommend iron supplements if your levels are too low to be corrected by diet alone or you have symptoms of iron deficiency. Iron supplements provide much higher doses than found in your diet. There are different types of iron supplements, with different levels of elemental iron.

To know how much iron can be used by the body, look on the label for the amount of elemental iron. Iron supplements are available in tablets, enteric-coated tablets, slow-release tablets, capsules, liquids, and drops. The liquids could temporarily stain your teeth. Enteric-coated tablets will have fewer gastrointestinal side effects but are not as well absorbed. For best absorption, take between meals on an empty stomach; however, you may experience more side effects on an empty stomach, so you can adjust your routine as required.

Did You Know?

Know Your Limits
Iron storage levels can be measured by a test called serum ferritin. To raise your iron level, you will need to eat iron-rich foods and take iron supplements. Too much iron in the blood is also not good, so don't supplement your diet without first knowing your levels. You may feel better before your levels are back to the normal range, but don't stop taking the iron supplements until a blood test confirms this is so. The upper level (UL) is the maximum amount of iron you should have from supplements and food combined. The UL for adults 19 years of age and older is 45 milligrams.

Types of Iron Supplements

This chart provides an example of some of the more common iron supplements available.

Type of Iron Supplement	Example of Brand Name	Percentage of Elemental Iron	Comments
Carbonyl iron (U.S. only)	• Ferralet 90	100%	• Microparticles of highly purified elemental iron.
Ferric ammonium citrate	• Iron Citrate	18%	• Less bioavailable than ferrous forms
Ferrous bisglycinate (U.S. only)	• Ferrochel	20%	• Relatively high bioavailability
Ferrous fumarate	• Nephro-Fer • Palafer (Canada)	33%	• Similar tolerance and efficacy as ferrous sulfate
Ferrous gluconate	• Fergon • Floradix	12%	• Similar tolerance and efficacy as ferrous sulfate
Ferrous sulfate	• Fer-In-Sol	20%	• Commonly recommended, given tolerance, effectiveness, and low cost
Ferrous sulfate (dried)	• Slow-FE	30%	• Commonly recommended, given tolerance, effectiveness, and low cost
Heme iron polypeptide	• Proferrin	100%	• Made from red blood cells from pigs • Well tolerated
Polysaccharide iron complex	• Niferex • Triferexx (Canada)	100%	• Similar bioavailability to ferrous sulfate

Source: *Pharmacist's Letter/Prescriber's Letter*. 2008 Aug;24(240811).

Poor Absorption

The amount of iron you absorb from food depends on how much iron you have stored in your body. People with low iron levels absorb more. The amount of iron you absorb also depends on the type of iron you eat. Heme iron is well absorbed. Non-heme iron is not as well absorbed. There are side effects associated with iron supplements, including nausea, vomiting, constipation, diarrhea, dark-colored stools, and/or abdominal distress. For more information on the different types of iron supplements, which is best for you, and tips to help with absorption, consult with your pharmacist.

Guidelines for Improving Iron Absorption

❶ Take iron throughout your day in two to three doses. The amount that can be absorbed from the supplement decreases with the higher doses.

❷ Do not take your iron supplements while you drink coffee and tea, because the oxalic acid in these drinks can reduce absorption. Dairy products and calcium supplements also reduce the absorption of iron.

❸ Eat foods high in vitamin C at each meal to derive the most non-heme iron from foods. Vitamin C–rich foods include bell peppers, oranges, broccoli, Brussels sprouts, strawberries, grapefruit, snow peas, orange and grapefruit juices, and fruit juices with vitamin C added.

❹ Eat foods that contain heme iron to help you absorb non-heme iron. Examples of food combinations that help you get the most iron include chili con carne (beans provide non-heme iron and ground beef provides heme iron); iron-fortified breakfast cereal (non-heme iron) with orange juice (vitamin C); hummus (non-heme iron) and roasted red peppers (vitamin C).

❺ Cook with cast-iron or stainless steel cookware.

❻ See Part 4 for recipes that are high in iron.

Source: HealthLink BC.

Megaloblastic Anemia

This type of anemia is the result of a deficiency of folate or vitamin B_{12}.

Folate Deficiency

Folate is one of the B vitamins: B_9. In its naturally occurring form it is called folate; in its synthetic form, in a fortified food or supplement, it is called folic acid.

In this type of anemia, the bone marrow produces large, abnormal immature red blood cells instead of the normal healthy ones. These defective blood cells cannot carry sufficient oxygen to the body's cells. Symptoms include a feeling of fatigue, lightheadedness, and pale skin, as well as a sore tongue, diarrhea, anorexia, upset stomach, headaches, and forgetfulness. If left untreated, your symptoms will worsen and heart problems may ensue.

> **Survivor Wisdom**
>
> *I had a friend who had breast cancer, and I swear she was taking more supplements than food. Moderation and common sense should prevail.*

Recommended Daily Allowance of Folate

The RDA for men and women aged 19 to 70 is 400 micrograms (mcg) of folate per day. The upper level of folate for adults aged 19 and older is 1000 micrograms per day. Most food labels do not list a food's folate content.

Folic Acid Fortification Program

The FDA and Health Canada have established regulations requiring the addition of folic acid to breads, cereals, flours, corn meals, pastas, rice, and other grain products. These folic acid–fortified products help address the low level of folate in the Western diet.

Food Sources of Folate and Folic Acid

Items marked with an asterisk (*) are fortified with folic acid as part of the folic acid fortification program.

Food	Serving	Folate or Folic Acid
Breakfast cereals fortified with 100% of the DV*	¾ cup (175 mL)	400 mcg
Beef liver, braised	3 oz (90 g)	185 mcg
Cowpeas or black-eyed peas, immature, cooked	½ cup (125 mL)	105 mcg
Breakfast cereals fortified with 25% of the DV*	¾ cup (175 mL)	100 mcg
Spinach, frozen, cooked	½ cup (125 mL)	100 mcg
Great Northern beans, cooked	½ cup (125 mL)	90 mcg
Asparagus, cooked	4 spears	85 mcg
Rice, enriched long-grain white, parboiled, cooked*	½ cup (125 mL)	65 mcg
Baked beans, vegetarian, canned	1 cup (250 mL)	60 mcg
Spinach, raw	1 cup (250 mL)	60 mcg
Green peas, frozen, cooked	½ cup (125 mL)	50 mcg
Broccoli, frozen chopped, cooked	½ cup (125 mL)	50 mcg
Egg noodles, enriched, cooked*	½ cup (125 mL)	50 mcg
Broccoli, raw	2 spears, each 5 inches (12.5 cm) long	45 mcg
Avocado, raw, sliced	½ cup (125 mL)	45 mcg
Peanuts, dry-roasted	1 oz (30 g)	40 mcg
Romaine lettuce, shredded	½ cup (125 mL)	40 mcg
Wheat germ	2 tbsp (30 mL)	40 mcg
Tomato juice, canned	6 oz (175 mL)	35 mcg
Orange juice, fresh or from concentrate	¾ cup (175 mL)	35 mcg

Food	Serving	Folate or Folic Acid
Orange	1 small	35 mcg
Bread, white or whole wheat*	1 slice	25 mcg
Egg	1 large	25 mcg
Cantaloupe	¼ medium	25 mcg
Papaya, cubed	½ cup (125 mL)	25 mcg

Source: National Institutes of Health.

Vitamin B_{12} Deficiency Anemia

Another cause of megaloblastic anemia is low levels of vitamin B_{12}. This vitamin is found only in animal products: meat, shellfish, milk, cheese, and eggs. B_{12} deficiencies can be determined by a blood test. Your physician may recommend B_{12} supplements in a tablet form or by injection. Increasing your intake of foods containing B_{12} is also recommended. Vegans (strict vegetarians) will experience this type of anemia more than nonvegans.

B_{12} requires a protein called intrinsic factor for its absorption. Since intrinsic factor is produced in the stomach, cancer patients who have had all or part of their stomach surgically removed (total or partial gastrectomy) can be at risk for developing B_{12} deficiency. This does not necessarily happen right away because the body can store B_{12} for two years. B_{12} is also absorbed in a part of the small intestines called the ileum. Any surgery or disease in this part of the intestines can result in B_{12} deficiency. Some drugs can also cause B_{12} deficiency.

> **Survivor Wisdom**
>
> *The only treatment I had was surgery. I have had a poor appetite since then. I can go all day, and it's 4 p.m., and I say, "Why am I so tired?" And then I realize I haven't eaten all day. When I eat, it has to be easy, nutritious and flavorful.*

Recommended Daily Allowance of Vitamin B_{12}

The amount of vitamin B_{12} we need depends on our age and life stage.

Patient	Vitamin B_{12} RDA	UL (upper limit)
Men or women, 19 years or older	2.4 mcg	Unknown. Vitamin B_{12} is not toxic at high amounts because our bodies remove what is not needed.
Pregnant women, 19 years or older	2.6 mcg	
Lactating women, 19 years or older	2.8 mcg	

Source: EatRight Ontario.

Food Sources of Vitamin B12

Because B12 is found only in animal sources, the best food choices will be seafood, meats, eggs, and dairy products. Vegetarian products can be fortified with B12, and nutritional yeast is used by some vegetarians as a source of this essential vitamin. This is different from the yeasts used to make bread or in brewing. Nutritional yeast is an inactive form of the same species of fungi, called *Saccharomyces cerevisiae*. Some brands of nutritional yeast contain folic acid and iron in addition to B12.

Food	Serving	Vitamin B12
Clams, canned	2½ oz (75 g)	74.2 mcg
Beef liver, cooked	2½ oz (75 g)	53.0 mcg
Mussels, cooked	2½ oz (75 g)	18.0 mcg
Red Star T6635+ Nutritional Yeast	2 tbsp (30 mL) large-flake or 1½ tbsp (22 mL) mini-flake	8.0 mcg
Sardines, canned in oil, drained	2½ oz (75 g)	6.7 mcg
Meatless deli slices	5 oz (150 g)	6.0 mcg
Trout, cooked	2½ oz (75 g)	5.6 mcg
Salmon, pink, canned, with bones	2½ oz (75 g)	3.7 mcg
Soy burger	5 oz (150 g)	3.6 mcg
Beef rump roast, cooked	2½ oz (75 g)	2.3 mcg
Ground beef, regular, pan-fried	2½ oz (75 g)	2.3 mcg
Tuna, light, canned in water, drained	2½ oz (75 g)	2.2 mcg
Salmon, Atlantic farmed, cooked	2½ oz (75 g)	2.1 mcg
Cottage cheese (2%)	1 cup (250 mL)	1.7 mcg
Eggs, boiled	2 large	1.1 mcg
Milk (1%)	1 cup (250 mL)	1.1 mcg
Soy or rice beverage	1 cup (250 mL)	1.0 mcg
Pork loin chop/roast, roasted	2½ oz (75 g)	0.9 mcg
Yogurt (flavored or plain)	¾ cup (175 mL)	0.8–1.0 mcg
Cheese (16% to 30% milk fat)	1½ oz (50 g)	0.4 mcg
Chicken breast, skinless, roasted	2½ oz (75 g)	0.3 mcg
Chicken, whole leg, with skin, roasted	2½ oz (75 g)	0.2 mcg

Source: HealthLink BC.

Appetite Loss, Anorexia, and Cachexia

When I worked in home care, it was very common for me to arrive at someone's home and be met by the caregiver at the front door. The caregiver would be overwhelmed with concern that their loved one was not eating. They would say something like, "Tell them they have to eat."

At first glance, loss of appetite would not be considered a serious illness, but loss of appetite during cancer treatment is a serious concern and, unfortunately, a very common issue for people with cancer. Although one or more of your cancer treatments may exacerbate it, the cancer itself can also cause a reduction in your appetite.

Anorexia, Early Satiety, and Aversion

The medical term for loss of appetite is "anorexia." Usually coinciding with loss of appetite is a sensation of feeling full quickly — even with only small amounts of food. This is called early satiety. A third issue is food aversion, which occurs in 30% to 55% of patients receiving chemotherapy or radiation. The "offensive" foods tend to be red meat, vegetables, caffeinated beverages, chocolate, and high-fat foods. Together, anorexia, early satiety, and food aversions pose a serious problem for cancer patients and their caregivers.

Poor appetite generally leads to poor nutritional intake and weight loss. This may make a person more prone to infection and complications. If you become too weak, you may have to miss treatments or reduce the dosage of your treatments.

Nutrient Deficiency and Weight Loss

Appetite problems during your cancer treatments, and later during your recovery, can result in mild to serious malnutrition and dangerous weight loss. These complications need to be tackled head on.

Malnutrition

Malnutrition is the condition that results when your body does not receive sufficient calories (energy malnutrition) or protein (protein malnutrition). Your body will start to use its stored form of calories and protein, and you will notice loss of both fat and muscle. A dangerous by-product of fat breakdown called ketones may be produced by your body. If you are malnourished, your degree of malnutrition can be assessed by your registered dietitian at your cancer center and will include a detailed diet history, weight history, various body measurements, and blood tests. An individualized treatment plan will be prescribed for you.

Weight Loss Red Flags

Your weight loss is considered severe if you have lost more than 10% of your original body weight. For example, if you weighed 200 pounds (90 kg), 10% of this would be 20 pounds (9 kg). If your original weight was 125 pounds (56 kg), then 10% would be 12.5 pounds (5.6 kg).

Patients with pancreatic and gastric cancers appear to be at the greatest risk of severe weight loss. Patients with non-Hodgkin lymphoma, breast cancer, acute non-lymphocytic leukemia, and sarcomas generally have the lowest weight loss.

Losing a large amount of weight can put your lungs under stress because they lose the muscle tone required to maintain good function.

Dangerous Weight Loss

Weight loss is considered severe if you have unintentionally lost:

- 5% of your body weight in 1 month or
- 10% of your body weight in 6 months

To calculate your percentage weight loss, use this formula:

$$\% \text{ weight loss} = \frac{\text{usual body weight} - \text{current body weight}}{\text{usual body weight}} \times 100$$

For example, if you normally weigh 175 pounds (80 kg) and you now weigh 163 pounds (74 kg), that would be:

$$175 - 163 = 12$$
$$12 \div 175 = 0.068$$
$$0.068 \times 100 = 6.8\%$$

If you lost this weight in 1 month or less, then the weight loss is classified as severe because it is above the 5% guideline. If you lost the weight in 6 months or less, it is not classified as severe.

Eating Schedule

To combat poor nutrition and weight loss, patients and caregivers must make an unyielding commitment to eating well every day. As you gain weight, your nutritional status will likely improve — and vice versa. When it comes to gaining weight, meeting your nutrition goals every day is essential. This includes days you are out of the house for medical appointments or treatment. Even when you eat well 5 days out of the week and miss only a couple of days, weight gain is compromised.

To help manage your weight, follow a schedule. You can also use the Liquid and Soft Foods Plan on page 138. Most people find that when their appetite is low, liquids are more appealing and less intimidating than solid foods. A registered dietitian can help you plan an individualized eating schedule.

Guidelines for Establishing an Eating Schedule

Eating sporadically will not help your appetite return, but keeping a regular eating schedule will help. It is better to eat a small meal or snack than to skip eating, even if what you actually consume is meager. For a variety of breakfast, lunch, dinner, and snack ideas, see the recipes in Part 4.

❶ *Breakfast:* Eat within 1 hour of waking up. This can be a challenge, because many cancer patients start the day with a handful of medications that can fill them up. Furthermore, some medications may require you to wait some time before eating, but don't delay breakfast beyond what is required by your medications; otherwise, breakfast is so late that it becomes the morning snack. Given that your appetite is low, breakfast may be pretty small, which is fine, but don't skip it.

❷ *Morning snack:* Eat something, even if it is small, between breakfast and lunch. Remember to pack a morning snack to take with you if you will be out of the house.

❸ *Lunch:* As with all the meals, try to choose a time you can stick to most days of the week. Ideally, eat a meal that balances foods from three to four food groups — vegetables and fruits, grains, meat and meat alternatives, and dairy products. The components of a balanced meal can be combined into a single soup, smoothie, or other dish. If you have an aversion to red meat, try other sources of protein, such as fish, chicken, eggs, and cheese.

4 *Afternoon snack:* Try for a balance of carbohydrates (fruit, milk product, or grain) and proteins (meat or meat alternative or dairy product) — for example, an apple and a handful of nuts, half an egg salad sandwich, or a yogurt smoothie.

5 *Dinner:* Aim to eat another balanced meal. As with lunch, the food groups could be separate, such as chicken with rice and vegetables, or combined in a stew or soup.

6 *Evening snack:* If you suffer from heartburn (acid reflux) or have difficulty sleeping, plan this snack carefully. Don't eat your snack too close to your bedtime. If you can wait 2 to 3 hours after dinner and 1 hour before you go to bed, that will allow you enough time to digest dinner before eating again and allow time for the snack to digest before going to sleep.

FAQ

Q. *How do I know if I'm eating enough food to gain weight and prevent nutrient deficiencies?*

A. To ensure you receive adequate calories and nutrients in your diet, follow one of the national food guides: Eating Well with Canada's Food Guide, from Health Canada; MyPlate, from the United States Department of Agriculture (USDA); or the Eatwell Plate, from the British National Health Services.

FAQ

Q. *How do I rebuild muscle after my treatments?*

A. Building muscle is a two-part process. First, you must work the muscle by doing resistance training. This could be isotonic (the body part being worked is moving) or isometric (the body part is holding still). Working with weights (weight training) is a popular form of isotonic exercise. Consult with a physical therapist, kinesiologist, or certified personal trainer to develop a personalized muscle-building program. Do not take exercise into your own hands. You also need to provide your body with the right type of fuel at the right time. A registered dietitian who is familiar with sports nutrition can customize an effective nutrition plan.

Guidelines for Eating to Build Muscle

1 Don't work out on an empty stomach. You should have something to eat within 4 hours of your workout. Aim to eat about 35 grams of carbohydrates and about 6 grams of protein before a workout.

2 Stay well hydrated during your workout.

3 Within 2 hours of completing your workout (the sooner the better), eat more carbohydrates and protein to replace glycogen stores (the storage form of carbohydrate). Protein is particularly important after the workout because it will provide the building block that will repair the muscle that you worked during your session.

Clinical Supplements and Procedures

If your nutrition and weight loss become serious, there are supplements you can use.

Meal Replacements

Liquid meal supplements and meal replacements have been available in hospitals for decades. In the last 10 years or so, they have been readily available in pharmacies and grocery stores. The brands you have likely seen are Ensure and Boost; however, there are hundreds of different specialty formulas available. Many are "nutritionally complete," meaning that you would receive 100% of your nutrient needs if you consumed about 5 servings a day. They are portable, easy to find, come in a variety of flavors, and you can drink them cold over ice, which is appealing for most people with cancer.

These supplements can be useful for reversing malnutrition and for regaining weight and strength, especially in more serious cases. In cases of mild malnutrition, the effect is not as dramatic, but the supplements provide you with a convenient source of additional calories, protein, and nutrients. If you're not sure if you should use them or which formula is right for you, speak with the registered dietitian at your cancer center. As a word of caution, you can develop taste fatigue with these products, so you may prefer to save them for days when you are not able to eat regular food.

Did You Know?

Visual Appeal

In a recent study of appetite and food presentation, patients were given a brownie to eat on a napkin, on a paper plate, or on a nice piece of Wedgwood china. Then they were asked what they thought of the brownie. If they ate it from the napkin, they said, "Wow, this is really good." Of a paper plate, they said, "This is really, really good." And if they ate it off Wedgwood china, they said, "This is the greatest brownie I've eaten in my entire life."

Now is the time for the best china, flatware, and table settings. Make the meal or snack as visually appealing as possible.

(Source: *Nutrition Action Health Letter*, May 2011.)

Enteral Nutrition

Enteral nutrition, or tube feeding, is another strategy for gaining weight and preventing malnutrition. Tube feedings can be used as short-term nutrition support to provide you with necessary nutrition as you recover from a phase of your treatment. For example, after surgery for head or neck cancer, you may be temporarily unable to swallow; you may be given a tube feeding until it is safe for you to take food and fluids again.

When the tube feeding is expected to be temporary, it is provided through a small, flexible tube that is inserted through your nose, down your esophagus, and into your stomach. While this tube is in place, you can still eat and drink foods that you tolerate and enjoy, but the tube feeding is providing the nutrition you need. As your nutrition improves, the tube can be removed easily. This is called an NG tube, which stands for naso-gastric (nose to stomach).

For longer-term situations, a feeding tube can be inserted through a small opening in the stomach. For the insertion procedure, you will likely be given a local anesthetic to mask any pain. The end of the tube can rest either in the stomach or be directed farther down your digestive system into a part of the small intestines called the jejunum. When the end of the tube rests in your stomach, it is called a G tube (G stands for gastric). When the end of the tube rests in your intestines, it is called a J tube (J stands for jejunum).

You may still be allowed to eat and drink with the tube in your stomach or jejunum. Track your tolerance to the tube feeding so that you can advise your dietician if you have any problems with your bowels or other side effects. Your dietitian can advise you on how to adjust the tube feeding regimen to improve your tolerance.

FAQ

Q. *What are branched chain amino acids, and can they help me?*

A. Amino acids are protein building blocks. "Branched chain" refers to the chemical structure of certain amino acids, which have a branch that is joined by an atom of carbon. The three branched chain amino acids are leucine, isoleucine, and valine. They are part of the family of essential amino acids — nine amino acids that humans cannot make and must therefore get from diet. When the use of branched chain amino acid supplements was studied in patients with cancer in the liver, researchers noted a reduced hospital stay, more rapid recovery of liver function, reduced illness and improved quality of life, but no difference in death rates.

Appetite Medications

A number of medications are designed to stimulate the appetite and promote weight gain, but they are not all that effective and come with their own side effects. Discuss these options with your doctor or dietitian.

Drug or Compound	What Is It?	Test Results with Cancer Patients
ß-Hydroxy ß-methylbutyrate (HMB)	• Made from leucine (an amino acid) • Shown to reduce loss of muscle • Not yet regularly prescribed	• When combined with certain amino acids, increased muscle mass in cancer patients • More testing is likely, due to positive results to date
Anabolic steroids (corticosteroids)	• Used to treat anorexia and cachexia in AIDS patients • Mimics the male sex hormone testosterone	• Contraindicated in patients with cancer due to its growth-promoting potential, as well as potential to interact with your chemotherapy
Cyproheptadine	• Antihistamine used to treat allergy symptoms • Used to stimulate appetite in underweight patients	• Produced only a slight improvement in appetite and did not significantly prevent weight loss in cancer patients with anorexia
Dronabinol Marinol	• Man-made cannabis (synthezied THC) • Used to treat loss of appetite, as well as severe nausea and vomiting from chemotherapy when other medications have been unable to control these side effects	• Not successful in stopping weight loss in cachectic cancer patients • Not tested with cancer patients on active treatment but does seem appropriate for a palliative patient to improve appetite
Eicosapentaenoic acid (EPA)	• Fish oil, available over the counter without a prescription	• Anti-tumor and anti-cachectic effects • Clinical trials have had mixed results when EPA was started too late
Ghrelin	• Neuropeptide released by the stomach when you become hungry to prompt you to eat • Not currently prescribed as an appetite stimulant	• Some preliminary animal trials have shown positive results • Shown to improve calorie intake in cancer patients, but the study wasn't long enough to see changes in body weight
Glucocorticoids Dexamethasone Prednisolone Methylprednisolone	• Improves quality of life, but not shown to increase body weight	• Can increase appetite, food intake, and feelings of well-being, but should be limited to end-stage disease for a few weeks of use, due to loss of skeletal muscle

Drug or Compound	What Is It?	Test Results with Cancer Patients
Megestrol acetate Megace and Megace ES Apo-Megestrol and Megace OS (in Canada)	• Most common appetite stimulant for cachexia • Synthetic progestin that acts in the body in a similar way as the naturally occurring hormone progesterone	• Weight gain mostly from an increase in body fat, not an increase in muscle, with no improvement in quality of life or physical abilities • Patients showed an inferior response to chemotherapy and a trend for a shorter survival
Mirtazapine	• Antidepressant used in cancer-related weight loss, with modest success	• Effectiveness in the cancer population has not been confirmed • Side effects include dizziness, blurred vision, sedation, malaise, dry mouth, and constipation
Thalidomide	• Banned in the 1960s due to birth defects, now being investigated as an appetite stimulant • Not yet prescribed as an appetite stimulant	• Allowed patients to maintain their muscle mass in one study and gain weight and muscle in another versus those who were given a placebo • Further study required.

Sources: Kumar NB, Kazi A, Smith T, et al, Cancer cachexia: Traditional therapies and novel molecular mechanism-based approaches to treatment, *Curr Treat Options Oncol*, 2010 Dec;11(3–4):107–17; and Tisdale MJ, Mechanisms of cancer cachexia, *Physiol Rev*, 2009 Apr;89(2):381–410.

EPA, the Standout

Of the appetite stimulants in the chart above, the one you may want to try first is the omega-3 fatty acid EPA (eicosapentaenoic acid), which has limited side effects and the potential for good results. EPA not only reduces inflammation but also increases appetite and enables weight gain. Most studies have shown that EPA allows cancer patients to stabilize their body weight and stimulates their appetite. One pilot trial was conducted with 36 cancer patients who had experienced unplanned weight loss of 5% of their body weight within the past 3 months. The patients were given a prescription version of omega-3 fats called Lovaza. The patients were able to increase their carbohydrate and fat intake and maintain their protein intake. Blood measures of protein (albumin and transferrin) rose and their activity level increased.

EPA has also been shown to prevent loss of muscle mass in cases of cancer cachexia. The key to breaking the cycle of cachexia using the omega-3 supplement is to start early and not wait until the cachexia is too advanced. Using fish oil in combination with a high-calorie, high-protein diet and physical activity are key to achieving success.

EPA is available in fatty fish and in fish oil supplements found in most pharmacies and health food stores. There currently is no recommended dietary allowance (RDA) for fish oils, but there is an "average intake" (AI) recommendation of 1600 milligrams per day for men and 1100 milligrams per day for women. In the case of cachexia, you would need fish oils with the highest amount of EPA, so read the labels. As with any supplement, discuss this with your cancer care team first.

Constipation

During cancer treatment, constipation can occur as a side effect of chemotherapy drugs; reduced activity, especially after surgery; and dehydration. Constipation can also occur if there is a tumor in your colon blocking the passage of stool, in which case you have a narrowing, or partial obstruction. A complete bowel obstruction is a medical emergency for which you must seek immediate help. The recommendations for treating these two different types of constipation are opposite, so you need to take special care to avoid compounding the problem.

Constipation Without Obstruction

Everyone's body works at its own pace. You are considered to be experiencing constipation if your bowel movements are less frequent than normal for you, if they are hard to pass, or if you have the feeling that you aren't able to release all the fecal material when you go to the bathroom. To prevent constipation, the goal is to have larger and softer stools. Fiber, fluids, and exercise can help achieve this goal.

Guidelines for Treating Constipation Without Obstruction

❶ Increase your fiber intake. Aim to increase intake gradually from your current level until your bowels are regular.

❷ Increase your fluid intake. Aim to drink 64 ounces (2 L) of fluid throughout the day. If this is much more than you are drinking right now, increase your fluids gradually as tolerated. Adding additional fiber without fluid can make constipation worse.

❸ Increase your physical activity level.

Fiber Action

Fiber can help alleviate constipation in three ways. First, the fiber itself adds weight to the stool. Second, the fiber holds on to water, which adds to the weight and softens the stool. Third, the fiber is fermented by colonic bacteria, which increases the bacterial mass of the stool. Soluble fiber will help to hold water and make the stool softer and easier to pass, and insoluble fiber will add bulk to the stool to keep it moving through your system. Wheat bran is best at adding bulk to the stool. Putting yourself on a regular eating and toileting schedule will also be beneficial.

Recommended Dietary Allowance for Fiber

Age	RDA for Fiber
Women	
19–50 years	25 g per day
≥50 years	21 g per day
Men	
19–50 years	38 g per day
≥51 years	30 g per day

Source: Eat Right Ontario.

Most food labels will tell you the amount of fiber per serving but will not tell you how much is soluble and how much is insoluble. Both are important, so try to have sources of both types of fiber in your diet. For more information on these two kinds of fiber, see page 109.

Track not only your fiber intake, but also your fluid intake, exercise, and bowel movements. This will help you to establish how much fiber, fluid, and activity you need each day to keep yourself regular. Eating soup is a great way to get fluid and fiber together. You will find plenty of appealing soup recipes in Part 4.

Food-Based and Medicinal Laxatives

Increasing fiber, fluid, and activity are the main recommendations for relief of constipation, but many plant foods — such as dates, figs, prunes, and rhubarb — also have a reputation for being particularly helpful. Look for recipes labelled "Recommended for constipation" in Part 4.

Food Sources of Fiber

For items with an asterisk (*), check the Nutrition Facts table on the product for exact amounts.

Food	Serving	Fiber
Soy nuts, roasted	¾ cup (175 mL)	15 g
All-bran cereals	⅓–½ cup (75–125 mL)	10–13 g*
Black beans, cooked, or canned baked beans	¾ cup (175 mL)	9–10 g*
Kidney beans, dark red, cooked	¾ cup (175 mL)	9 g
Chickpeas or lentils, cooked	¾ cup (175 mL)	6 g
Edamame, cooked and shelled	¾ cup (175 mL)	6 g
Green peas, cooked	½ cup (125 mL)	6 g
Pear, with skin	1 medium	5 g
Almonds, roasted	¼ cup (60 mL)	4 g
Blackberries or raspberries	½ cup (125 mL)	4 g
Mango	1 medium	4 g
Split peas, cooked	¾ cup (175 mL)	4 g
Sunflower seeds, hulled	¼ cup (60 mL)	4 g
Bread, sprouted grain	1 slice	3–5 g*
100% natural wheat bran	2 tbsp (30 mL)	3 g
Apple, with skin	1 medium	3 g
Brussels sprouts	4	3 g
Flax seeds, ground	1 tbsp (15 mL)	3 g
Kiwifruit	1 large	3 g
Mixed vegetables, cooked	½ cup (125 mL)	3 g
Peanuts, dry-roasted	¼ cup (60 mL)	3 g
Stewed rhubarb	½ cup (125 mL)	3 g
Oatmeal (large-flake), prepared	¾ cup (175 mL)	2–3 g*
Banana	1 medium	2 g
Corn, carrots, or broccoli, cooked	½ cup (125 mL)	2 g
Dates, dried	3	2 g
Popcorn, popped	2 cups (500 mL)	2 g

Source: HealthLink BC.

There are different classes of medications to treat constipation. Laxatives include bulking agents, fermented fiber, stool softeners, stimulants, lubricants, osmotic agents, and enemas. They are all called laxatives, but they work differently.

Bulking Agents

These laxatives contain soluble fiber, usually psyllium or bran. An example is Metamucil. They must be taken with additional water or other fluid. They result in a larger and softer stool by forming a gel with the soluble fiber and water. The softer stool is easier to pass. They can take 12 to 72 hours to take effect.

Fermented Fiber

Fiber supplements can be made from inulin (chicory root) and oligofructose. They are fermented by bacteria that live in the colon and add bulk to the stool by increasing the microbial mass.

Stool Softeners

These medications allow additional water and fats to be incorporated into the stool, making it softer and easier to pass. An example is docusate (Colace). They take effect in 12 to 72 hours.

Stimulants

Medications that stimulate the nervous system to increase intestinal movement (motility) and secretion, thereby increasing stool passage, include senna, aloe, and cascara.

Lubricants

Mineral oil is used to make the stool slippery so it slides through the intestines more easily. Lubricants take 6 to 8 hours to work. They can cause dependency, so you do not want to use them for long periods of time.

Osmotic Agents

These agents increase the fluid content of the stool by drawing water into the intestines via osmosis. Lactulose, polyethylene glycol (PEG) and magnesium citrate are all examples of osmotic agents. They work in 30 minutes to 6 hours.

Enemas

Fluids injected into the bowel to stimulate a bowel movement work very quickly and tend to be reserved for more advanced causes of constipation.

Constipation Due to Obstruction

If your constipation is due to a tumor mass, you must follow a low-fiber or low-residue diet. You should not follow a high-fiber diet. The range of fiber restriction varies depending on the size and position of the tumor.

Eat in a relaxed manner, because tension during eating can lead to tension in the bowel, which further restricts the passage of food matter. Eat solids in the early part of the day and soft foods and liquids for the evening meal. Avoid coffee, alcohol, prune juice, and bulk-forming laxatives.

Fiber Restrictions

- *Low-fiber diet:* Avoid foods with 2 grams of fiber or more per serving.
- *Minimal-fiber diet:* Avoid all whole grains, fruits, vegetables, nuts, seeds, and legumes. You can drink juices, with the exception of prune juice.
- *Fluid diet:* Only fluids are allowed, no solid food.
- *NPO:* In cases of complete bowel obstruction, you would need to be fed through a feeding tube or IV. Your diet order would be NPO — an abbreviation derived from the Latin nil per os, or nothing by mouth. In the UK, this is called NBM — nil by mouth.

Sources: American Dietetic Association and Dietitians of Canada.

Depression

Depression is not so much a side effect of cancer treatment as a condition that can occur at any time before, during, or after your cancer diagnosis, treatment, or recovery. It can affect the person with cancer or the caregiver. It is not a sign of weakness or a shortcoming.

The American Institute for Cancer Research describes the connection between cancer and depression this way: "As you or your loved one begins treatment, you may find yourself on an emotional roller coaster. Hope for a cure, joy at each success, and a determination to get life back to normal, alternate with fear that treatment will fail, frustration at physical limitations, and sadness when treatment brings changes in physical appearance. Powerful anticancer drugs, radiation therapy, surgery, biological therapy, and hormone therapy sometimes cause unpleasant side effects that may lead to irritability and depression."

Did You Know?

Degrees of Depression
There are various degrees of depression. People with mild to moderate depression can experience persistent sadness, decreased energy, irritability, and loss of appetite, which interfere with work, sleep, eating, and activities that were once pleasurable. These symptoms occur most days, all day, for more than 2 weeks. Since mild or moderate depression can lead to more serious depression involving personal injury, thoughts of suicide, hallucinations, and delusions, it should be treated by a qualified health professional and not left to you to self-medicate.

Guidelines for Managing Depression

The American Institute for Cancer Research makes these recommendations:

❶ Be gentle with yourself. Be careful not to get angry at yourself for all those emotions. They are natural reactions.

❷ Talk it out. Sometimes expressing your fears to a trusted family member or friend helps relieve anxiety.

❸ Learn to tell others what you need. Family, friends, and physicians often take their cues from patients. Ask questions about the cancer and its treatment, and ask for help when you need it.

❹ Don't be afraid to ask for support. Most cancer patients need emotional support from individuals other than family members and friends. Nurses, social workers, and dietitians are among the professionals that are available through support groups, local hospitals, health-care agencies, and mental health centers.

❺ Take good care of yourself. Fill your days with activities that are important to you, but don't overextend yourself physically. It's easier to feel hopeful when life is balanced with rest, nutritious meals, recreation, and meaningful work.

❻ Educate yourself. Often, what you imagine causes greater fear than the facts. Read materials from reputable cancer sources, such as the American Institute for Cancer Research and others listed in the Resources (page 306).

❼ Be positive and proactive. Take charge of your health and medical care.

Source: American Institute for Cancer Research.

Survivor Wisdom

I definitely went through depression. I couldn't take any pills because of my bleeding ulcer, so I looked into foods that would help my mental health.

Food and Mood

As you might suspect, there is a connection between your mood and your nutrition. Some specific adjustments to your diet may help stabilize your mood.

Blood Sugar Control

Controlling fluctuations in blood sugars will help level out the hormones insulin and glucagon, which can translate into more stable levels of the brain neurotransmitter serotonin. There are several strategies to limit fluctuations in your blood sugar:

- Choose low glycemic carbohydrates and combine a carbohydrate with a protein at all meals and snacks.
- Reduce your intake of sweets like soft drinks (soda pop), candies, and other sweet treats. When you do have them, take them after a meal and not on an empty stomach. That way, they will have a slower impact on your blood sugar level.
- Eat smaller meals more often throughout the day and try not to go longer than 4 hours between meals or snacks.

Omega-3 Fatty Acids

There is evidence that the docosahexaenoic acid (DHA) and eicosapentaenoic acid (EPA) in omega-3 fats can have a positive benefit on mood. DHA and EPA are found in several food sources, including cold-water fish such as salmon, mackerel, herring, anchovies, and sardines. Omega-3 is also present in some fortified products, such as omega-3 eggs. There are also plant sources of omega-3 in a different form that may still be helpful. This type is found in ground flax seeds, walnuts, canola, and soy oil. For more information on omega-3 fatty acids, see page 105.

B Vitamins

There is some evidence that some of the B vitamins — namely folate (or folic acid), vitamin B_{12}, and vitamin B_6 — may help improve mood. Folic acid is found in fortified whole-grain breakfast cereals and folate is found in lentils, black-eyed peas, soybeans, oatmeal, mustard greens, beets, broccoli, sunflower seeds, wheat germ, and oranges. Sources of vitamin B_{12} include shellfish, wild salmon (fresh or canned), fortified whole-grain breakfast cereal, lean beef, low-fat dairy, and eggs. Sources of vitamin B_6 include fish, beef liver, meat, poultry, whole grains, nuts, peas, and dried beans and lentils.

Vitamin D

Vitamin D can improve mood, particularly if your mood is low during the winter months, when you don't receive enough ultraviolet light from the sun to make sufficient vitamin D in the body. Because vitamin D–rich foods are limited, it may be beneficial to take a daily supplement. It is estimated that Americans receive 200 IU per day from their diet and Canadians receive 300 IU per day. The new public health recommendations for North Americans, released in the fall of 2010, are that children and adults from 9 to 70 years of age require 600 IU (15 mcg) per day, and adults over 70 require 800 IU (20 mcg). The tolerable upper intake is set at 4000 IU (100 mcg) per day. You should not exceed this amount from food and supplements combined. There is evidence of harm at intakes of 10,000 IU or more per day.

Treating the Whole Self

Exercise is a proven tool to release endorphins, which are the body's natural mood boosters. Sleep is also essential. If you are not sleeping well, you need to address this with your cancer-care team and get some help. Getting out in nature, spending time with a pet, or finding a person in whom you can confide are all parts of a depression recovery plan. But the solution

---

Did You Know?

Mediterranean Diet
In a study of diet and depression conducted with a large cohort of more than 10,000 people, participants kept records of what they ate and any experience of depression. The diets of those who developed depression were compared with those who did not. Participants who followed a Mediterranean diet pattern were less likely to have developed depression. The Mediterranean diet is high in olive oil, vegetables, grains, fish, legumes, fruits, and nuts. It is moderate in dairy, milk, and alcohol and low in meat and meat products.

Food Sources of Vitamin D

- Fortified milk
- Fortified margarine
- Fortified soy beverage
- Fortified yogurt
- Egg yolks
- Fatty fish (salmon, tuna, mackerel)
- Beef liver
- Cheese
- Mushrooms
- Certain brands of orange juice
- Canned salmon (if you consume it with bones)

for many is likely a combination of diet, exercise, talk therapy, and medication.

There are many prescription medications designed to help with depression, as well as many complementary therapies. For more information on complementary therapies, see page 90.

Diabetes

Many people newly diagnosed with cancer will have preexisting diabetes. Diabetes and cancer have a reciprocal relationship. Preexisting diabetes appears to modestly increase the risk of certain types of cancer, including liver, pancreas, colorectal, kidney, bladder, endometrial, and breast cancers, as well as non-Hodgkin lymphoma. Cancer treatments can affect diabetes treatment adversely, especially in the case of corticosteroid treatment and pancreatic surgery, and some cases of diabetes may be caused by pancreatic cancer.

It is unclear how diabetes and cancer are linked, but high blood sugar (hyperglycemia) or high insulin levels (hyperinsulinemia) may be the culprits. Impaired glucose tolerance, sometimes referred to as prediabetes, is also associated with increased cancer risk.

Two Types of Diabetes

There are two distinct types of diabetes, type 1 and type 2. Type 1 is less common and typically affects younger people when the pancreas no longer produces any insulin. With this type of diabetes, the treatment is lifelong use of insulin by injection. Type 1 diabetes is most strongly linked to stomach, endometrial, and cervical cancers.

Type 2 diabetes is more common and is linked to lifestyle, with obesity and inactivity being strong risk factors. This type of diabetes can be treated with lifestyle changes or oral medication, but some people will require insulin. This type of diabetes is linked to breast, pancreatic, colorectal, and kidney cancers.

Treatment Adjustments

The goal of diabetes management is to achieve and maintain optimal blood sugar control. During your cancer treatment, however, the target for your blood sugar control and other aspects of your diabetes management may change. This may mean a change from oral medication to insulin or changes in the amount or timing of your medication or insulin. It will very likely mean that you are required to test your blood sugars more often to assess the effects of the cancer and its treatment on your blood sugar control.

Did You Know?

Sun Source

The sun provides a source of vitamin D through exposure to ultraviolet (UV) light. This exposure will be diminished by cloud cover, darker skin pigment, shade, severe pollution, and use of sunscreens with an SPF (sun protection factor) of 8 or more. It is estimated that you can receive enough light for your body to make vitamin D from 5 to 10 minutes of sun exposure to the face, arms, legs, or back between 10 a.m. and 3 p.m. at least twice a week without sunscreen; however, it is important to balance your sun exposure because of the risk of skin cancer.

Glucometer Tests

Although many people may think that they know where their blood sugar levels are just by "feeling," this feeling may very well be off while you are unwell. It is best to know for sure by testing with a glucometer. Blood sugars greater than 288 mg/dl (16 mmol/L) are too high and should be managed with the input of your doctor. If you have type 2 diabetes, test again in about 10 minutes to see if your blood sugar is going up or down. If it is on its way down, you can encourage this by going for a walk and drinking some water. If it is going up, then don't exercise, just rest. If you are type 1, then you should test your urine for ketones. Depending on the instructions you have received from your diabetes-care team, you may be required to give yourself additional fast-acting insulin.

Side Effects

One of the challenges with managing diabetes during cancer treatment will be dealing with the side effects, especially changes in appetite and food intake.

High Blood Sugar

You might assume that since you are not eating much, you should reduce your insulin or medication, but the cancer or treatment may actually cause your blood sugar to go up. To lower blood sugar, you may need to adjust your meal plan by eating fewer carbohydrates and drinking extra water. Be sure to test more often to track which way the blood sugar is going, and call your diabetes-care team if you are having difficulty getting it into the normal range. Unexpected high blood pressure could be caused by an infection. Discuss this with your doctor.

Low Blood Sugar

If your blood test reveals that your blood sugar is too low — less than 72 mg/dl (4 mmol/L) — you need to treat this by eating a fast-absorbing, high glycemic form of sugar. Be careful not to overtreat. Usually, about 15 grams of sugar is all you need. This is equivalent to 1 tablespoon (15 mL) of sugar, ¾ cup (175 mL) of juice, a regular soft drink, 6 candies, 1 tablespoon (15 mL) of honey, or the preferred choice, which is glucose tablets (read the label to see how many tablets you need to get 15 grams of glucose). Then relax for 10 to 15 minutes and check your blood sugar again. If it is still below 72 mg/dl (4 mmol/L), you need to take another 15 grams of fast-acting sugar, wait, and test again.

Did You Know?

Normal Levels
Americans measure blood sugar using mg/dl (milligrams per deciliter), whereas Canadians and Britons use mmol/L (millimoles per liter). Normal blood sugar levels are 72 to 108 mg/dl fasting and before meals, and 90 to 144 mg/dl two hours after a meal, which is equivalent to 4 to 6 mmol/L fasting and 5 to 8 mmol/L two hours after a meal.

Did You Know?

Red Flags
Call your doctor or another member of your care team if you have diabetes and are ill for more than 24 hours, test results show high blood sugar levels and urine ketones are moderate to high, you have a fever for more than 1 day, you vomit twice within 4 hours, or your blood sugars are below normal (less than 72 mg/dl or 4 mmol/L) and you cannot eat or drink enough to get them into the normal range.

Fluid Diet for Sick Days

If you are feeling too ill to eat your regular diet, change your meal plan to fluids containing carbohydrates. Consume 15 grams of carbohydrate every hour; for example, ¾ cup (175 mL) fruit juice, 1 cup (250 mL) milk, ½ cup (125 mL) regular Jell-O (not sugar-free), ½ cup (125 mL) ice cream, ½ cup (125 mL) regular soda (not diet), 1 cup (250 mL) soup (not broth), 1 regular Popsicle (not sugar-free), or 7 soda crackers. You may be nervous about eating the sugar-containing foods on this list, but this is only a temporary menu until you are able to consume regular foods.

Coordinating Care

You will likely be working with two different care teams, one that specializes in your cancer care and another that specializes in your diabetes care. Make sure to take notes of your meetings with members of your care teams so that you can keep each team informed about any changes in your treatment plans. It would likely be best if you can have someone with you during your appointments to make notes and remind you of questions that you have. Don't be afraid to ask the various team members to communicate with each other. All they need is your consent to share information, so once you give this, then the different specialists can communicate with each other about your care.

Here are some questions to ask before you begin treatment:

For your cancer-care team
- What effect do you expect this treatment to have on my blood sugars?
- Is this treatment compatible with the medication I am currently taking for my diabetes?
- As you know, a person with diabetes needs to take special care of their eyes, kidneys, blood vessels, and nerves. How will this treatment affect those organs? Is there anything I can do to protect them from damage during treatment?

For your diabetes-care team
- What is the goal for my blood sugar control during cancer treatment?
- How often and when should I test my blood sugar during treatment?
- How would you like me to record my blood sugars, food intake, and symptoms?
- Can I call you if I have questions about my blood sugar control or diabetes medications, and if so, how do I reach you and when can I call?

Diarrhea

Diarrhea can occur during cancer treatment as a side effect of chemotherapy drugs, radiation to the abdominal area, certain surgeries, medications, infection, impaction, or food intolerances. About 20% of patients taking antibiotics during treatment experience diarrhea, and radiation to the abdominal region can cause radiation-induced enteritis and colitis in 80% of patients.

Causes of Diarrhea

Try to determine the cause of the diarrhea so that appropriate medical treatment can be prescribed:

- Compromised immune system: During cancer treatment, your immune system can be compromised, which can put you at higher risk of bacterial infection from contaminated food or water and viral or parasitic infections. This is why attention to hygiene and food safety practices is so important (see page 141).
- Food allergies or intolerances: These can also account for diarrhea but are usually preexisting and not caused by having cancer, although the stress of cancer may exacerbate preexisting intolerances.
- Anxiety: Anxiety can manifest with a variety of symptoms, including diarrhea.

Diarrhea Treatments

Regardless of the cause, the dietary treatment of diarrhea for the cancer patient is the same.

Helpful Bacteria in Food

While not all probiotics have been shown to help with diarrhea, the bacteria in food products that have been shown to help with diarrhea are:

- *L. casie* DN-114001: found in DanActive fermented milk
- *L. acidophilus* CL1285: found in Bio-K+, along with a supplement of *L. casei* Lbc80r

Helpful Bacteria in Supplements

You can also consider a probiotic supplement — capsule or powder — which you can purchase at a pharmacy or health food store. Probiotic supplements have been reported to treat three types of diarrhea: antibiotic-associated, traveler's, and infectious diarrhea.

> **Did You Know?**
>
> **Stool Leakage**
> Impaction or obstipation may result in liquid stool leaking out around impacted stool. It is evidenced by continued low-volume leakage of stool.

> **Did You Know?**
>
> **Difficult to Control**
> *Clostridium difficile* is a spore-forming, Gram-positive bacterium that is part of normal intestinal flora and present in 3% of healthy adults and 15% to 30% of hospitalized patients. *C. difficile* is also a dangerous bacterium that can cause severe diarrhea if uncontrolled. You may get *C. difficile* if you take antibiotics, or it can be passed to you from another person. It can cause a type of colitis — inflammation of the colon in which toxins are released. *C. difficile* infection can cause diarrhea that may contain blood or pus, abdominal cramps, fever, and dehydration. In rare cases, it can perforate the bowel.

Guidelines for Dietary Treatment of Diarrhea

1 Make sure you are replacing the fluid and electrolytes that are lost as a result of the diarrhea. This should be 64 to 80 ounces (2 to 2.5 L) per day. Sip fluids throughout the day and don't chug them. The best fluids are water, weak tea, broth, diluted juice, sports drinks, commercially prepared electrolyte replacement drinks, or homemade electrolyte replacement drinks such as the one provided on page 301.

2 Choose foods that can help make a more solid stool. These include smooth peanut butter, short-grain white rice, oatmeal or oat bran bread. Also make sure to choose foods that won't aggravate diarrhea. Low-fat, low-spice protein foods — such as eggs, skinless chicken, and lean fish — are recommended.

3 Replace high-fiber foods with low-fiber foods, such as white bread, white rice, soda crackers, and boiled peeled potatoes.

4 Avoid raw fruits and vegetables, with the exception of ripe bananas. Fruit that has been cooked, such as applesauce, is okay.

5 Add probiotic foods to your diet. For example, choose a probiotic yogurt, especially one that is not too high in sugar, because too much sugar could aggravate the diarrhea. It is best if you can find a plain rather than a sweetened or sugar-free (artificially sweetened) yogurt.

Did You Know?

Radiation Enteritis

This is the name given to inflammation of the digestive tract following radiation treatment. It usually occurs 5 to 8 days after the initial treatment of 8 Gy or more. It can occur anywhere in the gastrointestinal (digestive) tract. It results from inflammation of the mucous membrane. The inflammation results in changes to the intestines similar to Crohn's disease and results in malabsorption diarrhea.

Studies on other specific probiotic bacteria have yielded positive results when it comes to fighting diarrhea caused by infections or antibiotic use.

Reduced duration of diarrhea
- *L. rhamnosus GG (ATCC 53103)*

Reduced complications from antibiotics
- *Saccharomyces cerevisiae boulardii*
- *L. casei NG-114001*
- *L. acidophilus CL 1285* plus *L. casei Lbc80r*
- *L. rhamosus GG* when tested with the antibiotics erythromycin, penicillin, and ampicillin

There have also been studies that look at using probiotic supplements to minimize or prevent diarrhea caused by radiation treatment. The product used, VSL#3, resulted in fewer cases and lower severity of radiation-induced diarrhea versus a placebo. Consult your cancer care team to see if this product would be appropriate for you.

Lactose Intolerance

Lactose is the sugar naturally present in milk and milk products. To be digested in the small intestine and absorbed into the bloodstream, lactose requires the enzyme lactase. This enzyme can be swept away by repeated bouts of diarrhea, leaving the intestines temporarily intolerant to lactose. When the lactose cannot be digested in the small intestine, it carries on to the large intestine (colon), and bacteria that live in the colon start to ferment the lactose. The by-product of this fermentation is gas. In addition, the high sugar content of the colon draws water into the colon to help dilute the sugar. This fluid and gas makes you feel bloated and uncomfortable and can result in more diarrhea. In some patients with diarrhea, lactose can be swept through the gastrointestinal system before the food value from milk can be absorbed.

Symptoms may develop soon after consuming lactose or a few hours later. Symptoms can vary from mild to severe, depending on how much lactase enzyme you actually have and how much lactose you consumed.

Guidelines for Managing Lactose Intolerance

1 If you suspect that you may have developed a temporary lactose intolerance as a result of your medications or diarrhea, you should avoid milk and milk products that are high in lactose. Many people with lactose intolerance will tolerate small amounts of lactose in the diet, so super-strict regimens are not usually required.

2 Aim to keep your lactose intake below the level at which you would experience symptoms. For severely lactose intolerant people, this would be about 3 grams of lactose a day, and for the mildly lactose intolerant it would be 12 grams a day. This should be spread out throughout the day and not taken all at once.

3 In addition to limiting the amount of lactose in your diet, consider consuming a pill version of the lactase enzyme. These are available over the counter in most pharmacies. You can also purchase these in drop form so that you can add it to your milk 24 hours before you drink it. Lactose-reduced milk is also readily available in most grocery stores. This is milk that has been treated with the lactase enzyme and does not contain lactose, but rather glucose and galactose. It can taste sweeter than regular milk but does not have more sugar, just a different version of it.

Lactose Content of Common Foods

Food or Beverages	Serving	Lactose
Milk (whole, low-fat, or skim) or buttermilk	1 cup (250 mL)	12 g
Nonfat dry milk	⅓ cup (75 mL)	12 g
Goat's milk	1 cup (250 mL)	11 g
Plain yogurt (low-fat)	1 cup (250 mL)	8 g
Ice cream	½ cup (125 mL)	5 g
Fruit-flavored yogurt (low-fat)	1 cup (250 mL)	4–5 g
Condensed milk (whole)	2 tbsp (30 mL)	4 g
Evaporated milk	1 oz (30 g)	3–4 g
Cottage cheese	½ cup (125 mL)	3 g
Pudding (ready-to-eat)	½ cup (125 mL)	2 g
Cream cheese	2 tbsp (30 mL)	1–2 g
Processed American cheese	1 oz (30 g)	1 g
Sour cream	2 tbsp (30 mL)	1 g
Butter or margarine	1 tbsp (15 mL)	trace
Cream (5%, 10%, 18%, or 35%)	2 tbsp (30 mL)	trace
Swiss, Cheddar, Parmesan, blue, or mozzarella cheese	1 oz (30 g)	trace
Whipped cream topping (pressurized in a can)	2 tbsp (30 mL)	trace

Source: www.lactaid.com.

Did You Know?

Age Matters

As a general rule, the older the cheese, the lower the lactose content. Aged cheese, such as Cheddar, would be low in lactose, but unaged cheese, such as cheese curds, cottage cheese, and fresh cheese, would be higher. Yogurt is generally well tolerated by people with lactose intolerance because of its probiotic bacteria.

Foods to Avoid with Diarrhea

To manage your diarrhea, you should avoid many foods:

- Fatty, spicy foods
- Coffee, tea, cola, alcohol, energy drinks
- Candies, cakes, soft drinks (soda pop), full-strength juices
- Sweeteners known as sugar alcohols (sorbitol and mannitol) found in sugar-free foods
- Dates, figs, prunes
- High-fat dairy products (butter, cheese, ice cream)
- Foods high in insoluble fiber (whole-grain breads, cereals, fresh fruits and vegetables).

This is a short-term diet only, and once the bowels return to normal, all forms of fiber, including whole grains and fresh fruits and vegetables, should be gradually reinstated as tolerated.

Dry Mouth

Dry mouth (xerostomia) is common following radiation or surgery of the mouth for oral cancers. Chemotherapy can also cause dry mouth, as can other medications. Dry mouth is caused by damage to the salivary glands. There are three main glands and hundreds of minor glands in the mouth area that produce saliva. Radiation causes the most damage to saliva glands. After radiation, the saliva flow can be reduced by 95% and may stop almost entirely within 5 weeks.

Symptoms

Dry mouth can make it very difficult to eat because you feel as if food is too dry to swallow. Because of the lack of saliva in your mouth, your teeth are more prone to cavities and demineralization. It can even affect your ability to talk. Other symptoms of dry mouth include bad breath, a sticky or sore mouth, cracking at the corners of the mouth, red mouth, blisters, mouth ulcers, a pebbled look to the tongue, difficulty eating dry or spicy foods, waking up with a dry mouth at night, decreased sense of taste, difficulty swallowing, and dry lips.

> **Did You Know?**
>
> **Artificial Saliva**
> You can purchase artificial saliva in a variety of forms from your pharmacy: spray bottles that you use to spritz your mouth, toothpaste, gel, oral rinse, and even a gum. Don't use regular mouthwash — these contain alcohol and are too strong for you right now.

Guidelines for Dietary Treatment of Dry Mouth

1. Consume moist and wet foods.
2. Add butter, margarine, mayonnaise, broth, yogurt, milk, and water to foods to keep the moisture level high.
3. Dunk or soak dry foods in liquids.
4. Take frequent sips of water.
5. Rinse your mouth with water before eating.
6. Limit drinks with caffeine, such as coffee, tea, and cola drinks.
7. Sip on soda water to help loosen thick saliva.
8. Limit salty and spicy foods.
9. Avoid alcohol and tobacco.

Source: Canadian Cancer Society.

The American Cancer Society recommends this mouth rinse for dry mouth and sore mouth: 1 teaspoon (5 mL) baking soda plus 1 teaspoon (5 mL) salt mixed into 1 quart (1 L) of water.

Medications

Several medications have been developed to treat dry mouth during cancer treatment.

Amifostine

In medical language, dry mouth is called xerostomia. You can ask your oncologist about a medication called amifostine, which has been used to help protect the mouth from xerostomia during radiation treatment.

Xylitol

You can purchase gum or mints containing xylitol to treat dry mouth and prevent cavities. Xylitol is a sweetener that is often called a "sugar alcohol" because of its chemical structure. It is derived from plant fibers of berries, cornhusks, and birch trees. You will often see it on the ingredient list of foods, gums, and liquids labeled "sugar free." A study done in Finland in 1970 showed that it can help reduce dental cavities. There are several companies that sell xylitol products (gum, gel, toothpaste, liquid, and mouthwash) you can use while you are experiencing dry mouth. Some dentists have samples of these you can try. Use caution with these products if you are experiencing diarrhea.

Preventive Dentistry

Protect your teeth before, during, and after treatment.

Before Treatment

If possible, see your dentist one month before your treatment begins, especially if you are beginning radiation or chemotherapy to the head or neck areas. Your dentist can detect any underlying dental infection that could delay or compromise your treatment.

If you need teeth removed, have this done before the mold is made for your radiation treatment so that your facial contour is not changed. The removal of infected teeth before radiation prevents the possible formation of radiation-induced bone decay, called osteoradionecrosis. Allow 2 weeks for recovery before you begin your cancer treatment.

To protect your teeth from cavities, you should have a fluoride application before cancer treatment. A thorough dental scaling and polishing before treatment to eliminate gingivitis (gum disease) will help keep your mouth as healthy as possible before treatment begins.

During Treatment

Dental work should be avoided during chemotherapy unless absolutely necessary. You may be predisposed to oral infections around the gum when your white blood cell counts are low.

After Treatment

Cancer treatment will put you at higher risk of dental cavities in the future. Arrange to see your dentist after you have completed all of your treatments, for instructions on a more rigorous prevention program. For the first 6 months after radiation treatment to the head and neck, you may be advised to see your dental hygienist every 4 to 6 weeks for scaling and evaluation of your dental routine. In addition to brushing with fluoride toothpaste, a fluoride varnish or gel may be recommended. If you experience bleeding gums, use a soft-bristled toothbrush, softened in warm water, and avoid flossing the areas that are bleeding.

Fatigue

Feeling tired is a common complaint among cancer patients. Fatigue can be caused by the cancer itself or occur as a result of surgery, chemotherapy, and especially radiation. In general, the larger the radiation field, the greater the fatigue that may result. Daily radiation treatments over a period of time can be grueling for patients and families, depending on the distance to your

---

Did You Know?

Hunger-Free

In a study of 31 terminally ill cancer patients, thirst and dry mouth, not hunger, were the most common complaints. These conditions were managed with ice chips, small amounts of food and water, and lubrication of the lips. Dehydration results in a concentration of the blood, which can produce a sedative effect on the brain.

Guidelines for Dietary Treatment of Fatigue

❶ Don't skip meals. Keeping a regular schedule of meals and snacks is important to maintain your energy levels. Even though your radiation treatment may only last 30 seconds, by the time you get to the cancer center and then get back home, it may take you the better part of the day. Chances are, this routine interferes with at least one meal or snack. The same goes for chemotherapy, but in this case, the treatments are usually much longer.

❷ Be prepared and take some healthy portable snack items with you. Although it may feel out of place to be eating away from home, if you wait until you are back home, you may be compromising your nutrition. Given that many cancer treatment programs can last for months, if your nutrition is suboptimal for the entire time, you may be adding to your fatigue.

❸ Balance your intake of carbohydrate and protein at every meal and snack. This helps with energy levels by regulating fluctuations in blood sugar levels. Healthy carbohydrates include fruits, grains, starches, milk, and yogurt. Protein includes nuts, seeds, eggs, cheese, meat, fish, poultry, milk, yogurt, tofu, soy beverages, and protein powders. An example of this would be to eat a fruit (carbohydrate) with some nuts (protein) at a snack. You can eat a yogurt by itself because it contains both carbohydrate and protein.

cancer center. Good nutrition, including carbohydrate-protein balancing (see point 3, page 67), combined with a regular exercise routine and good sleep, can help maintain your energy levels during cancer treatment.

Carbohydrate-Protein Balancing

Here are some examples of carbohydrate-protein combinations:

Carbohydrate	Protein
Whole-grain crackers	Cottage cheese
Oatmeal	Protein powder
Fruit	Cheese
Whole-grain bread	Tuna
Whole-grain tortilla	Peanut or almond butter

Food Aversion

Research indicates that 30% to 55% of patients receiving chemotherapy or radiation experience food aversion. Common aversions include meat (especially red meat), vegetables, caffeinated beverages, and chocolate. Aversion is usually restricted to two or three foods, and can last anywhere from a few weeks to a few months.

Acquired Food Aversion

If you experience nausea and vomiting from your treatment, avoid eating your favorite foods prior to the time you are likely to feel sick. Any food eaten before the onset of nausea or vomiting can develop into an "acquired food aversion." This means you will lose your appetite for this food because you remember eating it before being sick. Save your favorite food for a time when your nausea and vomiting are well controlled.

Scapegoating

There is a technique called scapegoating that can be used prior to chemotherapy or radiation treatment. This involves eating a strongly flavored unhealthy food before treatment; a good example would be candies. Choose something new to you. Eat the new candy just before treatment or before you anticipate being sick. If you develop an aversion to this new food, your nutrition does not suffer — and you eliminate an unhealthy food that was never part of your eating routine.

Heartburn

Heartburn can occur if the esophagus is damaged during radiation of the neck or chest for cancers of the esophagus, breast, lymph nodes, stomach, and bone.

Reflux

The esophagus is the tube that transports food from the mouth to the stomach. At the base of the esophagus is a "doorway" called the lower esophageal sphincter. This muscular device allows food to pass from the esophagus into the stomach and then seals off the opening so that strong stomach acid and other contents do not back up into the esophagus. This backup, or reflux, is commonly called heartburn because of the burning sensation felt in the lining of the esophagus near the heart. Heartburn is more accurately called gastroesophageal reflux disease, or GERD. During radiation treatment, the lower esophageal sphincter can be damaged, resulting in acid reflux.

Guidelines for Dietary and Lifestyle Treatment of GERD

❶ Eat small, frequent meals. When your stomach is full after a large meal, it exerts extra pressure on the lower esophageal sphincter.

❷ Reduce foods that may trigger symptoms, such as spices, peppermint, chocolate, citrus juices, onions, garlic, tomato products, alcohol, and caffeine.

❸ Keep a food and symptom record so you can determine which foods or ingredients aggravate the discomfort. You don't need to avoid foods unless they worsen your symptoms.

❹ Sit upright while eating and for 45 to 60 minutes following a meal. If you eat while you are reclined, it is easier for stomach acid to reflux.

❺ Avoid eating too close to nap times or bedtimes.

❻ If you haven't quit smoking already, consider quitting now, because smoking makes heartburn worse.

❼ Avoid clothing that is tight around the waist.

Source: Dietitians of Canada.

Heart Disease

Heart disease and cancer are both relatively common conditions, so it is not unusual for people newly diagnosed with cancer to have pre-existing heart disease. When that is the case, one must balance the sometimes conflicting nutritional advice that accompanies each of these conditions. Heart disease is not one single condition but many different conditions that affect the structure or function of the heart, including angina, arrhythmia, atherosclerosis, coronary artery disease, heart attack, heart failure, and high blood pressure, among several others. Because heart disease is strongly linked to lifestyle, there are many diet, exercise, and behavior recommendations to prevent or reverse heart disease.

With a new diagnosis of cancer combined with heart problems, you may be somewhat frightened and highly motivated to implement all the heart-healthy recommendations all at once. Just like the children's fable of the tortoise and the hare, however, slow and steady wins the race. Systematically structure your life so you are able to live a smoke-free life that includes regular exercise, successful stress management, and a healthy diet. A heart-healthy diet is consistent with a diet to reduce cancer risk.

Guidelines for Managing Heart Disease During Cancer Treatments

1 Be smoke-free.

2 Be physically active.

3 Know and control your blood pressure.

4 Eat a healthy diet, such as the Mediterranean diet or DASH diet, that is lower in fat, especially saturated and trans fats.

5 Achieve and maintain a healthy weight.

6 Manage your diabetes.

7 Limit alcohol use.

8 Reduce stress.

9 Visit your doctor regularly and follow your doctor's advice.

Source: Heart and Stroke Foundation of Canada.

The Mediterranean Diet

If you have high cholesterol levels, you may already be following a Mediterranean diet. In addition to heart disease, there is evidence that this diet reduces cancer risk. The Mediterranean diet involves:

- Eating high intakes of fruits, vegetables, whole grains, legumes, nuts, herbs, and spices.
- Replacing butter with olive oil.
- Limiting red meat to a couple of times a week.
- Eating fish and poultry at least twice a week.
- Drinking red wine, in moderation. Ask your oncologist if red wine would still be acceptable during treatment.

The DASH Diet

DASH stands for Dietary Approaches to Stop Hypertension, and "hypertension" is another word for high blood pressure. This diet features a high intake of foods containing fiber, calcium, potassium, and magnesium and a low intake of sodium (salt). Specifically, the DASH diet includes on a daily basis:

- 4–5 servings of fruit
- 4–5 servings of vegetables
- 7–8 servings of grains (mostly whole grains)
- 2–3 servings of low-fat or no-fat dairy products
- 2 or fewer servings of lean meats, poultry, or fish (and 4–5 servings per week of nuts, seeds, and dried beans)
- 2–3 servings of fats and oils
- 2300 milligrams of sodium (in some cases, a lower sodium intake is recommended)

Low Blood Pressure Caution

You can continue the DASH diet during your cancer treatment, but the cancer treatment could cause changes in your blood pressure and adjustments to your medication may be required. If you lose weight as a result of your cancer or its treatment, you may need to have your blood pressure medication reduced.

Signs that your blood pressure is too low include feeling dizzy or lightheaded when you stand up or move from lying down to sitting. If you measure your blood pressure, a systolic count less than 90 mmHg or a diastolic count less than 60 mmHg would indicate that your blood pressure is too low. If you are experiencing low blood pressure and are not on medications for blood pressure, then adding salt to your diet would likely be recommended. For some people, this may seem contradictory to what you've been advised by your heart specialist, but you need to prioritize two different medical conditions and make the dietary change that is appropriate for the situation at hand; in this case, adding salt to your diet to correct low blood pressure would be the priority.

Weight Loss

If you are experiencing weight loss during your cancer treatment and recovery, and it is causing you to be underweight, you may need to make some changes to your heart-healthy eating plan:

- Add more protein to your diet by eating larger servings of meats or eating meat more often.
- Add more fat to your diet by eating olive oil, avocado, nuts, cheese, ice cream, and higher-fat yogurts.

Did You Know?

Potassium
Potassium is a mineral that helps the body maintain normal blood pressure. It is also an important electrolyte, helping the body retain fluid when recovering from dehydration. Adults need 4700 mg (4.7 g) of potassium a day. Good sources of potassium include dried beans and lentils, milk, yogurt and fish. Fruit and vegetable sources include bananas, honeydew melons, oranges, papayas, prunes, avocados, beets, baked potatoes, spinach, squash and tomato paste.

Did You Know?

Dizzy
The dizzy feeling you experience when you stand up or change from lying to sitting is due to low blood pressure, which is caused by dehydration. If you are taking medication to lower your blood pressure, this may need to be reduced or stopped and you should contact your health-care team.

Although you may be nervous about making these changes, you need to decide which concern is the priority. For example, if you experience unintentional weight loss during cancer treatment and have a history of high cholesterol, your priority will likely shift from cholesterol lowering to regaining the lost weight, especially if your weight is now below normal. Likewise, if you are anemic as a result of your cancer treatment, you may need to eat iron-rich foods, such as red meat and organ meats, that are not recommended on a healthy-heart diet.

Insomnia

Insomnia is a frequent problem for people with cancer. Insomnia is defined as difficulty falling asleep, staying asleep, or achieving a restful sleep. It is a common side effect of chemotherapy, often accompanied by frequent urination, nausea and vomiting, pain, and night sweats. For those in a hospital or other care setting, the noise, light, and change in surroundings can also affect your sleep.

Guidelines for Dietary and Lifestyle Treatment of Insomnia

1. Keep a normal bedtime routine with consistent sleep and wakeup times.
2. Avoid long or late afternoon naps.
3. Use the bedroom for sleep and sexual activity only.
4. If possible, try to stay active or exercise a little each day.
5. Drink warm, noncaffeinated drinks (such as warm milk) before sleep and avoid caffeinated drinks late in the day.
6. Avoid drinking alcohol close to bedtime.
7. Go to sleep in a quiet setting.
8. Try relaxation exercises, listening to soothing music, darkening the room, or massage before bed.
9. Keep sheets clean, neatly tucked in, and as free from wrinkles as possible.
10. Have extra covers handy in case it gets cold.
11. Talk about fears and concerns during the day to help decrease fear and free the mind at night, which can help with more peaceful sleep.
12. Report symptoms, such as pain, that may be causing problems with sleep.
13. Talk to the health-care team about medications to help with sleep.
14. Take medications for sleep, pain, or other symptoms as prescribed before trying to sleep.
15. Try complementary therapies, such as cognitive behavior therapy, healing touch, or massage.

Source: Canadian Cancer Society.

Mouth Sores

Mouth sores are common as a result of radiation to the mouth and exposure to many chemotherapy drugs. This side effect of radiation therapy is known as mucositis, which refers to inflammation of the mucous membranes that line the mouth, throat, esophagus, and intestines. Stomatitis refers to inflammation of the mouth, gums, tongue, cheeks, and lips.

These sores make chewing and swallowing painful. They can interfere with your ability to take in nourishing food and, if severe, can lead to nutritional deficiency that will affect the outcome of your treatment.

Dietary Care

Soft foods are best when you have a sore mouth. Avoid extremely hot or extremely cold foods or drinks, and limit salty, acidic, and spicy foods to prevent irritation to an already sore mouth.

Mouthwashes

You may be prescribed a special mouth rinse or told to rinse with baking soda and water to prevent mouth sores. Do not use commercial mouthwashes because they contain alcohol, which can be an irritant. If you see white buildup on the tongue or in the throat, you may have a yeast infection called thrush or candidiasis, which can be treated with an antifungal medication. For pain control, a "magic mouthwash" containing anesthetic may be prescribed.

Glutamine Therapy

Glutamine is an amino acid (a protein building block) that has been shown to be effective in treating mouth sores. Some studies use oral glutamine, while others use glutamine as part of a "swish and swallow" therapy. Talk to your cancer-care team about whether glutamine might be appropriate for you.

Oral Cryotherapy

This involves holding ice chips in the mouth before chemotherapy and every 30 minutes after chemotherapy. It is thought to help by constricting blood vessels in the mouth, thereby reducing their exposure to chemotherapy drugs.

> **Did You Know?**
>
> **Trismus**
> You can exercise your mouth to prevent trismus, which is an inability to open the mouth as a result of radiation treatment. The exercise involves opening your mouth as far as possible and closing it, 20 times, three times a day.

> **Survivor Wisdom**
>
> *I was intubated for my surgery, and my voice didn't recover for 2 months. I had a sore throat, and Popsicles were very soothing.*

Nausea

Nausea is a well-documented side effect of chemotherapy, but it can also be caused by radiation, surgery or the cancer itself. Nausea is also associated with gastrointestinal obstruction, liver metastases, gastric surgery, brain cancers, and anxiety. It has a direct impact on nutrition. If you have severe nausea, it will be difficult to eat. If you avoid food for too long, you may lose weight, which can weaken your immune system. On the other hand, some people with mild nausea continually graze throughout the day, which could inadvertantly lead to unwanted weight gain. A proper balance is necessary.

Types of Nausea

There are different types of nausea, classified by when they occur. Anticipatory nausea is something you experience before you even receive your chemotherapy. It is a learned response to chemotherapy that occurs in 30% of cancer patients by their fourth chemo cycle. If you experience anticipatory nausea, this cannot be treated by medication, but rather by using behavioral strategies, such as relaxation. A second type is immediate nausea, which occurs in the first 24 hours after treatment. Delayed nausea, also called post-chemotherapy nausea, occurs 24 hours or more after chemotherapy.

Treatment Strategies

Treatments vary according to the type of nausea you experience.

Immediate Nausea

There are many effective medications for treating nausea. Your oncology team will work with you to determine the best medication to control your nausea. Depending on your chemotherapy, you may receive an antinausea medication before your first treatment. Be sure to communicate to your care team if your nausea is not well controlled.

Anticipatory and Delayed Nausea

For treatment of anticipatory and delayed nausea, these treatments have shown benefits:

- Acupuncture and acupressure
- Progressive muscle relaxation training plus meditation or imagery
- Behavioral interventions (hypnosis, biofeedback, relaxation)
- Exposure to fresh air, relaxing music, a darkened room, a cool wash cloth on the face, loose clothing, and a sniff of fresh lemon
- Anti-anxiety medications, such as low-dose alprazolam (Xanax) and lorazepam
- Dietary treatment (see box on page 75)

Guidelines for Dietary Treatment of Nausea

1 Stay well hydrated. If you become dehydrated, the nausea may become worse and can create other problems, such as constipation. In addition, dehydration can make it difficult for nurses to start an IV.

2 Eat small meals and snacks throughout the day. An empty stomach can make the nausea feel worse.

3 Try dry foods, such as crackers, toast, dry cereal, and pretzels, that may appeal to you. Alternate these with fluids.

4 Avoid oily or fatty foods, which will take longer to leave your stomach. Also avoid spicy or strong-smelling foods.

5 Eat cold or room temperature foods, which have less aroma.

6 Drink through a straw or using a cup with a lid, to help limit food odor.

Food and Cooking Odors

Because the odor of cooking food can trigger nausea, aim to minimize cooking odor. In some houses, cooking smells may be difficult to confine to the kitchen, so the entire family may need to make some changes to assist the person in the household undergoing treatment.

When you do cook, turn on the kitchen exhaust fan and open windows to ventilate the kitchen. Cook outside on the barbecue, but be sure that odors do not come back into the house. You can also confine cooking to times when the patient is sleeping or out of the house. This is an area where support from friends and family comes in handy. They can prepare meals at their home that the cancer patient's family can eat.

If you don't feel like cooking at all, consult the shopping list on page 140 to get ideas for convenient foods you can have on hand. These will help you maintain good nutrition without triggering nausea due to cooking smells.

Smells such as perfume can also trigger nausea. You may need to make your home scent-free during treatment.

Dietary Ginger

Since the 1500s, ginger has been used in Indian (Ayurvedic) and traditional Chinese medicine to treat nausea and flatulence. In North American folklore, it is said to relieve nausea, vomiting, and motion sickness.

Did You Know?

To the Point
The acupressure point for nausea is on the inside of your wrist. In a study of breast cancer patients, acupressure was found to reduce the amount of vomiting and the intensity of nausea for those experiencing delayed nausea and vomiting following their chemotherapy treatments. Acupressure was found to be a safe and effective treatment to be used along with medications. You can purchase "sea bands" — wrist bands that apply pressure to the correct point on the inside of your wrist.

Ginger Capsules

In a review article, the authors reported that powdered ginger taken in capsule form helped control nausea and vomiting during pregnancy and in post-surgical patients, but the benefits were less pronounced in treating chemotherapy-induced nausea and vomiting. In another study, patients given 0.5 g and 1.0 g of powdered ginger in capsule form showed improvement in nausea versus placebo.

Before beginning a treatment of ginger capsules, make sure you speak with your oncologist. It is not recommended for everyone and may be a problem for those with bowel disease or on blood-thinning medication.

Positive Thinking

Be conscious of your expectations about nausea and your chemotherapy. Being positive may be a way for you to counter the severity of your side effects. Monitor and correct your thoughts around this. If you find yourself saying, "This is going to be bad," correct this negative self-talk using coaching strategies, such as "My body will respond well to this treatment and my side effects will be minimal," or "My cancer experience is unique; my side effects will be minor." The mind is a powerful tool, and you should use all the tools at your disposal.

Taste Changes

Alterations in your taste (dysgeusia) can occur as a result of chemotherapy or other drugs, as well as radiation in the mouth area. Some people lose their sense of taste entirely, while others experience alterations in their taste. Sweetness and saltiness can become amplified, you may experience a strong metallic taste, and familiar foods just don't taste like they used to.

There are five main flavors we can taste: sweet, sour, salty, bitter, and umami. "Umami" is the Japanese word for "savory" or "meaty," and foods with this flavor include meat, as well as aged cheese, beets, broccoli, cabbage, green tea, soy sauce, truffles, and walnuts, among others.

Use one or two seasonings to try to get the food to taste normal or at least palatable for you. For example, if your food tastes too bitter, try adding sweet and fat to your cooking. For a bitter-tasting vegetable, you could try adding cheese sauce, peanut sauce, or something sweet, like a sweet barbecue sauce or a yogurt sauce. Using a sour flavor, such as lemon juice, along with sweet flavors can work well for bitter or metallic tastes. Part 4 contains tips on how to adjust many of the recipes to suit your taste buds.

Guidelines for Dietary Treatment of Taste Changes

❶ Rinse your mouth before and after eating to help clear your taste buds. Club soda or a solution of $\frac{1}{2}$ teaspoon (2 mL) of salt mixed with 1 cup (250 mL) of water may help. Your treatment center may also have a suggested recipe for you to follow.

❷ Keep your mouth and teeth clean. If your mouth is sore, your dentist or hygienist can suggest gentle ways of cleaning your teeth.

❸ Try foods or beverages that are different from the ones you usually eat.

❹ Serve foods cold or at room temperature to reduce strong tastes and smells.

❺ Use plastic cutlery and glass cooking pots if foods taste metallic.

❻ If they appeal to you, experiment with seasonings and spices, which can make food taste better.

❼ Suck on lemon candies or mints or chew gum to help get rid of unpleasant tastes that remain after eating. Choose those with xylitol if you also have a dry mouth.

❽ Drink plenty of fluids while eating.

❾ Chew slowly.

Glutamine, Zinc and Vitamin D Supplements

These supplements have been tested for their effectiveness in helping with taste alterations during cancer treatment. In one study, 21 adults received glutamine and 20 received a placebo before treatment with taxane-based chemotherapy. There was no benefit to those taking the glutamine. There have been mixed results with patients taking zinc sulfate. Vitamin D supplements may improve taste changes in those who are deficient in this vitamin. Speak with your health-care team to see if glutamine, zinc or vitamin D supplements might help you develop less severe taste alterations and encourage your taste to return to normal more quickly.

Vomiting

Vomiting can occur with and without nausea. If you vomit for more than 24 hours or notice blood or bile in your vomit, you should contact your health-care team. Bile is produced by the liver and functions to help the body digest fat. If you vomit bile, it can appear green, greenish yellow, or dark yellow. If you see bile, it means your vomiting has cleared out all the food matter that was in your system and now the remaining contents of your small intestines are being expelled from the body. If this continues, dehydration and malnutrition can result.

Guidelines for Dietary Treatment of Vomiting and Dehydration

1 Take small sips of fluids throughout the day. Start with 1 teaspoon (5 mL) every 10 minutes and then gradually increase this amount. These fluids could include ice chips, flat ginger ale, sports beverages, frozen treats like Popsicles or freezies, and electrolyte repletion beverages. These are also known as "clear fluids."

2 If clear fluids are tolerated for a day, you can advance to lower-fat "full fluids." These fluids include skim milk, gelatin, frozen yogurt, or sherbet.

3 When you think you are able, try dry starchy foods, such as crackers and dry toast.

4 Be careful with carbonated beverages because they could make you feel full or bloated or cause burping, which can stimulate vomiting.

5 Introduce foods that are high fat or high fiber gradually.

Dehydration

Vomiting can lead to dehydration, especially if you are also experiencing diarrhea. Dehydration can make it difficult for your body to get rid of the toxic by-products of chemotherapy and other medications. It can also cause constipation, which can make nausea and vomiting worse, so that you enter a vicious cycle of nausea, vomiting, and constipation, each making the other worse. Maintaining the body's fluid levels becomes a priority.

Signs of Dehydration

Mild Dehydration
- Increased thirst
- Infrequent urination
- Urine that is dark in color

Moderate Dehydration
- Dry mouth
- Sticky saliva
- Dry, sunken eyes
- Dizziness when you stand up

Severe Dehydration
- Extremely dry mouth and eyes
- Little or no urine being passed for 12 or more hours
- Loss of alertness and an inability to think clearly
- Weakness, dizziness, inability to stand, and fainting
- Loss of the turgor, or elasticity, in your skin

Did You Know?

Turgor Testing
You may experience a loss of the turgor, or elasticity, in your skin. You can test this by using your thumb and first finger to make a tent out of the skin on the forearm of your opposite hand. When you let go, the skin should return to place quickly. If you are dehydrated, it will return slowly. This test is less reliable on the elderly because they have naturally lost some of the skin's elasticity.

FAQ

Q. *Should I eat before my chemotherapy?*

A. Eating before chemotherapy is a good idea. Because chemo can often result in nausea that can be most intense for a couple of days right after treatment, eating before your treatment can provide an opportunity for needed wholesome nutrition. Having some food in your stomach may also help with the nausea. During and after your chemo, focus on increasing your fluid intake, because the body will need to process the by-products of the powerful chemo drugs and excrete them.

Severe dehydration is a medical emergency. Contact your doctor or emergency services immediately.

Dental Erosion

When you vomit, very strong stomach acids travel up the esophagus and come in contact with the mouth and teeth before being expelled by the body. This exposure of the teeth to stomach acid can lead to dental erosion. Although your mouth will have a strong, unpleasant taste in it after an episode of vomiting, it is best not to brush your teeth right away. When you do this, you are scrubbing the erosion-causing acids into the teeth. Instead, rinse your mouth with warm water or warm water mixed with baking soda. You can brush your tongue right away, but wait about an hour before brushing your teeth. Make a note that you will need to see your dentist once your cancer treatment has finished to have your teeth assessed.

Weight Gain and Obesity

The relationship between cancer and being overweight or obese has several layers. First, being overweight or obese puts you at higher risk of developing some types of cancer. Second, being overweight or obese may be associated with a poorer prognosis. Third, some cancer treatments have the side effect of weight gain, and people who gain weight after their treatment may have a higher risk of recurrence of cancer and a reduced rate of survival.

Miscalculations

Most patients think that their cancer treatment will result in weight loss; however, for some treatments, weight gain is the norm. Excessive weight gain can lead to a poorer prognosis in some clinical situations. Research shows that weight gain of $4\frac{1}{2}$ to 9 pounds (2 to 4 kg) is common with some

---

Did You Know?

Electrolytes
Dehydration is not effectively treated by drinking water alone. When you are dehydrated, you lose important salts from your system. Dehydration is best treated by taking salt-containing beverages, such as soda water, broths, and electrolyte solutions. There is a recipe for a homemade electrolyte drink on page 301.

Did You Know?

A 2-Pound (1 kg) Limit
If you were overweight before being diagnosed with cancer, weight loss should be one of your goals. Aim to lose weight at a maximum of 2 pounds (1 kg) a week. When you lose faster than this, you risk losing beneficial muscle mass.

---

chemotherapy regimens, including CMF (cyclophosphamide, methotrexate, and fluorouracil) and CEF (cyclophosphamide, epirubicin, and fluorouracil). In early-stage resected breast cancer, weight gain after diagnosis may increase the risk of a cancer recurrence and decreased survival.

How Body Fat Leads to Cancer

When you eat more calories than your body uses for energy, the excess calories are at first stored in your existing fat cells, which get bigger. When they are full, your body creates new fat cells to fill up. Every body is different: some can keep making more fat cells; others cannot, so they look for new places to store fat. Excess fat may be stored in muscles, the heart, the liver, or the abdominal cavity, packed around the stomach, liver, intestines, kidneys, and pancreas. This misplaced fat is responsible for a condition called insulin resistance, which leads to diabetes. Excess abdominal fat also leads to low levels of chronic inflammation, the starting point for cancer cell development.

Toxic Fat

People with excess body fat have elevated levels of certain hormones and pro-inflammatory factors that promote cancer cell growth. Body fat is associated with cancers of the esophagus, pancreas, colorectum, breast (in post-menopausal women), endometrium, and gallbladder.

Not All Fat Is Equal

Fat is distributed differently in different people. It is found beneath the skin (subcutaneously) in the upper arm, buttocks, belly, hips and thighs. It is also found in the abdominal cavity. A person's distribution of fat is largely based on genetics.

Visceral Fat

Visceral fat is located in the abdominal cavity, packed around the stomach, liver, intestines, kidneys, and pancreas. This fat is associated with type 2 diabetes, heart disease, insulin resistance, and inflammatory disease. This type of fat puts you at a greater risk of cancer.

Subcutaneous Fat

This type of fat is located below the skin. Women typically store subcutaneous fat in the hips, thighs, and buttocks, thanks to higher levels of female hormones. After menopause, with a shift in hormone levels, women tend to store more abdominal fat. Interestingly, before menopause, high body fat is associated with lower rates of breast cancer; after

Name That Fat

The two types of fat go by many different names.

Visceral Fat
- Abdominal fat
- Ectopic lipid
- Intra-abdominal fat
- Central obesity
- Organ fat
- Apple shape
- Belly fat
- Android distribution

Subcutaneous Fat
- Peripheral fat
- Pear shape
- Gynoid distribution

menopause, excess body fat is linked with a higher risk of breast cancer. This may be due to the fact that before menopause the excess fat is located in the hips and thighs, while after menopause it is in the higher-risk abdominal area. Also, premenopausal women who are obese may not ovulate regularly, leading to lower levels of estrogen.

Breast Cancer and Excess Weight

Most of the data discussing excess body weight and cancer deals with breast cancer patients, but more information is emerging for colon and prostate cancers. From this population, we know that weight gain after diagnosis is common in some cancer patients. The research shows this is especially true among breast cancer patients receiving chemotherapy or hormone therapy after their surgery or radiation. This is a summary of information on obesity and breast cancer:

- More studies than not see a higher risk of recurrence and lower survival with women who are overweight and obese (some don't see this relationship).
- Obese patients with lymph-node-negative and estrogen-receptor(ER)-positive breast cancer benefited from tamoxifen therapy as much as lighter-weight women.
- Women with a body mass index (BMI) between 20 and 25 had the lowest risk of recurrence and death; those with a BMI lower than 20 or greater than 25 had an increased risk of recurrence and death.
- Women with more abdominal obesity showed higher mortality.
- Weight gain after diagnosis increased recurrence risk and decreased survival rates.

Measuring Risk

There are several ways to estimate your risk for weight-related diseases (heart disease, diabetes, cancer, joint problems) that are based on your weight and body fat. To determine a healthy weight for you, you can use the body mass index (BMI) or the waist circumference method.

Body Mass Index

BMI is the most popular measure of healthy and unhealthy weight. You can make the calculations on a hand calculator or at a BMI site on the Internet.

❶ First, calculate your height in meters squared. To do this, record your height in meters. If you don't know your height in meters but in inches, take the number of inches

---

Did You Know?

Overindulgence
For many patients, a diagnosis of cancer may be seen as an opportunity to indulge in eating high-fat, high-sugar treats. Coupled with this, friends and family will give you tempting treats and comfort foods as gifts. While dealing with the stress and emotional aspects of your cancer, you need to enlist new ways of coping, such as peer or group support, meditation, relaxation, and other complementary therapies, and not use food indulgence for comfort. Keep your home safe from unhealthy foods by shopping carefully, and ask friends to bring only healthy foods into your home.

---

and multiply by 0.0254. For example, if you are 66 inches tall, multiply the total inches by 0.0254 (66 × 0.0254) = 1.676 meters. Square your height by multiplying this number by itself 1.676 × 1.676 = 2.81.

❷ Second, determine your weight in kilograms. If you don't know your weight in kilograms but in pounds, take your weight in pounds and divide by 2.2. For example, if you weigh 200 pounds, divide the total pounds by 2.2 (200 ÷ 2.2 = 91 kilograms).

❸ Third, divide body weight in kilograms by height in meters squared: 91 ÷ 2.81 = 32.

❹ Fourth, interpret your results:
• A BMI below 18.5 is classified as underweight.
• A BMI of 18.5 to 24.9 is classified as normal weight.
• A BMI of 25.0 to 29.9 is classified as overweight.
• A BMI of 30.0 to 39.9 classified as obese.
• A BMI of 40+ is classified as morbidly obese.

There are some limitations with BMI. If you are holding a lot of fluid in your body, the excess weight may classify you as overweight or obese when in fact you may not be. If you have very little muscle mass, you may be classified as normal weight but could still have too much body fat.

Waist Circumference

To measure your waist circumference, use either inches or centimeters. Use a soft, flexible measuring tape that a tailor or seamstress might use. Locate your upper hip bone and place the measuring tape halfway between the upper hip bone and the bottom of your rib cage. Make sure the tape is horizontal and isn't twisted or being put over bulky clothing or a belt. It should be snug but not constricting.

Health Risk	Waist Circumference	
	Men	Women
Low risk	≤37 inches (93 cm)	≤31½ inches (79 cm)
Substantially high risk	≥ 40 inches (102 cm)	≥35 inches (88 cm)

Source: World Health Organization, 2007. **Note:** The World Health Organization suggests cut-offs for people of Mexican and Asian descent be lower than those for people of European descent due to greater risk of disease with modest increases in intra-abdominal fat.

Weight Management

Achieving and maintaining a healthy body weight is recommended by the American Institute for Cancer Research to reduce your risk of developing an initial cancer or a recurrence of cancer. Your weight loss nutrition and exercise program should be consistent with other recommendations for cancer risk reduction. A low-carb diet, for example, would not be recommended, because with this type of diet you avoid whole grains, fruits, and many vegetables and eat more meat. Long-term success is more likely when you enroll yourself in some type of program that offers accountability for the long term — at least a year. Combinations of nutrition, exercise, and behavioral changes are best versus just one program alone.

> **Did You Know?**
>
> **Liposuction**
> Liposuction, while it will reduce your waist circumference, will not reduce your health risk, as it removes subcutaneous fat and not the more metabolically active visceral fat.

Guidelines for Dietary, Activity, and Behavorial Treatment of Weight Gain and Obesity

Diet

❶ Enlist people to help you. Include a combination of a nutrition professional, such as a registered dietitian, and an exercise professional, such as a certified personal trainer, and always include support people, such as family and friends.

❷ Set short-term and long-term goals for yourself and make them SMART (specific, measureable, achievable, realistic, and timely). Write them down.

❸ Choose the best time to begin a weight loss program; you may want to wait until after the initial cancer therapy is completed.

❹ Eat breakfast, always.

❺ Eat at regular times, with no more than 4 hours between meals and snacks.

❻ Balance snacks with carbohydrate and protein.

❼ Balance meals with at least one-third of the plate filled with vegetables, one-quarter to one-third with whole grains, and one-quarter to one-third with lean protein.

❽ Drink plenty of water every day. Make it your main beverage. Avoid soft drinks (soda pop).

❾ Exercise every day. Walking is fine.

❿ Eat mindfully. Eat slowly while paying attention to the experience of all your senses — taste, smell, appearance, temperature, and texture.

⓫ Don't watch TV or a computer screen or another distraction while eating.

⓬ Stop eating when you are satisfied.

⓭ Choose small dinner plates: 9 inches (23 cm) across is a good size.

⑭ Repackage large containers of food into smaller ones.
⑮ Chew your food well.
⑯ Keep your home free of unhealthy foods by shopping carefully. Ask friends to bring only healthy snacks with cancer-fighting ingredients into your home.
⑰ Treat food like medicine. Ask yourself, "Will this food serve me well?"

Activity

❶ Begin or continue with an exercise program. Although you will very likely need to change the type and intensity of your program, you should continue to be active every day, or at least more days than not.
❷ Set a reasonable goal, such as to get through your treatment while maintaining your body weight. If you were overweight at the time of your diagnosis, a long-term goal should be to lose some of that excess weight.
❸ Don't do it alone. Get a network of support people.

Behavior

❶ Reduce your reliance on food as a stress reliever.
❷ Address your fears and worries about having cancer by seeking out support through peer or group support, meditation, relaxation, visualization, massage, and the many other complementary treatments.
❸ Tell yourself every day that "I can do this" and "My body is responding well" and "I enjoy nourishing, healthy food" and "I love to move my body and experience its full potential" and other positive affirmations.
❹ If you miss a workout or eat in a way that is not conducive to weight loss, just move on, don't dwell on it.

Wound Healing

Several factors can influence wound healing. Your age, for example, is one predictor of your wound-healing progress. In general, the older the patient, the slower the wound heals. Although age may delay wound healing, it does not prevent good-quality healing. Exercise has been shown to improve healing in older adults. Because of the beneficial effects of the female hormone estrogen, women tend to heal better than men. People with diabetes, because of damage to many of the systems involved in wound healing, tend to heal more slowly or be prone to impaired wound healing.

The use of glucocorticoid steroids, nonsteroidal anti-inflammatories, and chemotherapy drugs, such as Adriamycin and bevacizumab, can impede wound healing, as can alcohol consumption, smoking, poor nutrition, and being overweight or obese.

Nutritional Aid for Healing

Nutrition is important for wound healing. In the cancer population, wounds are most likely from post-surgical incisions. The main nutrients involved with healing are zinc, vitamin C, and protein. Nutritional deficiencies are associated with delayed wound healing. Optimizing your nutrition prior to surgery may help you avoid complications and longer hospital stays.

Zinc

Zinc is required by your body in small amounts every day and has been shown to aid in wound healing and maintaining a strong immune system. There are a wide variety of dietary sources of zinc. It is abundant in red meats; certain seafood; seeds; beans, peas, and lentils (pulses); and whole grains.

Zinc Deficiency

People at risk of being deficient in zinc include patients with sprue (celiac disease), Crohn's disease, short bowel syndrome, and sickle cell disease, as well as vegetarians and alcoholics.

Zinc is available in many food sources (see page 86), but you may need to take a supplement. Speak with your dietitian to see if you would benefit from a zinc supplement. If you take an iron supplement, you should take it between meals. When iron is taken with a meal, it reduces the absorption of zinc. If you have been advised to take a zinc supplement to aid in wound healing, do not take it for more than 3 months.

Vitamin C

Vitamin C (ascorbic acid) is an essential nutrient, which means that we cannot make it ourselves in our bodies and we must obtain it from our diet. Fortunately, it is easy to obtain vitamin C from fruits and vegetables (see page 87). Deficiencies of this vitamin are not common.

Vitamin C plays a significant role in the formation of collagen, an important component of skin and other tissues. Because of this, vitamin C is needed for the healing of wounds. Vitamin C is also an antioxidant and therefore has a role in reducing the risk of cancer and other chronic diseases and strengthening the immune system.

Patients may be tempted to take high doses of vitamin C during cancer treatments because of its wound-healing and antioxidant properties. It is suspected that vitamin C might have the unwanted effect of protecting tumor cells from cancer treatments, but eating dietary sources of vitamin C after your surgery should help with wound healing.

Signs of Infection in the Surgical Wound

- Fever of 100.4°F (38°C)
- Redness or swelling around the wound that gets worse
- Yellow or greenish fluid leaking from the wound
- Foul odor from the wound

Did You Know?

Processed Depletion Zinc is found in a wide variety of foods, including the germ and bran portions of grains, but as much as 80% of the total zinc can be lost during the making of white flour. Many breakfast cereals are enriched with zinc. Choose whole grains or fortified grain products. Use zinc supplements if needed to meet the RDA, but only for a maximum of 3 months.

Food Sources of Zinc

The RDA for adults is 8 milligrams per day for women and 11 milligrams per day for men. The tolerable upper intake level (UL) for adults is 40 milligrams per day. The requirement for zinc may be as much as 50% greater for strict vegetarians, whose major food staples are grains and legumes. The daily zinc requirement is also higher in alcoholics, 30% to 50% of whom have a low zinc status. Food labels, however, are not required to list zinc content unless a food has been fortified with this nutrient. Foods providing 20% or more of the % DV are considered to be high sources of a nutrient.

Food	Serving	Zinc
Oysters	6 medium	76.7 mg
Beef shanks, cooked	3 oz (90 g)	8.9 mg
Crab, Alaska king, cooked	3 oz (90 g)	6.5 mg
Pork shoulder, cooked	3 oz (90 g)	4.2 mg
Chicken leg, roasted	1 leg	2.7 mg
Lobster, cooked	3 oz (90 g)	2.5 mg
Pork tenderloin, cooked	3 oz (90 g)	2.5 mg
Baked beans, canned	½ cup (125 mL)	1.7 mg
Cashews, dry-roasted	1 oz (30 g)	1.6 mg
Fruit-flavored yogurt (low-fat)	1 cup (250 mL)	1.6 mg
Chickpeas, cooked	½ cup (125 mL)	1.3 mg
Raisin bran	¾ cup (175 mL)	1.3 mg
Swiss cheese	1 oz (30 g)	1.1 mg
Almonds, dry-roasted	1 oz (30 g)	1.0 mg
Cheddar or mozzarella cheese	1 oz (30 g)	0.9 mg
Chicken breast, skinless, roasted	½ breast	0.9 mg
Milk	1 cup (250 mL)	0.9 mg
Kidney beans, cooked	½ cup (125 mL)	0.8 mg
Oatmeal, instant	1 packet (35 g)	0.8 mg
Peas, cooked	½ cup (125 mL)	0.8 mg
Flounder or sole, cooked	3 oz (90 g)	0.5 mg

Source: National Academy of Sciences.

Food Sources of Vitamin C

The recommended intake is 75 milligrams per day for adult women and 90 milligrams per day for adult men. Smokers need an additional 35 milligrams per day. The upper limit of vitamin C is 2000 milligrams per day. You can see from this chart that it is easy to receive the recommended 75 to 90 milligrams per day.

Food	Serving	Vitamin C
Red bell pepper, raw	½ cup (125 mL)	95 mg
Orange juice	¾ cup (175 mL)	93 mg
Kiwifruit	1 medium	71 mg
Grapefruit juice	¾ cup (175 mL)	70 mg
Orange	1 medium	70 mg
Green bell pepper, raw	½ cup (125 mL)	60 mg
Broccoli, cooked	½ cup (125 mL)	51 mg
Strawberries	½ cup (125 mL)	49 mg
Brussels sprouts, cooked	½ cup (125 mL)	48 mg
Grapefruit	½ medium	39 mg
Tomato juice	¾ cup (175 mL)	33 mg
Cantaloupe	½ cup (125 mL)	29 mg
Cabbage, cooked	½ cup (125 mL)	28 mg
Cauliflower, raw	½ cup (125 mL)	23 mg

Source: National Institutes of Health.

Protein

Along with carbohydrates and fat, protein is a macronutrient. It helps build healthy tissue and heal wounds. Consuming sufficient protein post-surgery will help the body heal.

The amount of protein you need is based on your body weight. The average person requires 0.39 grams of protein per pound (0.86 g per kg) of body weight. However, after surgery, your protein needs will be increased and you will likely require 0.54 grams of protein per pound (1.2 g per kg) of body weight. So, if you weigh 175 pounds, for example, you need to consume 94.5 grams of protein per day (175 x 0.54 = 94.5).

If you are overweight or obese, this calculation will overestimate your protein needs. In this case, rather than your actual body weight, you should use your adjusted body weight. A dietitian can help you with this.

> **Did You Know?**
>
> **Wound Hygiene**
> Preventing infection is important, so don't touch your wound directly and use proper technique when dressing the wound. Proper dressing is important to heal a wound from the outside in, and proper nutrition is important for healing the wound from the inside out.

You can track your protein intake by keeping detailed food records, paying close attention to portion size. You can get the protein content of the food from the nutrition facts panel on the food label or use the table below to help you add up your protein intake.

Food Sources of Protein

Food	Serving	Protein
Meat, fish, or poultry	2½ oz (75 g)	21 g
Firm tofu	5 oz (150 g)	21 g
Eggs	2 large	13 g
Cheese	1½ oz (50 g)	12 g
Dried beans, peas, or lentils, cooked	¾ cup (175 mL)	12 g
Milk	1 cup (250 mL)	9 g
Peanut butter or other nut spread	2 tbsp (30 mL)	8 g
Yogurt	¾ cup (175 mL)	8 g
Nuts or seeds	¼ cup (60 mL)	7 g
Fortified soy beverage	1 cup (250 mL)	6–8.5 g
Bread	1 slice	3 g
Cereal, hot	¾ cup (175 mL)	3 g
Pasta or rice, cooked	½ cup (125 mL)	3 g

Source: HealthLink BC.

FAQ

Q. *I am experiencing nerve damage as a result of my chemotherapy. Do you have any recommendations for this?*

A. Peripheral neuropathy is a symptom arising from the damage to nerves because of chemotherapy, which can result in painful feet and legs, as well as weakness, numbness, tingling, a loss of sensation, cramps, spasms, or twitching in the muscles. Treatment may include vitamin E and glutamine supplementation, calcium and magnesium infusions, nortriptyline (an antidepressant), carbamazepine (an anticonvulsant drug), glutathione (an antioxidant), and acupuncture. However, none of these treatments has been studied with sufficient scrutiny to be endorsed. Check with your cancer-care team about their current recommendations. In addition, you may wish to speak to a physical therapist about using a cane, orthotic brace, or splint to improve alignment and balance and prevent injury.

FAQ

Q. *What is the difference between a dietitian and a nutritionist?*

A. One of the biggest differences between the two professions is the amount of education required. In the U.S., Canada, and the UK, dietitians have earned a minimum four-year degree in dietetics, food service management, or nutrition and have completed supervised practical training through a university program or in an approved hospital or community setting. They must then pass a certifying exam. Dietitians must be registered with state or provincial regulatory bodies, and they are the only professionals who can use the titles Registered Dietitian, Professional Dietitian, or Dietitian, which are protected by law. They are accountable to state or provincial regulatory bodies for their professional conduct and the care they provide. They must also participate in professional continuing education.

Although some states and provinces regulate use of the word "nutritionist" or "dietitian-nutritionist" through registration or licensing, in most areas anyone with an interest in nutrition can call him- or herself a nutritionist. There is no specific level of education, training or certification required.

Chapter 3

Complementary Cancer Care

A number of complementary therapies have been studied for their ability to help improve the effectiveness of conventional therapies and reduce adverse side effects. This practice of complementing conventional therapies with other treatment modalities is known as integrative oncology.

The study of the effectiveness and safety of complementary therapies is an emerging field; however, well-designed research studies have demonstrated the safety and effectiveness of clinical nutrition and physical activity. Research is emerging in other areas.

Alternative therapies differ from complementary treatments in that they are meant to replace conventional practices rather than support them. These therapies tend to be higher-risk remedies and can involve delaying or avoiding conventional treatments, and although some of these practices are quite old, their traditional healing values have not been subject to the same scientific rigor and scrutiny that conventional therapies have.

Complementary Treatment Categories

According to the U.S. National Institutes of Health, there are five main categories of complementary medicine: whole medical systems, energy medicine, mind-body practices, physical manipulation practices, and biologically based medicine.

Not all complementary practices have a direct application to cancer treatment and side effects. As you read this summary of complementary practices, see what therapies resonate for you. Be sure to discuss with your oncologist any therapies you may be considering. Although some may be innocuous, others may obstruct conventional therapies and be downright dangerous. When you are researching a particular treatment, ensure that the source of information is not only the manufacturer or advertiser of the treatment. The Resources (page 306) will give you a good start in searching for more information on these remedies.

Did You Know?

CAM Facts

According to the National Cancer Institute, people with cancer turn to complementary and alternative medicine (CAM) to support their conventional treatments for several reasons:

- To help treat or cure their cancer when conventional treatments are failing to do so
- To help cope with the side effects of conventional cancer treatments, such as nausea, pain, and fatigue
- To comfort themselves and ease the worries of cancer treatment and related stress
- To feel that they are doing something themselves to help with their own care

Introduction to Complementary Medicine

Medical System	Practices	What Is It?
Whole medical systems	Ayurvedic medicine (traditional Indian medicine)	A traditional form of medicine from India that emphasizes balance among body, mind, and spirit. It views people as complex combinations of elements, which are called *doshas*, or bioforces. The mixture of bioforces is called *prakruti*. Ayurvedic practitioners analyze your *prakruti* and recommend a plan to rebalance your bioforces.
	Traditional Chinese medicine (TCM)	Based on the view that health is a balance in the body of two forces called *yin* and *yang*. Acupuncture is a common practice in traditional Chinese medicine that involves stimulating specific points on the body to promote health or to lessen disease symptoms and treatment side effects.
	Homeopathy	The principle of homeopathy is that like cures like. In this practice, very diluted doses of substances are used to trigger the body's ability to heal itself. The more diluted a product is, the stronger homeopaths consider it to be. It can be diluted to the point that levels of the original product are undetectable by laboratory instruments.
	Naturopathic medicine	Practiced by naturopathic doctors, who are the "family doctors" of natural health care. They treat the same conditions as family doctors and are not considered specialists in any particular area. Naturopathic doctors use six different treatment modalities: nutrition, acupuncture, botanical medicine, physical medicine, lifestyle counseling, and homeopathy.
Energy medicine	Tai chi	Involves slow, gentle movements, breath control, and meditation to reduce stress.
	Qigong	Uses breathing techniques, gentle body movement, and focused intention to cleanse, strengthen, and enhance the natural flow of energy in the body, called *qi*, or *chi* (pronounced *chee*).

Medical System	Practices	What Is It?
Energy medicine (continued)	Reiki	Designed to restore the natural flow of energy in the body and provide a relaxing experience and an improved sense of well-being. A trained practitioner places his or her hands on or near a patient to restore misaligned energy fields.
	Therapeutic touch	As with reiki, a trained practitioner uses his or her hands to assess and realign a patient's energy field, using light touch or working close to the body without touching.
	Polarity therapy	Therapists balance the energy flow between the positive and negative poles of your body to calm nerves, relax muscles, and open natural healing pathways.
Mind-body practices	Meditation	Focused breathing or repetition of words to quiet an anxious, racing mind.
	Biofeedback	A computerized device measures muscular tension, pulse, and temperature to determine a person's level of stress. It is used to help patients learn to relax and practice their relaxation techniques.
	Aromatherapy	Aromas from essential oils are inhaled or massaged into the skin. Scent receptors in the nose send messages to the brain that affect mood, blood pressure, heart rate, or breathing, or assist with other side effects of your cancer treatment.
	Hypnosis	A psychologist or hypnotherapist induces a trance state in the patient by focusing on a specific feeling, idea, or suggestion to aid in healing.
	Yoga	One of the most widely used complementary therapies for managing illness, yoga is a combination of breathing techniques, physical poses, and meditation that has been practiced for over 5,000 years.
	Imagery	Involves imagining positive scenes, pictures, or experiences to help the body heal. For example, cancer patients may visualize the immune system attacking and destroying cancer. Used to prepare for chemotherapy, control stress, and work through emotional distress.
	Positive affirmations	Use of positive, uplifting words to change the way you perceive a situation and manifest real change. In her bestselling book *You Can Heal Your Life*, Louise Hay recommends this affirmation for those dealing with cancer: "I lovingly forgive and release all of the past. I choose to fill my world with joy. I love and approve of myself."
	Creative therapies	Bringing art, music, dance, drumming, and creative writing to bear on healing cancer to achieve a lower stress level and improve emotional and physical well-being.

Medical System	Practices	What Is It?
Mind-body practices (continued)	Psychotherapy	Classical psychotherapy involves talking with a trained therapist about coping with cancer.
	Group therapy	Groups are led by professionals or trained volunteers, usually cancer survivors, and can be specific as to type of cancer or cancer stage (for example, metastatic stage), or they can be based on social groupings, such as teens, single parents, women, and gay men. The goal is to provide a safe and confidential setting in which participants share their challenges, fears, and successes.
	Prayer (belief)	Faith-based practices to provide support. Science is examining the benefits of prayer on healing.
Physical manipulation	Massage	Registered therapists use long, smooth stokes, kneading, and other movements to affect superficial muscles.
	Reflexology	Type of massage used to stimulate pressure points in the hands or feet to clear any blockages in the nervous system.
	Chiropractic	Performed by a licensed doctor of chiropractic medicine (DC) who manipulates the joints and other tissues, particularly those of the spinal column, with the goal of relieving any interference with the normal functioning of your nervous system.
	Physical activity	Evidence that physical activity can delay cancer development and enhance treatment is strongest for colon cancer, followed by post-menopausal breast, endometrial, lung, pancreas, and pre-menopausal breast cancers.
Biologically based medicine	Vitamins, minerals, herbs, foods	These treatments make use of natural products, including dietary supplements, herbs and foods.
	Special diets	Use of special diets to reduce cancer risk and manage symptoms. Some diets can be fads, with little evidence backing them up, while others are well substantiated.
	Clinical nutrition	Dietary strategies suggested by a registered dietitian after conducting an individualized nutrition assessment.

Support Agencies

There are many cancer support agencies that can provide guidance during your cancer journey. This may include support for your caregiver, as well as exercise and cooking classes. The Cancer Support Community in the United States is one such group. The Wellspring Organization in Canada and Maggie's Centres and the Paul D'Auria Cancer Support Centre in England provide similar services. There are links to these agencies and others in the Resources on page 306.

Survivor Wisdom

Be open to support groups. They can benefit your appetite, your vitality, and the healing process.

Two Complementary Therapies to Consider

With so many complementary therapies out there, you might not know where to begin. You may be most comfortable starting with those that have the most scientific evidence behind them. Physical activity and nutrition are two to consider.

Physical Activity

In the past, a person with cancer was advised to rest and take it easy. Physical activity was not part of any treatment or recovery plan. However, exercise has been shown to help keep cancer at bay. Exercise is not only linked to better weight management, which is a strong predictor of cancer risk, but is also thought to be helpful in a number of other ways. It reduces insulin resistance, reduces body fat, alters hormone levels, reduces chronic inflammation, and speeds up the digestive system to keep your bowels more regular.

According to researchers at the University of Alberta, physical activity reduces the risk of developing some cancers, helps cancer survivors cope with and recover from treatments, improves the long-term health of cancer survivors, possibly reduces the risk of recurrence, and extends survival in some cancer populations.

Levels of Exercise

- Light physical activity has only minor effects on the heart rate and breathing.
- Moderate physical activity increases the heart rate to around 60% to 75% of its maximum.
- Vigorous physical activity increases the heart rate to 80% or more of its maximum.

FAQ

Q. *What are mind-body practices?*

A. Mind-body therapy is based on the belief that your mind and body are strongly linked and that the mind is able to affect change in the body. There is some evidence to support the use of mind-body exercises in treating cancer survivors. In a study of 181 breast cancer survivors (3 to 11 months post-diagnosis), women participated in either a standard support group that provided an outlet for problem solving, sharing, and support or a complementary therapy support group that also included body awareness, meditation, affirmations, imagery, spirituality, and diet and lifestyle interventions. At the end of the 12-week programs, both groups showed improvements in their quality of life and spiritual well-being. Their test scores showed a decrease in anxiety, depression, and psychiatric drug use.

Moderate Exercise

According to the American Institute for Cancer Research (AICR), cancer patients should aim to be moderately physically active, equivalent to brisk walking, for at least 30 minutes every day. As your fitness improves, aim for 60 minutes or more of moderate exercise or for 30 minutes or more of vigorous physical activity every day. Longer or more intense activity has added benefit, so think of these as minimum levels.

Physical activity includes household, work, and leisure activities, as well as getting around your community. In combination with more activity, aim to limit sedentary habits, such as watching television.

Nutrition

As this book will attest, diet is an important part of cancer treatment, recovery, and ongoing survival. Chapter 4 provides detailed information about nutrition and cancer risk reduction. Make sure to check with your medical team before beginning any biologically based treatment, particularly if it involves medicines, tinctures, teas, supplements, injections or a change to your diet. In addition to your oncologist, the pharmacist, nurse, and dietitian at your cancer center are important resources for you to seek out and question about potential interactions from these therapies. To investigate claims that sound too good to be true, visit the U.S. Federal Drug Agency (FDA) website, which lists 187 fake cancer "cures."

FAQ

Q. *What is the alkaline diet, and should I follow it during treatment?*

A. Advocates of this diet believe that when a person eats meat, dairy products, and grains, too much acid forms in the body. This excess acid leads to cancer, as well as osteoporosis, obesity, heart disease, depression, and even death.

Acidic foods are limited to 20% of the diet and include blueberries, cranberries, plums, amaranth, barley, bread, wheat flour, oatmeal, rice, all beans and legumes (chickpeas, kidney beans, etc.), meats, dairy products, vegetable oils, alcohol, cocoa, coffee, and many, many other foods.

Alkaline foods should comprise 80% of the diet and include barley grass, beet greens, broccoli, cabbage, dulce, fermented vegetables, garlic, apples, blackberries, fresh coconut, almonds, chestnuts, whey protein powder, and alkaline antioxidant water, among many other foods, mostly fruits and vegetables.

Although this diet provides very detailed food lists of what can be eaten and what cannot, one thing it does not provide is evidence. It is not recommended to follow the alkaline diet for cancer risk reduction or cure.

FAQ

Q. *Before my cancer was diagnosed, I followed the blood type diet. Should I continue this diet during treatment?*

A. This diet first appeared in Eat Right for Your Type, by Peter D'Adamo. The diet specifies foods to be avoided and to be included in your diet based on your blood type: A, B, AB, or O. On a practical level, this would mean that members of the same family may need distinct and often conflicting diets if their blood types are different. To date, there is no evidence that this diet provides benefit in reducing cancer risk, and it may have the disadvantage of unnecessarily eliminating healthy foods from the diet.

Survivor Wisdom

Cancer affects physical, emotional, and spiritual sides of a person. Food addresses all these areas too. These three aspects affect our appetite for food, so you get into a positive cycle.

Reading Food Labels

One place to find information on nutrition is the food label now required on food packages. Food labels list the ingredients and provide nutrition facts. At first sight, these labels look like a foreign language, but once you crack the code, they are extremely useful.

Ingredients

Ingredients are listed in order of weight from highest to lowest. Look for good ingredients, such as whole grains, and limit problematic ingredients, including trans fats, nitrites, sugars, and sodium.

The ingredients and facts you pay particular attention to will depend on your specific nutrition issue. If you are trying to gain weight, make sure the item has lots of calories and protein. If you are trying to lose weight, look for limited calories and fat but lots of fiber and protein. If you have high blood pressure, look for high potassium but low sodium content. If you have constipation, high fiber is beneficial.

Ingredients to Limit

Trans fats

This unhealthy fat is usually described as "partially hydrogenated oil" or "shortening."

Nitrites

This ingredient is used to preserve processed meats and give cured meats their distinctive color and flavor. Nitrites can be converted to N-nitroso compounds in the meat or in our stomachs. These are known carcinogens.

Sugars

According to Health Canada, the following terms are synonymous with sugar:

- Brown sugar
- Cane juice extract
- Corn syrup
- Demerara or Turbinado sugar
- Dextrose
- Evaporated cane juice
- Fructose
- Galactose
- Glucose
- Glucose-fructose
- High fructose corn syrup
- Honey
- Invert sugar
- Lactose
- Liquid sugar
- Maltose
- Molasses
- Sucrose
- Syrup
- Treacle

Hint: Words ending in "ose" are likely sugars.

FAQ

Q. *Does sugar feed cancer?*

A. Sugar alone does not promote cancer. Consuming small amounts of sugar as part of an overall healthful diet is fine, but large amounts of sugar may indirectly raise cancer risk in two ways.

First, diets high in sugar may lead to elevated blood sugar levels, which can raise insulin levels. Routinely high levels of insulin may, in turn, increase the risk of colon cancer and perhaps other cancers. This indirect chain of events is seen most commonly among people who are overweight and sedentary or those who have insulin resistance or diabetes in the family.

Second, high sugar consumption may lead to weight gain. High-sugar foods are typically high in calories, and over time a high-calorie diet leads to excess weight. And excess weight is linked to a greater risk of several types of cancers, namely cancers of the esophagus, pancreas, colon and rectum, edometrium, kidney and breast (in postmenopausal women).

Q. *How much sugar can I eat?*

A. A 2009 press release from the American Institute of Cancer Research recommends that adults reduce their consumption of added sugars (table sugar, honey, corn syrup, molasses, syrups and other sugars added to processed foods) to 25 grams (6 tsp/30 mL) per day for women and 28 grams ($6^{1}/_{2}$ tsp/32 mL) per day for men.

Q. *Is there a type of sugar that is less harmful?*

A. One way to classify sugar is to use a scale called the glycemic index, a tool developed by Dr. David Jenkins at the University of Toronto in 1981. The glycemic index ranks the quality of a carbohydrate as either fast-absorbing (high glycemic) or slow-absorbing (low glycemic). For more about the glycemic index, see page 113.

FAQ

Q. *What is a detox diet, and should I do one?*

A. There are many detoxification (detox) and cleansing diets available on the Internet, from health food stores, and from nutrition practitioners. They usually have two components: herbal preparations and a diet that ranges from eliminating a few "unhealthy" foods (such as wheat, dairy, meat, sugar, caffeine, and alcohol) to an almost complete fast for a specified number of days. The herbal preparations usually claim cleansing and detoxifying attributes, but in reality are natural laxatives and diuretics.

Detox diets claim to rid the body of unwanted toxins, permit weight loss, flush fat, remove cellulite, eliminate body odor and bad breath, and cure headaches, nausea, and fatigue. However, there is no evidence that these diets are beneficial; in fact, fasting can lead to the production of ketones — which are a toxin. Our bodies have a natural way to get rid of toxins, a function performed by the liver and kidneys. Cleaning up your diet by reducing your consumption of refined sugars, excess saturated fat and alcohol, and processed foods is a great idea. But there is no evidence that you will achieve additional benefit by going to the extreme of fasting and using laxatives and diuretics.

Survivor Wisdom

Food is really a social event. It's community, it's love, it's family, it's friends. It's a big thing. In a lot of cultures, it's a huge thing. You show your visitors they're welcome by the meal you serve them. When you aren't eating well, you become more aware of the deeper meaning of food.

Sodium

According to Health Canada, about 77% of the sodium in the typical North American diet comes from processed food products. Only 5% comes from the salt we add to our food at the table. (Sodium chloride is the name for table salt.) Salt is used to add flavor and as a preservative. These terms indicate that sodium is present in your food:

- Baking powder
- Baking soda
- Brine
- Celery salt
- Disodium phosphate
- Garlic salt
- Monosodium glutamate (MSG)
- Onion salt
- Salt
- Sodium alginate
- Sodium benzoate
- Sodium bisulfate
- Sodium proprionate
- Soy sauce

Not all cancer patients need to avoid sodium. If you have low blood pressure, are dehydrated, or have experienced vomiting and/or diarrhea, you may, in fact, need additional sodium in your diet.

Serving Size

Look at the serving size to determine if the nutrition information provided is for a specific measure, which may be less than the entire package.

FAQ

Q. *What is colonic irrigation?*

A. Colonic irrigation (also simply called "a colonic") is promoted by alternative practitioners as a way to cleanse the colon, ridding the body of toxins and treating a variety of medical conditions. The procedure is performed at a colonic center, sometimes called a hydrotherapy center or clinic. It involves passing warm water into the colon by way of a rubber tube inserted through the rectum. Some clinics use herbal preparations, coffee, enzymes, wheat grass extract, or other additives in addition to the water.

There are many dangers associated with colonic irrigation, the most serious being the risk of colon perforation. Others include bacterial infection from unsterilized equipment, cramping, pain, heart failure, and electrolyte imbalance. Needless to say, the procedure is not recommended, and any claims that it can reduce your cancer risk are unsubstantiated.

Percent Daily Value

The percent daily value (% DV) is the measure of a specific nutrient in a serving that is needed to meet 100% of the recommended daily allowance. A 5% DV or less is a little and a 15% DV or more is a lot. For some nutrients, such as calcium, iron, fiber, and vitamins A and C, you will want a high % DV, but for others, such as saturated fat, trans fat, and sodium, you want a low % DV.

These are the reference values for % DV of common nutrients:

- Calcium: 1100 mg
- Iron: 14 mg
- Fiber: 25 g
- Vitamin A: 1000 IU
- Vitamin C: 60 mg
- Fat: 65 mg
- Saturated and trans fat: 20 g
- Sodium: 2400 mg

> ### Survivor Wisdom
> *First, I prayed every day, then I did visualization. I did yoga and tai chi. I didn't want to just stay in the house and be lonely. I joined a support group called Healing Journey.*

Daily values do not account for the increased nutrient needs of women who are pregnant or breastfeeding. In these cases, consult with your physician or dietitian.

Information Overload

Part of your cancer experience will likely include research and reading about your type of cancer and the different treatment options. This should help you feel sufficiently knowledgeable and empowered to ask your health-care team informed questions. But it can also be too much of a good thing. You may be feeling overloaded, overwhelmed, anxious, and burdened with the amount of information you have found. You may be putting undue pressure on an already stressful situation.

Get to know your tolerance for gathering information. When it is no longer constructive, give yourself a rest from the pressure of seeking to find answers. Ultimately, you need to get yourself into a treatment environment in which you feel comfortable with your caregivers, trust your caregivers, and feel optimistic that your treatment is the right one for you. If this isn't the situation for you, then look for a second opinion.

Some patients may read very little and follow only the conventional treatment outlined by their oncologist. Others may participate in many of the complementary therapies available. Each diagnosis of cancer is as unique as are the people experiencing the cancer. Know that there is no right way to go through treatment. Trust your instincts and your inner guidance and make decisions that feel right for you.

FAQ

Q. *How do I know the nutrition information that I am getting is reliable?*

A. When searching for information on the web, be skeptical when the site is trying to sell you a product. Avoid sites that claim to offer the cure for cancer or present a conspiracy theory; for example, doctors know the cure for cancer but won't let you have it because they would lose their jobs.

The best place to find reliable nutrition information is from national, provincial, or state cancer organizations; for example, the American Cancer Society (www.cancer.org) or the Canadian Cancer Society (www.cancer.ca). There are also several authoritative research organizations, such as the National Cancer Institute at the National Institutes of Health (www.cancer.gov) and the American Institute for Cancer Research (www.aicr.org).

Some organizations, such as the Leukemia and Lymphoma Society (www.lls.org), focus on specific cancers. The American Dietetic Association (www.eatright.org) and Dietitians of Canada (www.dietitians.ca) also provide reliable nutrition information. Many not-for-profit support agencies have good information and links to credible sites. See the Resources (page 306) for more reputable sites you can visit.

Part 2

Keeping Cancer at Bay

2

Chapter 4

Your Nutrition Toolbox

Anticancer Eating

The recommendations in this chapter can be summarized as follows:

❶ Eat a plant-based diet with lots of fruits, vegetables, whole grains, legumes, nuts, seeds, herbs and spices.

❷ Consume sources of omega-3 fatty acids and reduce your intake of omega-6 sources.

❸ Limit your intake of refined sugars and red meat, and avoid processed meats and alcohol.

While you are receiving treatment, your first priority should be to focus on getting through this stage as best you can. Follow the guidelines in chapter 2 to manage any treatment side effects. When you are ready to begin the next stage of your recovery and move on to lifelong healthy eating practices, implement the information you'll find in this chapter. If you have a good appetite during your treatment and are ready to introduce new foods or new ways of eating, then by all means get started right away. The dietary strategies described in this chapter are based on the latest evidence on foods and food components that have been shown to improve the immune system and/or interfere with the life of cancer cells.

The disciplines of nutrition and immunology came together in the 1970s to form the field of nutritional immunology. Research in this area is helping us understand the role that good nutrition plays in keeping the many cells of the immune system strong. Boosting the immune system and reducing inflammation are two goals that should be a priority for every cancer patient.

When there is short-term, or acute, inflammation in the body, the immune system reacts swiftly and effectively to the injury, resulting in healing and repair. But with chronic inflammation — which could be caused by stress, cigarette smoke, environmental pollutants, viruses, bacteria, or excess body fat — the immune response is a long, drawn-out degenerative process that changes the types of immune cells present in a particular area of the body. This new microenvironment allows cancer cells to survive,

FAQ

Q. *Is there one particular food that is best for fighting cancer?*

A. While some foods have higher levels of natural disease-fighting components, there is no superfood that guarantees results. But eating foods that are anti-inflammatory, high in fiber, and low on the glycemic index will help you put up a good fight. Also look for foods that are rich in nutraceuticals, phytonutrients, and antioxidants. These nutrients are available in a diet focused on plant foods, including fruits, vegetables, whole grains, nuts, seeds, dried legumes (pulses), herbs, and spices.

grow, multiply, and invade. At this point, many cancers are able to suppress the immune cells so they cannot eliminate the cancer cells.

The nutritional strategies presented in this chapter can help you reduce inflammation and support cancer risk reduction.

Beneficial Foods
Anti-inflammatory Foods

It is estimated that inflammation contributes to the development of about 15% of all cancers. However, certain foods and nutrients have the chemical makeup to reduce inflammation and thereby support the immune system.

Immune Cells

The immune system is large, complex, and dispersed throughout our bodies, with 25% to 75% of immune agents found in our intestines. The role of the immune system is to protect the body from internal and external invaders. It is very sensitive to changes in our nutrition.

There are many different types of cells in the immune system. Some, including macrophages, neutrophils, and natural killer cells, we are born with. Macrophages, meaning "big eaters," engulf and digest foreign cells. Neutrophils are the dominant white blood cells in our bodies. Like macrophages, they can swallow up invading cells. They can also release toxic granules to attack viruses and bacteria. Natural killer cells kill invading tumor and virus cells by releasing small toxic particles. There are also immune cells that we acquire after birth. These include T-cells, B-cells, and cytokines.

Did You Know?

Chronic Connection

Chronic inflammatory diseases can contribute to the onset and development of cancer. Patients with inflammatory bowel disease (Crohn's disease and ulcerative colitis), for example, have a higher risk of developing colon cancer. People with gastric ulcers caused by *Helicobacter pylori* bacteria in their stomach have a higher risk of cancer in the stomach. Patients with hepatitis have a higher risk of liver cancer.

Tests for Inflammation

The presence of chronic inflammation in the body can be detected through the use of blood tests. Among these tests, three are used most often: C-reactive protein (CRP), high-sensitivity C-reactive protein (hsCRP), and serum amyloid A (SAA). These tests are run in research labs but not routinely in cancer centers.

CRP has been used for several years to quantify the risk of heart disease and more recently to measure the risk for cancer and determine the prognosis in those diagnosed with certain types of cancer. Although measures of SAA and CRP are not commonly used for prognosis, they show potential for this use.

Diets rich in anti-inflammatory foods have been associated with lower serum CRP levels. The relationship of this to cancer risk has not been clearly established, but there are many molecular pathways that lead to cancer that may be affected by an anti-inflammatory diet.

The Top 20 Anti-inflammatories

Researchers have developed an index that ranks the anti-inflammatory potential of various food components. This is a simplified version of the top 20, from highest to lowest.

Food or Nutrient	Description	Food Sources
Omega-3 fatty acids	Essential fatty acid	Cold-water fish, walnuts, flax seeds
Turmeric (curcumin)	Polyphenol	Dried root used as spice in curries and curry powders
Tea	Polyphenol (catechins)	Green and black tea
Fiber	Non-digestible carbohydrate	Whole grains, dried legumes (pulses), fruits, vegetables, nuts, seeds
Garlic (allicin)	Phytochemical	Raw or cooked root used as a food or spice
Ginger	Phenol	Raw, cooked, or dried root used as spice
Saffron	Glycoside	Dried spice from a species of crocus
Protein	Amino acids	Meat, poultry, dairy products, dried legumes
Caffeine	Alkaloid	Coffee, tea, cocoa
Magnesium	Mineral	Halibut, almonds, cashews, soybeans, spinach
Genistein	Isoflavone	Soybeans and soy products
Quercetin	Flavonol	Citrus, apples, onions, parsley, tea, red wine
Luteolin	Flavone	Celery, green peppers, thyme, perilla, chamomile tea, carrots, olive oil, peppermint, rosemary, navel oranges, oregano
Vitamin E	Fat-soluble vitamin	Wheat germ, vegetable oils, nuts, seeds
Vitamin C	Water-soluble vitamin	Citrus fruits, red and green peppers, kiwifruit, broccoli, strawberries
Zinc	Mineral	Oysters, beef, chicken, fortified cereals, Great Northern beans, cashews
Vitamin B_6	Water-soluble vitamin	Chickpeas, beef liver, yellowfin tuna, salmon, chicken, enriched cereals
Niacin	Water-soluble vitamin (B_3)	Dairy products, eggs, enriched breads and cereals, fish, lean meats, dried legumes (pulses), nuts, poultry
Daidzein	Isoflavone	Soybeans and soy products
Riboflavin	Water-soluble vitamin (B_2)	Milk, cheese, leafy green vegetables, legumes

Adapted with permission from the Office of Dietary Supplements; and Cavicchia PP, Steck SE, Hurley TG, et al, A new dietary inflammatory index predicts interval changes in serum high-sensitivity C-Reactive protein, *J Nutr*, 2009 Dec;139(12):2365–72.

Anti- and Pro-inflammatory Fatty Acids

Two essential fatty acids play a central role in inflammation and cancer. Omega-3 fatty acids are anti-inflammatory, while omega-6 fatty acids are thought by some to be pro-inflammatory.

Omega-3 Fatty Acids

Omega-3 fatty acids include docosahexaenoic acid (DHA), eicosapentaenoic acid (EPA), and alpha linolenic acid (ALA). These three fats are anti-inflammatory and have been shown to protect against chronic inflammation and cancer.

EPA and DHA are naturally present in our food supply, specifically in fatty fish such as sardines, herring, mackerel, salmon, and rainbow trout. ALA is found in plant sources, specifically in walnuts, flax seeds, walnut oil, canola oil, soybeans, and green leafy vegetables.

If you are not eating fatty fish a couple of times a week, you could consider an omega-3 supplement, available at pharmacies and health food stores. When buying a supplement, make sure it contains both DHA and EPA, because research has not yet determined which is more important for strengthening the immune system. Do not supplement with omega 3-6-9 capsules, which are very popular but contain omega-6 and -9, which are already plentiful in the diet.

Omega-3 supplements appear to be not only safe but actually beneficial during chemotherapy. One therapeutic study of breast cancer patients where DHA was combined with the chemotherapeutic drugs epirubicine, cyclophosphamide, and 5-fluorouracil provided promising results. The DHA allowed the patients to take up more of the chemotherapy drugs, which resulted in slower progression of the tumor and longer survival in the patients. There are currently several studies looking at the combination of DHA and chemotherapy. Make sure you tell your oncologist about all the supplements you are taking or would like to take during your treatment.

Omega-6 Fatty Acids

The chief omega-6 fatty acids in our Western diet are linoleic acid (LA) and arachidonic acid (AA). Some researchers refer to them as pro-inflammatory because these fatty acids are used by the body to make compounds that are involved in inflammation. Linoleic acid is found in vegetable oils made from safflower, grape seeds, poppy seeds, sunflower seeds, hemp, and corn; arachidonic acid is naturally present in meat, eggs, and dairy foods.

Did You Know?

Semi-vegetarian or Pescetarian Diet
If you are thinking about adopting a vegetarian diet, given the high omega-3 content of fish and fish oils, you might consider a semi-vegetarian or pescetarian diet. This would allow you to eat DHA- and EPA-rich fish two to three times a week. You could also consume the ALA form of omega-3 by adding flax seeds, walnuts, canola oil, soybeans, and tofu to your diet. As an added benefit, flaxseed is also a source of lignans, which are phytoestrogens. These compounds may reduce the risk of breast cancer.

FAQ

Q. *What is the difference between grass-fed and grain-fed beef?*

A. In a study published in the Journal of Animal Science, beef cattle were given three different finishing diets. They were either fed corn, grass, or a 50:50 mixture of corn and grass. The meat from these animals was compared, and the grass-fed meat was higher in vitamin E content and significantly higher in omega-3 fatty acids.

Other studies have shown that grass-fed beef has a better omega-3 to omega-6 ratio (more omega-3 and less omega-6), as well as higher levels of vitamins A and E and other antioxidants (glutathione and superoxide dismutase). Grass-fed beef is also lower in fat content, with a shorter cooking time as a result. The meat has a distinct grass flavor, and the higher vitamin A content in the meat can make the fat appear somewhat yellow.

We do not need to avoid omega-6 fatty acids; rather, we should reduce their intake to achieve a better ratio of omega-6 to omega-3. In the Western diet, the current ratio of omega-3 to omega-6 is thought to be in the range of 1:10 to 1:30. In other words, for every gram of omega-3 we consume, we take in 10 to 30 grams of omega-6. The ideal ratio is thought to be 4:1. In other words, for every gram of omega-6, we should eat 4 grams of omega-3. Correcting this ratio may help correct the chronic inflammatory response in our bodies and bring our immune system back into balance.

To reduce your intake of omega-6 fatty acids, eat less red meat. When you do eat beef, try to buy grass-fed beef, which has a higher omega-3 level than conventional North American grain- and corn-fed beef. Limit dairy to two to three servings per day, and use olive and canola oil in place of other oils, which are higher in omega-6.

Herbs, Spices, and Tea

Since chronic inflammation at a cellular level leads to the initiation, growth, and invasion of cancer cells, it is sensible to consume a variety of foods with anti-inflammatory properties. Among the top anti-inflammatory foods are herbs and spices, specifically turmeric, garlic, ginger, and saffron. Using these herbs and spices will provide two benefits: you will add another anti-inflammatory component to your diet and you will use less salt to flavor your food. Another excellent anti-inflammatory is tea, which is growing in popularity around the world, thanks to its health benefits.

Turmeric

Turmeric is the top spice in the index of anti-inflammatory foods. Studies have shown that, in addition to being an anti-inflammatory, turmeric — or more specifically its active ingredient, curcumin — prevents cancer cells from proliferating, acts as an antioxidant, inhibits new blood cell formation by the cancer, and improves the immune response.

From the ginger family of herbs, turmeric is a key component of yellow curry, giving this preparation a distinctive yellow color and taste. The word "curry," often translated as sauce, soup, or stew, simply means a blend of spices. Turmeric may not be present in red and green curries.

You can purchase both turmeric and yellow curry in the spice section of most grocery stores. It is not expensive. When you purchase curry powder or paste, read the label. On the list of ingredients, it should say "turmeric." Some labels say only "spices." If you like a certain curry blend and are not sure whether it contains turmeric, you can always add more. That way, you are sure of receiving some of the anti-inflammatory spice in your meal. Also check to see if the curry blend contains black pepper, or add your own. Piperine, a component of black pepper, increases the body's absorption of curcumin. See Part 4 for several recipes using yellow curry.

Garlic

Garlic is a member of the allium family, which also includes onions, leeks, chives, and shallots. Garlic is rich in alliin. When a clove of garlic is crushed or chopped, the cell walls release an enzyme called alliinase that comes into contact with the alliin and then changes into allicin. Allicin is the compound responsible for the strong odor of garlic. Some believe that alliin is the source of its health benefits. Others believe that because allicin is unstable and quickly changes into more than 20 different compounds, it is likely that other compounds in garlic possess anticancer properties. Some of these compounds include diallyl sulfide (DAS) and diallyl disulfide (DADS).

Although the actual compounds responsible for garlic's cancer-fighting potential continue to be debated, you don't need to wait for the results to enjoy its health benefits. Or rather, you should wait only a short time: researchers have shown that, after you chop garlic, you should let it stand for 10 minutes before you eat it or heat it. This rest period maximizes its cancer-fighting potential.

Did You Know?

Weight Management
Achieving and maintaining an ideal body weight is another strategy for reducing inflammation in our bodies. Obesity is associated with inflammatory markers, including C-reactive protein (CRP), serum amyloid A (SAA), interleukin-6 (IL-6) and interleukin-1 (IL-1), and tumor necrosis factor (TNF-alpha). These markers have been shown to be higher in patients with early cancer and in patients with metastatic cancer than in patients without cancer. See page 83 for weight management guidelines.

Ginger

Ranked as the third spice on the anti-inflammatory index, ginger is native to South Asia but is now grown in East Africa and the Caribbean. The rhizome, or root, is eaten fresh or dried. To use it fresh, peel the fibrous outer skin with a vegetable peeler or the back of a spoon. You can dice it small for use in stir-fries or marinades, or leave it in big chunks or slices to make ginger tea. The dried ground ginger that you purchase in the spice section of the grocery store is generally what is used in baking.

Dried herbs and spices maintain the health benefits of the fresh spice, so don't think that you need to restrict yourself to only the fresh version. You were likely given flat ginger ale as a kid when you were sick, and this tradition stems from ginger's long history of use as a folk medicine for stomach and intestinal problems.

Saffron

Saffron is another spice that ranks high in anti-inflammatory potential. Saffron is made from the stigma of the saffron crocus. The stigma is the long, feathery, bright yellow part of the inside of this crocus flower. About 4,000 years ago, the stigma of this purple crocus was investigated for its medicinal properties. Since then, it has been used as medicine, clothing dye, perfume, body wash, and a cooking ingredient.

There is an emerging body of evidence that demonstrates saffron's ability to interfere with the life of the cancer cell. In addition to its anti-inflammatory properties, saffron has shown in the laboratory that it can kill malignant cells.

Tea

Tea has cancer-fighting ability because it contains catechins (part of the family of polyphenols called flavonols). These catechins appear to work by limiting the ability of the cancer cells to create new blood vessels for themselves. Tea is also anti-inflammatory, posing a "double threat" to cancer cells. Some sources recommend drinking three cups of Japanese green tea every day.

High-Fiber and Whole-Grain Foods

Another nutritional factor that has shown promise in reducing C-reactive protein levels is fiber. Fiber is found primarily in whole grains, as well as in vegetables and fruits, legumes, nuts, and seeds.

Fiber passes through our digestive system, providing benefits to our body along the way. First, it creates satiation, or the feeling of fullness, following a meal. This feeling of satiation is important for losing weight and for weight maintenance. Second, fiber can slow down the rise in blood sugar following a meal. The glycemic index, which measures this rise in blood sugar, is lower for higher-fiber foods.

Soluble and Insoluble Fiber

Most foods have a mixture of soluble and insoluble fiber. For example, wheat is higher in insoluble fiber, so wheat bran is often recommended to help with constipation because insoluble fiber helps increase the size of the stool, allowing it to pass through the digestive system faster. Bran muffins and bran cereal are long-standing remedies to help with constipation and regularity.

Oats and oat bran are higher in soluble fiber. As the name indicates, this type of fiber is soluble in water and will form a gelatinous mixture when mixed with water. Soluble fiber helps bind bile acids that hold cholesterol and remove it from the body. This is why you see oatmeal and oat bran recommended for cholesterol-lowering diets. Other soluble fibers include barley bran, psyllium, and pectin.

Fiber and Cancer

Most of the research on fiber and cancer focuses on colorectal and breast cancers, although prostate, stomach, and endometrial cancers have also been studied in this context.

Fiber and Colorectal Cancer

The results of studies examining cancer and fiber are mixed. Observational studies show that colon cancer rates are lower in countries where fiber intake is higher. Results of case studies have also shown that higher fiber intakes are associated with lower rates of colon and rectal cancers. Intervention studies, however, in which people were assigned to a high- or a low-fiber diet for three years, did not show a difference in colorectal adenomas.

When fiber reaches the large intestines, it is not digested but rather fermented by the good bacteria that live in our digestive tract. When this happens, products called short-chain fatty acids are released from the fiber. These short-chain fatty acids lower the pH and feed the healthy bacteria that live in the intestines. One of these short-chain fatty acids is called butyrate. In a laboratory study, butyrate was shown to stop the growth of cancer cells while providing energy to normal cells. Because of how it behaves in the laboratory, it is a reasonable hypothesis that fiber should protect the body against cancer.

Did You Know?

Fiber Intake
The recommended fiber intake is 25 grams per day for adult women and 38 grams per day for men. People following a typical Western diet consume less than this — about 14 grams per day. To increase your intake of fiber, eat more fruit, vegetables, whole grains, high-fiber breakfast cereals, dried legumes (pulses), nuts, and seeds.

Did You Know?

Fiber and Colorectal Cancer
Researchers from the U.S. National Cancer Institute tracked 489,000 men and women aged 50 to 71 to determine the role of fiber in colorectal cancer. When they controlled for other factors that may have an impact on colorectal cancer risk (such as red meat, dietary folate, or calcium intake), their analysis did not show that higher fiber intake was protective for colon cancer. When they analyzed whole-grain and not just fiber intake, however, they found that patients who had a higher intake of whole grains had a statistically reduced risk of colorectal cancer.

Fiber and Breast Cancer

In a study of 698 female breast cancer survivors, those with the higher intake of dietary fiber had lower levels of CRP (a measure of inflammation). Insoluble fiber intake by itself was associated with lower CRP levels.

Whole Grains

Whole grains are more than just fiber. The grain seed, kernel, or berry has three components: germ, bran, and endosperm. For a food product to be considered a whole grain, it must contain these three parts in the same proportion in which they exist in nature. This can include processed grains in which the three components are separated and then put back together.

Whole grains contain 75% more nutrients than refined grains and include phytochemicals, antioxidants, phytates, phytoestrogens, plant stanols and sterols, vitamins, minerals, and phenolic compounds. All of these have been linked to disease prevention. Another benefit of whole grains is their lower glycemic index, which means a slower blood glucose rise and more moderate insulin response. These improvements in the nutritional environment of the intestines may provide immune protection throughout the entire body.

Food Labels

When you purchase grains, make sure you are getting whole grains. This will require you to read your food labels carefully.

The USDA uses a whole-grain stamp with a picture of a sheaf of grain on a gold background. If you see the basic stamp on food labels, it means there are 8 grams of whole grains per serving, and if the stamp states "100% whole grains," this product has 16 grams of whole grains per serving. The stamp also includes the message "Eat 48 g or more of whole grains a day." Since the USDA started using this food labeling system, consumption of whole grains has improved in the United States.

In Canada, bread, flour, and other grain products can be labeled "100% whole wheat" and still have 5% of the grain removed. The parts removed are usually the germ and part of the bran. If you want 100% whole grain, look for "whole grain" and not "whole wheat" on the label. The first ingredient should be "whole grain whole wheat flour" or "whole grain whole wheat flour including the germ."

The Complete Whole Grains Cookbook from Robert Rose Inc. is an excellent source of information on whole grains.

Types of Whole Grains

There are many kinds of whole grains available to add variety to your diet. See Part 4 for some whole-grain recipes and help in preparing these grains.

Name of Grain	Details	Whole-Grain Versions	Refined Versions	Nutritional Value
Amaranth	Seeds from a spinach-like plant	• Amaranth seeds • Amaranth flour • Amaranth flakes		• Good source of magnesium and manganese
Barley	Kernel	• Hulled barley • Whole barley • Barley grits • Whole barley flour • Barley couscous	• Pearl barley • Pot barley (less refined than pearl, so a better choice)	• High in soluble fiber, manganese, and selenium
Buckwheat	Seeds from a rhubarb-like plant	• Buckwheat groats (kasha) • Buckwheat flour		• Gluten-free • Contains all the essential amino acids, making it high-quality protein
Corn	Sweet corn or field corn	• Hominy • Hominy grits • Stone-ground cornmeal • Stone-ground grits • Popcorn • Whole-grain cornmeal • Masa harina	• Corn flour • Cornmeal	• Gluten-free • Contains carotenoids, beta-carotene, lutein, and zeaxanthin
Job's tears	Seeds from a tropical plant native to Asia	• Premium hato mugi	• Sold in Asian markets, the refined version is more common than the whole-grain version	• Gluten-free • Whole-grain versions can be found online and by mail order
Millet	Possibly the world's oldest grain	• Millet grains • Millet flour • Teff grains • Teff flour		• Good source of magnesium
Oats	Very popular grain, used to make oatmeal and in baking	• Oat groats • Steel-cut oats • Rolled oats • Oat flour		• High in soluble fiber (beta-glucan) • Good source of manganese

Name of Grain	Details	Whole-Grain Versions	Refined Versions	Nutritional Value
Quinoa	Seeds from a spinach-like plant	• Quinoa seeds (red, yellow, or black) • Quinoa flour		• Complete protein (contains all essential amino acids)
Rice	Staple grain in Asia	• Brown, red, or black rice • Parboiled (converted) brown rice • Brown rice flour • Brown rice pasta	• White rice	• Good source of manganese, magnesium, and selenium
Rye	Popular in North America and Europe	• Rye berries • Rye flakes • Rye flour	• Many rye breads also contain mostly refined white flour	• Tends to be lower glycemic than wheat products
Sorghum (milo)	Round grain from a tropical plant popular in Africa and Asia	• Sorghum grain • Sorghum flour		• Sorghum flour is used to make bhakri (unleavened bread) in India
Teff	Variety of millet with darker color and stronger flavor	• Teff grains • Teff flour		• Major ingredient in injera (Ethiopian flatbread) • Gluten-free
Triticale	Hybrid of wheat and rye	• Berries • Flour • Flakes		• High in protein
Wheat	The main grain in North America, used to make bread, pasta, and cereals	• Bulgur • Whole wheat couscous • Farro • Emmer • Kamut • Spelt • Wheat berries, or kernels • Whole-grain pasta	• Couscous • Pearled farro (perlato) • Partially pearled farro (semi-perlato) • White flour • White pasta	• Good sources of manganese, selenium, phosphorus, and magnesium
Wild rice	Seed from an aquatic North American grass	• Wild rice		• Higher in protein than regular rice

Adapted with permission from Finlayson J, *The Complete Whole Grains Cookbook: 150 Recipes for Healthy Living*, Toronto: Robert Rose Inc., 2008.

Low Glycemic Index Foods

The glycemic index is a tool used to measure how quickly the sugar from a carbohydrate will enter the bloodstream. Carbohydrates, also called saccharides, provide energy in the form of sugar for the body. Carbohydrate foods include sweets (candies and pastries) but also all fruits, vegetables, grains, dried legumes (pulses), and dairy foods.

There are different types of saccharides — for example, monosaccharides, or single sugars, such as glucose. Disaccharides, or double sugars, include lactose, the sugar naturally present in milk and milk products. Another disaccharide is sucrose, also known as table sugar. Polysaccharides include starch, which is in corn, rice, pasta, bread, cereals, and other grains. Most carbohydrates are absorbed more slowly than glucose.

Glucose Circulation

After you consume a carbohydrate food, the sugar from the food is broken down into its smallest component part, which is glucose. Glucose is a small single sugar that can be absorbed through the wall of the intestines and enter the bloodstream quickly. Once in the bloodstream, glucose circulates through the body and goes to where it is needed to provide energy.

To leave the bloodstream and enter the cell of the body, insulin is required to open the door to the cell. A slow-rising blood sugar provides the opportunity for the body to clear the glucose from the bloodstream in an efficient manner and maintain a normal blood sugar level, even after meals. A fast-rising blood sugar can place stress on the pancreas, which is the organ that manufactures and releases insulin.

Benefits of Low GI

High glycemic index foods are quick to enter the bloodstream, while low glycemic index foods are slow to be broken down in your digestive tract and slower to enter the bloodstream. Foods that have a low glycemic index can be thought of as the "slow carbs" that provide you with many benefits. These benefits include achieving and maintaining weight loss, increasing your sensitivity to insulin, improving diabetes management, reducing the risk of heart disease, improving cholesterol levels, managing the symptoms of polycystic ovary syndrome, reducing hunger and feeling full for longer, and a prolonged ability for physical endurance.

Did You Know?

Reading the GI

On the glycemic index (GI), glucose is assigned a value of 100. High GI foods measure 70 or more, medium GI foods measure 56 to 69, and low GI foods measure 55 or less. The higher the number on the glycemic index, the faster that food enters the bloodstream. According to the glycemic index database hosted by the University of Sidney in Australia (www.glycemicindex.com), there are a few foods that rank higher than pure glucose on the GI scale. Unfortunately, there is no way to know the glycemic index of a food without looking it up on a database. There is no particular ingredient or food labeling system that can assist you (there is a voluntary food labeling system in Australia, but no other countries). A good rule of thumb is to consume fewer refined foods.

Glycemic Load

Some believe the glycemic load is a more useful measure of food value than the GI alone.

Glycemic Load Formula

The glycemix load formula is calculated by multiplying the GI of a food by its amount of carbohydrate in grams, then dividing that number by 100.

For example, the glycemic index of a ripe banana is 51 and the amount of carbohydrate in it is 25 grams.

$$51 \times 25 \div 100 = 12.75$$

This number can be rounded up to 13. Therefore, a banana has a glycemic load of 13.

An orange has an average glycemic index of 43 and contains 11 grams of carbohydrate.

$$43 \times 11 \div 100 = 4.73 \text{ (round up to 5)}$$

It's clear that the orange will have a smaller impact on the systems in the body that maintain normal blood sugar control. This is not to say that bananas are bad for you. There are many ways to measure how beneficial a food is — such as the vitamins, minerals, and other phytonutrients that it contains — but the glycemic load is another piece of the puzzle.

Most vegetables are low on the glycemic index, so you can eat them without limitation and enjoy the benefits of the antioxidants, nutraceuticals, and other beneficial plant compounds without any undue stress on your system to manage a rise in blood sugar. The exception to this is potato, which has a higher glycemic index score.

These recommendations for a low glycemic index diet are consistent with the recommendations from the American Institute for Cancer Research to reduce your cancer risk.

FAQ

Q. *Can eating low glycemic index foods affect cancer development, spread, and side effects?*

A. In one meta-analysis, 37 different studies were analyzed. Diets with a high glycemic index and high glycemic load increased the risk of breast cancer, type 2 diabetes, heart disease, gallbladder disease, and all diseases combined.

Glycemic Index of Common Carbohydrates

These foods are ranked according to their GI. The corresponding glycemix load (GL) is also calculated. This is not a complete list. If you are curious about the glycemic index score of any foods you are consuming, consult the glycemic index database online at www.glycemicindex.com.

High GI = 70 or higher
Medium GI = 56–69
Low GI = 55 or lower

Carbohydrate Source	Glycemic Index	Glycemic Load
Grains		
Whole wheat bread	69–78	8–10
Pasta and noodles	45–58	20–26
Pumpernickel bread	46–55	5–7
Bulgur (cracked wheat)	48–53	11–12
All-bran cereal	38–51	8–12
50% oat bran bread	44	8
Barley	27–29	9–11
Parboiled (converted) rice	38	14
Legumes		
Lentils (green)	30–37	4–5
Chickpeas	31–36	9–11
Split peas	25–32	3–6
Sweeteners		
Glucose (dextrose)	100	10
Sucrose (table sugar)	60–65	6–7
Maple syrup	54	10
Honey	44–52	8–11
Agave syrup	10–19	1–2

Source: www.glycemicindex.com. To calculate ranges, the highest and lowest from each category were removed. Foods manufactured in the U.S., Canada, and the UK were included; others were excluded.

Guidelines for Eating Foods Low on the Glycemic Index

The trick with the glycemic index is to incorporate it into your diet in a way that allows you to eat a healthy balanced diet without excluding otherwise healthy choices.

1. Choose one low glycemic index food per meal.
2. Reduce the portion size of rice, pasta, and potatoes.
3. Combine protein foods with carbohydrates at meals and snacks.
4. Eat your pasta "al dente" (don't overcook it).
5. Don't avoid carbohydrates or follow low-carbohydrate diets — these unnecessarily restrict healthy foods like whole grains and fruits.
6. Eat at least 5 servings of non-starchy vegetables and fruits every day.
7. Eat whole, unprocessed grains and limit refined starchy foods.

Therapeutic Nutrients

Anticancer Elements

- Vitamins
- Minerals
- Herbs
- Phytonutrients
- Antioxidants
- Probiotics
- Prebiotics

Food contains macronutrients (carbohydrates, proteins, and fat) and micronutrients (vitamins and minerals). For years, these have been the main dietary components by which the healthfulness of our diet has been measured. However, modern science is looking to traditional healing practices from many cultures to discover the healing powers of phytonutrients, antioxidants, probiotics, and prebiotics. While there are few clinical trials of these dietary elements in cancer patients, a number of laboratory studies show that these elements are capable of destroying cancer cells in a petri dish and in animals with cancer. The potential of these elements is exciting and gives cancer patients cause for hope that their dietary choices have the potential to alter their future.

Nutraceuticals

"Nutraceutical" is a term that combines "nutrition" and "pharmaceutical." Nutraceuticals are nutrients that provide medical or health "side" benefits beyond their basic nutritional functions. In the case of cancer, nutraceuticals can disrupt the development and spread of cancer cells, and some may reduce inflammation. Nutraceutical compounds include vitamins, minerals, herbs, phytonutrients, probiotics, and prebiotics. Nutraceuticals can be derived from plant, animal, marine, or microbial sources.

FAQ

Q. *What is glutamine, and can it help me?*

A. Glutamine is an amino acid (a building block of protein). It is made by the body and is therefore not an essential nutrient, but it can become essential when the body is overcome by illness — glutamine is used up by cancer cells, which can lead to a deficiency. Many studies have examined the use of glutamine supplements, given as an oral supplement or as part of enteral or parenteral nutrition formulas, during cancer treatment. These supplements have been shown to improve the metabolism and overall condition of a cancer patient without increasing the growth of the cancer itself. Speak with your cancer care team about taking glutamine, as tolerance is good and side effects are minimal.

Functional Foods

The quick and obvious definition is that functional food performs more than one function. The Institute of Medicine's Food and Nutrition Board defines it as "any food or food ingredient that may provide a health benefit beyond the traditional nutrients it contains." This would include phytochemicals, antioxidants, probiotics, and prebiotics. These foods are sometimes called bioactive compounds. Examples of functional foods would be probiotic yogurt, oats, cabbage, and omega-3-fortified eggs.

Therapeutic Action

Scientists at the University of Texas Cancer Center have studied how nutraceuticals interfere with the development of cancer cells. The formation of cancer takes many years and involves a chain reaction in which a damaged cell fails to participate in preprogrammed cell death and then grows, builds its own blood supply, and spreads. This is all encouraged by chronic inflammation. Nutraceuticals derived from spices, legumes, fruits, nuts, and vegetables have been shown in laboratory studies to stop the cancer cell at various points in its life cycle.

Fresh or Processed Foods

According to the American Institute for Cancer Research, produce at its peak of ripeness contains the highest levels of vitamins, minerals, and phytonutrients. After harvesting, these nutritional components begin to break down due to exposure to heat, light, time, and natural processes. Fresh is best, and buying local may be one way to achieve this goal. Frozen fruits and vegetables are flash frozen soon after harvesting, so the nutrients are preserved. In some cases, they may have higher levels of nutrients compared to "fresh" if that item is being

> **Did You Know?**
>
> **High-Quality Diet**
> Women who were three years post–breast cancer treatment showed better physical and emotional quality of life when their diet was of higher quality. Emotional quality of life also improved, included feeling peaceful, happy, and calm. Physical quality of life included feeling no pain, feeling full of pep and energy, and having no limitations in their social or work lives. When you improve your diet, not only are you mounting a defense against the cancer cells in your body, but you feel good about what you're eating, which makes you feel physically well.

FAQ

Q. *Are cooked vegetables still beneficial?*

A. The difference between raw and cooked vegetables and cancer risk has been studied. What these studies found was that both raw and cooked vegetables were associated with a lower risk of cancers but that the strength of that relationship may be stronger for raw vegetables. In one study that looked specifically at raw cruciferous vegetables and bladder cancer, investigators found that, after making adjustments for behaviors like smoking and other factors that had an impact on bladder cancer risk, only intake of raw cruciferous vegetables (broccoli, cauliflower, cabbage, Brussels sprouts, kale, turnip greens, collard greens and mustard greens) was associated with a reduced risk of bladder cancer. The study also looked at smokers in the group, because smoking is strongly linked to bladder cancer. The heavy smokers benefited the most from consumption of raw cruciferous vegetables.

In another study, researchers measured the amount of toxic metals and environmental pollutants in raw versus cooked foods. Results were mixed, in that some foods were lower when raw and some were lower once cooked, but in general, cooking procedures that released or removed fat from the food reduced the amount of contaminants in the cooked food.

eaten several days after harvesting. When produce is canned, it is heated to destroy any harmful organisms that could cause the item to spoil. This will reduce the amount of vitamin C but will increase the availability of the nutrient lycopene (in canned tomato products, for example). Whether fresh, frozen, or canned, aim to consume at least 5 servings of fruit and vegetables every day.

Phytonutrients

"Phyto" is a Greek word meaning "plant"; a phytonutrient, or phytochemical, is a plant nutrient with biological activity that supports human health. Phytonutrients are part of the larger group of nutrients known as nutraceuticals; however, phytonutrients are plant-based only, whereas nutraceuticals are plant-, animal-, marine-, or microbial-based. The main families of phytochemicals are polyphenols, terpenes, sulfur compounds, and saponins. These families are further divided into classes and subclasses, so the actual number of phytonutrients is about 4,000.

Most cultures in the world have a history of folk medicine, and these traditions form the basis of the modern study of phytonutrients. Thousands of phytonutrients have been isolated and cataloged from a wide range of plants, including fruits, vegetables, grains, legumes, nuts, seeds, herbs, and spices. They can have strong medicinal properties, and several phytonutrients are the basis of our modern pharmaceutical industry. White willow bark and the Pacific yew tree (*Taxus brevifolia*) were the forerunners of aspirin and Taxol, respectively.

Guidelines for Eating Phytonutrient-Rich Foods

1 Consume a generous amount and variety of different plant foods every day. Most food guides recommend a liberal intake of fruits and vegetables. The ChooseMyPlate food guide released by the United States Department of Agriculture advises that half of your plate should contain fruits and vegetables. Health Canada's Food Guide calls for adults to consume 7 to 10 servings of fruits and vegetables per day (7 to 8 for women and 8 to 10 for men) and to make at least half of your daily 6 to 8 grains choices whole grains. The National Health Service in the UK suggests eating at least 5 portions of fruits and vegetables every day and choosing whole grains whenever you can.

2 Aim to achieve this number of servings every day.

3 Since phytonutrients are responsible for the color of fruits and vegetables, choosing colorful plant foods is one way to ensure phytonutrient intake.

Put Color on Your Plate

While the chart on pages 120–122 provides excellent examples of how plants in our diets can help fight cancer, you don't need to know phytonutrient names to make the right choices. A simpler way to eat a cancer-fighting diet is to put color on your plate:

- **Green:** apples, avocados, green grapes, honeydew melon, kiwifruit, limes, artichokes, asparagus, broccoli, green beans, green bell peppers, leafy greens (such as spinach)
- **Orange and deep yellow:** apricots, cantaloupe, grapefruit, mangos, papayas, peaches, pineapples, carrots, sweet potatoes, yellow or orange bell peppers, yellow corn
- **Purple and blue:** blackberries, blueberries, plums, raisins, eggplant, purple cabbage, purple-fleshed potatoes
- **Red:** cherries, cranberries, pomegranates, red or pink grapefruit, red grapes, watermelon, beets, red bell peppers, red onions, rhubarb, tomatoes
- **White, tan and brown:** bananas, brown pears, dates, white peaches, cauliflower, mushrooms, onions, parsnips, turnips, white corn

Source: American Dietetic Association, *Eat Right with Color During Nutrition Month*, www.eatright.org.

FAQ

Q. *What is the raw food diet and should I follow it to help treat my cancer?*

A. This diet is also known as rawism, based on the belief that food should be uncooked, unprocessed, and organic. The thinking behind this diet is that enzymes and bacteria, which live on the surface of food, are destroyed when food is heated. To follow this diet, you would avoid any food that is heated above 104° F (40°C). Some raw foodists also advocate a vegan diet, while others include raw (unpasteurized) milk and milk products and raw meat. Because food can't be cooked, rice and grains are eaten after being soaked in water and sprouted. Sprouting is also recommended for nuts and seeds. Some proponents allow foods to be frozen, while others recommend against frozen food.

Although no studies to date have examined the raw food diet versus a typical or mixed diet, they do provide evidence that a diet that includes raw vegetables, specifically cruciferous vegetables, can be beneficial for some populations. At the present time, there is no evidence that an entirely raw diet is superior to a mixed diet for cancer risk reduction.

Guide to Anticancer Plant Nutrients (Phytonutrients)

This chart illustrates the benefits of various plant foods in the fight against cancer.

Phytonutrient	Food Source	Anticancer Action in Laboratory
6-gingerol	Ginger	• Antioxidant • Anti-inflammatory • Antiproliferative • Inhibits new blood cell formation
Allicin Diallyl sulfide (DAS) S-allylcysteine	Garlic, onions	• Anti-inflammatory • Antiproliferative • Inhibits new blood cell formation • Boosts immunity
Apigenin	Celery, parsley	• Antiproliferative • Inhibits cancer growth • Inhibits new blood supply • Encourages self-destruction of cancer cells
Beta carotene	Carrots, green leafy vegetables, pumpkin, red palm oil	• Antioxidant • Anti-inflammatory • Antiproliferative • Encourages self-destruction of cancer cells
Caffeic acid	Artichokes, pears, basil, oregano, thyme	• Anti-inflammatory • Antiproliferative • Inhibits new blood supply

Phytonutrient	Food Source	Anticancer Action in Laboratory
Capsaicin	Chile peppers	• Antiproliferative • Inhibits new blood supply • Encourages self-destruction of cancer cells
Curcumin	Turmeric	• Antioxidant • Anti-inflammatory • Antiproliferative • Inhibits new blood cell formation • Encourages self-destruction of cancer cells • Boosts immunity
Delpinidin	Pomegranates, strawberries	• Antioxidant • Inhibits new blood cell formation • Encourages self-destruction of cancer cells
Epigallocatechin-gallate (EGCG)	Tea (higher in green tea than black)	• Antioxidant • Anti-inflammatory • Antiproliferative • Antimutation • Inhibits new blood supply • Encourages self-destruction of cancer cells
Genestin	Alfalfa sprouts, chickpeas, peanuts, soy beans	• Antioxidant • Anti-inflammatory • Antiproliferative • Inhibits new blood cell formation • Encourages self-destruction of cancer cells
Geranoil Limonene	Cherries, citrus fruits, grapes	• Anti-inflammatory • Inhibits cancer growth • Inhibits new blood cell formation • Encourages self-destruction of cancer cells
Indole-3-carbinol	Cruciferous vegetables	• Antiproliferative • Inhibits new blood cell formation
Lutein	Spinach	• Antioxidant • Inhibits new blood cell formation • Encourages self-destruction of cancer cells
Luteolin	Carrots, celery, green peppers, olive oil, oregano, peppermint, rosemary, thyme	• Inhibits new blood supply
Lycopene	Oranges, papayas, tomatoes	• Antioxidant • Anti-inflammatory • Antiproliferative • Inhibits new blood cell formation • Boosts immunity

Phytonutrient	Food Source	Anticancer Action in Laboratory
Proanthocyanidins A2, B1, C1	Beans, berries, cocoa, nuts	• Antioxidant • Anti-inflammatory
Quercetin	Apples, berries, broccoli, onions, parsley	• Anti-inflammatory • Antiproliferative • Inhibits new blood supply • Encourages self-destruction of cancer cells
Resveratrol	Grapes	• Antioxidant • Anti-inflammatory • Antiproliferative • Inhibits new blood cell formation • Encourages self-destruction of cancer cells
Rosmarinic acid	Lemon balm, oregano, peppermint, rosemary, sage, thyme	• Inhibits new blood supply
Sulforaphane	Broccoli, Brussels sprouts, cabbage, kale, mustard greens, turnips, watercress	• Anti-inflammatory • Antiproliferative • Inhibits new blood cell formation
Tangeritin	Citrus peel	• Anti-inflammatory • Inhibits cancer growth
Ursolic acid	Apple peel, cranberries, prunes, basil, oregano, rosemary, thyme	• Antiproliferative • Inhibits new blood supply
Vanillin	Coffee, vanilla beans	• Inhibits new blood supply
Zeaxanthin	Cabbage, oranges, peas	• Antioxidant • Anti-inflammatory • Encourages self-destruction of cancer cells

Sources: Aravindaram K and Yang NS, Anti-inflammatory plant natural products for cancer therapy, *Planta Med*, 2010 Aug;76(11):1103–17; and Gupta SC, Kim JH, Prasad S and Aggarwal BB, Regulation of survival, proliferation, invasion, angiogenesis, and metastasis of tumor cells through modulation of inflammatory pathways by nutraceuticals, *Cancer Metastasis Rev*, 2010 Sep;29(3):405–34.

FAQ

Q. *Soy foods are phytonutrients, but are they safe to eat during my breast cancer treatment and while recovering?*

A. Soy contains isoflavones that have been shown to have strong cancer-fighting potential. Indeed, one of the reasons that soy came to the attention of cancer researchers is the large discrepancy in the high rates of breast and prostate cancer in North America compared with the much lower rates in soy-eating parts of the world, namely Japan and China.

    Despite this, many women diagnosed with estrogen-receptor-positive breast cancer and women using tamoxifen for treatment of breast cancer are concerned about consuming soy and soy products because they fear that soy, as a form of estrogen, will promote growth of their cancer. However, four recent studies show that there are no detrimental effects from soy consumption for women with estrogen-positive breast cancer, including those on tamoxifen; in fact, there is a benefit. All of these studies are cited in the References (page 310). If you are concerned about soy, you should discuss this with your cancer-care team.

Antioxidants

Although recent studies with antioxidant supplements have been disappointing, data shows that people with higher intakes of dietary antioxidants experience lower cancer risk, and demonstrate that a plant-based diet is a good defense. Recent studies have indicated that antioxidants in food are more effective in preventing and treating cancer than antioxidant supplements.

Oxidation

Oxygen is a molecule involved in a number of complex chemical reactions, including the chemical process of oxidation, within our bodies. Chemical substances contain electrons, and whenever possible, these substances strive to have a balanced number of electrons. Because oxygen (O_2) has two electrons that it can donate, natural chemicals in the body that contain oxygen are often involved in reactions called oxidation.

Free Radicals

When an electron is donated from one chemical to another, a product called a free radical can result. Free radicals can damage the genetic code of a cell (DNA) or kill the cell. Certain nutrients in our diet, known as antioxidants, neutralize the free radicals that can damage our cells. In this way, antioxidants are thought to protect our health.

Did You Know?

Antioxidant Caution
In a recent summary of all antioxidant-based research, the authors report that none of the trials have produced any results that would justify recommending antioxidant supplements to people trying to avoid cancer. Despite this research, antioxidant supplements can be purchased over the counter in many pharmacies and health food stores, as well as on the Internet. These supplements are not recommended by cancer professionals, including the American Institute for Cancer Research. Eat antioxidant-rich foods instead.

FAQ

Q. *Since antioxidants fight cancer, wouldn't it make sense to take a high-dose antioxidant supplement during my treatment to help fight the cancer?*

A. Most of the supplements available in pharmacies and health food stores have very high levels of antioxidants. Many cancer doctors advise against taking high-dose antioxidants during chemotherapy or radiation for fear that the antioxidants could repair the cellular oxidative damage done to the cancer cell, making the treatment less effective. Others, however, believe that the antioxidants help protect normal cells from treatment damage.

In sum, it is not clear whether there is benefit or harm from taking high-dose antioxidants during treatment. Until we know more about antioxidants during cancer treatment, keep your supplement dosages within the recommended dietary allowance (RDA). If you aren't sure what dosage that is, consult with the registered dietitian or pharmacist on your care team.

Food Sources of Antioxidants

Chief Antioxidants

- Vitamin C
- Vitamin E
- Selenium
- Lycopene
- Beta carotene

- Beta carotene is found in many foods that are orange in color, including sweet potatoes, carrots, cantaloupe, squash, apricots, pumpkin, and mangos. Some green leafy vegetables, including collard greens, spinach, and kale, are also rich in beta carotene.
- Lutein, best known for its association with healthy eyes, is abundant in green leafy vegetables such as collard greens, spinach, and kale.
- Lycopene is a potent antioxidant found in tomatoes, watermelon, guava, papaya, apricots, pink grapefruit, blood oranges, and other foods. Up to 85% percent of American dietary intake of lycopene comes from tomatoes and tomato products.
- Selenium is a mineral component of antioxidant enzymes. Plant foods, such as rice and wheat, are the major dietary sources of selenium in most countries. The amount of selenium in the soil, which varies by region, determines the

FAQ

Q. *Can vitamin D prevent or treat cancer?*

A. Many studies are currently under way to examine the role of vitamin D in the prevention and treatment of cancer. But for now there is no consensus on the recommended intake of vitamin D for high-risk cancer populations. There is potential for both harm and benefit, which may depend on dose, timing, duration of exposure, type of cancer, lifestyle factors, and genetics. Until the studies are concluded, follow the current recommendations for the general public (see page 57).

FAQ

Q. *I have heard that coconut oil is good for you. Is this true?*

A. The coconut is a source of food for people in tropical countries, providing "meat," oil, milk, and juice, and has been used in traditional medicine for a variety of ailments. Coconut oil is becoming more popular, with many health food stores now stocking it. It has a unique fatty acid profile in that it is high in lauric acid, a fat that is naturally found in human breast milk.

There is no conclusive evidence that coconut oil is protective against cancer, and it is quite high in saturated fat, which can promote heart disease. While it can be part of a healthy diet, it does not merit more than occasional use. The American Dietetic Association and Dietitians of Canada recommend that consumers aim to reduce their intake of saturated and trans fats and increase their intake of omega-3 fats.

amount of selenium in the foods grown in that soil. Animals that eat grains or plants grown in selenium-rich soil have higher levels of selenium in their muscles. In the United States, meats and bread are common sources of dietary selenium. Brazil nuts also contain large quantities of selenium.

- Vitamin A–rich foods include liver, sweet potatoes, carrots, milk, egg yolks, and mozzarella cheese.
- Vitamin C (ascorbic acid) can be found in high abundance in many fruits and vegetables and is also found in cereals, beef, poultry, and fish.
- Vitamin E (alpha-tocopherol) is found in almonds, in many oils (wheat germ, safflower, corn, and soybean oils), and in mangos, nuts, broccoli, and other foods.

Probiotics

Probiotics are defined by the Food and Agricultural Organization/World Health Organization (FAO/WHO) as "live microorganisms which when administered in adequate amounts confer a health benefit to the host." A Ukrainian scientist by the name of Elie Metchnikoff (1845–1916) is credited with making the connection between the consumption of live acidophilus-type bacteria in foods and an extended life span — a link that was the result of his observation that Bulgarian peasants who consumed milk fermented with lactobacillus bacteria lived long lives. In a review article published in 2004, researchers noted that a number of different probiotics improved the immune system. These probiotics were all lactobacillus bacteria, namely *L. casei*, *L. acidophilus*, *L. rhamnosus GG*, and *Bifidobacterium bifidus*.

Did You Know?

Naming and Numbering Probiotics
There are three parts to a bacterium's name. The first word is the genus, for example *Lactobacillus*, which is sometimes shortened to one letter, for example, L. The species name, such as *rhamnosus*, is next, and the strain is the last part of the name, for example, *GG*. Different strains have different effects in the body.

Probiotics are measured by their cfu, or colony forming units. Not all bacteria should be considered probiotic. First, the probiotic bacterium has to be a strain that can survive stomach acid and bile; second, it has to be present in a quantity large enough to colonize the intestines. For example, although all yogurt is made with a live bacterial culture, not all types would fit the WHO definition of probiotic.

Cancer Connection

Researchers have studied how probiotics might reduce cancer risk. First, probiotics enhance the immune system. Second, probiotics break down cancer-causing agents (carcinogens) and produce compounds that prevent cancer cells from mutating. Third, they reduce the pH environment of the colon and feces, which helps prevent cancer development. (pH is a scale used to measure acid and alkaline levels. When the colon has a lower pH, it may prevent the growth of putrefactive bacteria.) The cancers that have been studied and show positive results to probiotics to date are colon and bladder cancers.

Prebiotics

Prebiotics are the "food" eaten by probiotics, particularly the lactobacillus and bifodobacterium species. Prebiotics are fibers that the good bacteria ferment as a source of food. They have the added benefit to our digestive system of increasing the weight of the stool, reducing the pH of the colon, improving mineral absorption, and, most importantly, improving the

FAQ

Q. *What is a macrobiotic diet?*

A. Macrobiotic diets recommend eating foods from your local region, eaten in season. This diet also restricts refined or processed foods, foods from the nightshade family (tomatoes, peppers, potatoes, eggplant, spinach, beets, and avocados), tropical nuts (brazils, cashews, hazelnuts, macadamia nuts, and pistachios), all tropical fruits (bananas, coconut, dates, figs, mangos, papaya, pineapple, and citrus), red meat, poultry, dairy foods, sweeteners, coffee, tea, cold drinks, and tap water. Macrobiotics also addresses the manner of eating by recommending against overeating and requiring that food be thoroughly chewed before swallowing.

Although there have been claims that the macrobiotic diet can reduce cancer risk, there are no randomized controlled clinical trials that provide evidence for this claim. However, the restriction on many fruits and vegetables is contradicted by evidence that plant foods are beneficial in reducing cancer risk. Strict adherence to a macrobiotic diet is not recommended during cancer treatment and recovery.

immune system. Also known as fructans, they are a group of naturally occurring sugars found in onions, bananas, wheat, artichokes, and garlic. They are also extracted from chicory root (producing a substance called inulin) or manufactured from sucrose for use in the food industry. They are the basis of fiber supplements and are added to fiber-enriched foods.

Prebiotics and Cancer

Prebiotics have been shown to stimulate the growth and activity of beneficial bifidobacteria and lactobacilli while at the same time reducing the activity of harmful bacteria. In animal studies, rats who were fed prebiotics (oligofructose-enriched inulin) had fewer precancerous lesions. This was also true when prebiotics and probiotics were combined and given together. This treatment also resulted in an improvement in the immune system.

In human studies, 80 patients with a history of colon cancer or polyps were given prebiotic (oligofructose-enriched inulin) and probiotic (*Bifidobacterium lactis Bb12* and *Lactobacillus rhamnosus GG*) for 12 weeks. The people in this study experienced an increase in the number of beneficial bacteria in their colons and a reduced number of harmful bacteria. This resulted in less DNA damage to the colon and fewer polyps.

To obtain a prebiotic effect from your diet, aim to consume 2.5 to 5 grams of prebiotic fiber, such as inulin, in your diet every day. Eat more onions, bananas, wheat, artichokes, garlic, yogurt, and kefir.

Foods to Avoid or Limit

There is evidence that certain foods can promote the growth of cancer cells. These foods — including sugary drinks, energy-dense foods, red meat, processed meats, alcoholic beverages, and salt — should be avoided or limited.

FAQ

Q. *Should I avoid high-fructose corn syrup?*

A. There are different types of sugars in our food. Names of sugars end in the suffix "-ose". Sucrose is a combination of two single sugars called glucose and fructose. High-fructose corn syrup (HFCS) is made from corn syrup, which is normally mostly glucose, but an enzyme is added to the corn syrup that converts some of its glucose to fructose. Two different versions of HFCS (called glucose-fructose in Canada and the UK) are manufactured: HFCS-42 (42% fructose and 53% glucose) and HFCS-55 (55% fructose and 42% glucose).

There is no evidence linking HFCS with cancer, but studies have shown that a diet of food high in fructose can result in weight gain of visceral fat, increased insulin resistance, and higher triglyceride levels in the blood and liver. The American Cancer Society notes that "sugar increases calorie intake without providing any of the nutrients that reduce cancer risk. By promoting obesity and elevating insulin levels, high sugar intake may indirectly increase cancer risk. . . . Limiting high-sugar foods, such as cakes, candy, cookies, sweetened cereals, and high-sugar beverages such as soda, can help reduce sugar intake."

Avoid Sugary Drinks

These include soft drinks (soda pop) and juice-flavored drinks. Unsweetened fruit juice is fine but should be limited to 1 cup (250 mL) a day. Read food labels to make sure you are buying unsweetened fruit juice and not a fruit "drink," "punch," or "cocktail," which are all words used on a label to indicate the food has been sweetened.

Avoid Energy-Dense Foods

These are usually processed "junk" foods —including fast foods, doughnuts, cupcakes, cakes, candy bars, chips, and other salty snack foods — that contain added sugar and fat and very little fiber. The best way to avoid eating these foods is to ban them from your home. Keep your home, car, and workplace a safe place for you to be without the temptation of unhealthy foods.

Limit Red Meat

Eat only 18 ounces (510 g) of red meat a week. Red meat includes beef, pork, lamb, and goat meat, and this amount refers to the cooked weight of the meat.

Determine how many times in the week you plan to consume red meat. If you were to consume some type of red meat every day, you would need to restrict your serving to $2^1/_2$ ounces (70 g) daily. If you eat red meat 4 days a week, you should limit the daily portion to $4^1/_2$ ounces (125 g). Remember to include red meat you may have at lunch and dinner in your tally.

Raw meat usually loses 25% of the weight during cooking. When you eat in a restaurant and the menu lists an 8-ounce (225 g) steak, this refers to the raw weight of the meat. This is also true when you purchase raw meat in the supermarket. To determine if this fits within your weekly 18-ounce (510 g) limit, you can do an estimate of the cooked weight. For example, 6 ounces (170 g) of raw meat would cook down to about 4½ ounces (125 g).

Also consider how many people will be eating the meat. If there are three people in your home, and you are buying a package of ground meat that weighs 2 pounds (900 g), then divide this number by 3 to get an estimate of your portion. This would be about 10 ounces (300 g). Once this meat is cooked, it will lose another 25%, for a final cooked weight per portion of 7½ ounces (215 g).

FAQ

Q. *You recommend eating fish, but do I need to be concerned about toxins in fish, such as mercury and PCBs?*

A. Fish is an excellent source of protein, but like many foods today, it may have been exposed to contaminants. Two main contaminants discussed in relation to fish are methyl mercury and PCBs (polychlorinated biphenyls). Even though PCBs have been banned since the late 1970s, they remain in the environment.

Methyl mercury and PCBs work their way up the food chain, from bacteria to plankton and into small and finally large fish. Although PCBs cause hormone disruption, with some links to cancer, methyl mercury is a neurotoxin.

You can reduce your exposure to these contaminants by eating foods lower down on the food chain and choosing the proper cooking method. Limit your consumption of large predatory fish, such as shark, swordfish, fresh or frozen tuna, marlin, orange roughy, and escolar, to about 5 ounces (150 g) a week. When buying tuna in a can, limit your intake of albacore tuna, often labeled "white" tuna, and instead purchase yellowfin, skipjack, or tongol, often labeled "light" tuna.

Use a cooking method that allows the fat to leave the food. Broil, bake, boil, poach, or grill the fish, but avoid frying. Discard the inner organs and remove the skin and visible fat.

Fish and shellfish that are high in anti-inflammatory omega-3 fat and low in methyl mercury are sardines, mackerel, herring, anchovies, capelin, char, hake, mullet, pollock (Boston bluefish), rainbow trout, lake whitefish, blue crab, shrimps, clams, mussels, oysters, and salmon.

Other fish and seafood safe to eat, according to Health Canada, include cod, haddock, halibut, sole, scallops, squid, snapper, perch, bass, and tilapia.

For information on fish that you catch yourself, contact your state or provincial health authority.

FAQ

Q. *When I cook with vegetable oil, am I creating "bad" trans fats?*

A. No. In order to make trans fats, the oil must be heated to a very high temperature with the addition of hydrogen gas. You may, however, speed up the oxidation process when you heat the vegetable oil. To limit this, avoid burning and heating oils to their "smoke point" (the point at which they start to smoke). Oils have different heat tolerance, so gauge your heat accordingly. Here are some guidelines for cooking with oil:

1 For high-heat frying, up to 500°F (260°C), choose canola, almond, apricot kernel, peanut, or soybean oils.

2 For stir-frying and baking below 375°F (190°C), use canola, walnut, or light (untoasted) sesame oil.

3 For light sautéing and baking under 320°F (160°C), use olive oil or any of the higher-heat oils.

4 For use in sauces and salad dressing, where heating is not required, use flax, hemp, and wheat germ oil.

Source: Izakson O. Oil right: Choose wisely for heart-healthy cooking (Eating Right). *E: The Environmental Magazine,* 2003 Mar–Apr.

Did You Know?

Perimeter Shopping
To avoid buying problematic foods, shop the perimeter of the supermarket. When you shop the perimeter, you are buying foods from the produce, bakery, fresh meat, seafood, and dairy departments. The inside aisles of the supermarket tend to contain more processed foods higher in sodium.

Avoid Processed Meat

There is no weekly or daily limit for processed meat, but rather a recommendation to avoid it altogether because the preservative used in processed meat can lead to the development of cancer cells. Processed meat includes cold cuts, bacon, hot dogs, and sausages.

Limit Alcoholic Beverages

Limit yourself to 2 drinks a day if you are a man and to 1 drink a day if you are a woman. Drinking alcohol puts you at higher risk of cancer of the mouth, throat, larynx, esophagus, liver, and breast. Alcohol combined with smoking appears to be a particularly damaging combination. If you choose to drink, the nutraceutical content of red wine may make it a better choice, but the amount still needs to be restricted.

Limit Salt

Sodium (salt) is linked with a higher risk of cancer of the stomach. Keep your sodium intake below 2400 milligrams per day. Read food labels to keep yourself within this limit. Many restaurant meals are higher in sodium than meals you would prepare at home. Eating out at restaurants should be limited.

FAQ

Q. *Can I still eat barbecued or grilled meats during cancer treatments?*

A. Development of breast, pancreatic, and prostate cancers are associated with eating well-done or charred meat. When you barbecue or grill meat over coals, the high temperature melts the fat on the meat, which then drips onto the coals below. When it hits the hot coals, it forms a compound called polycyclic aromatic hydrocarbon (PAH). The smoke-containing PAH then rises up from the coals and attaches to the meat. You can reduce your exposure to these carcinogens by marinating your meat before grilling. Marinades that contain phytonutrients (healthy plant compounds) are best. These phytonutrients include garlic, olive oil, lemon juice, and herbs and spices. Here are some other guidelines for grilling meat:

❶ If the meat is leaner, there is less fat to melt and drip onto the coals, so choose lean meats.

❷ Select smaller and thinner meats because they will cook faster. You can also partially cook the meat in the oven first and then add it to the grill to finish the cooking.

❸ Flip the meat often.

❹ If there are charred pieces of meat, cut them off.

❺ Line your grill with foil and poke small holes in it. This will prevent smoke from attaching itself to the meat.

❻ Grill your meat to medium or under. When the meat is cooked to "well done," there is a higher amount of cancer-causing compounds. This is not true, however, for vegetables — when they get black on the grill, they are still safe to eat.

Genetically Modified Foods

Genetically modified (GM), genetically engineered (GE), or transgenic products are plants or animals that have had their genetic code altered by implanting a strand of DNA from another plant, animal, or bacteria in order for that plant or animal to take on a specific characteristic.

Advocates see GE crops that are resistant to pests as a benefit to farmers. Genetically engineered corn, for example, was developed to be resistant to insects — in this case, the European corn borer and root worm. The result is a reduction in the population of the corn borer. Genetic modification has not been shown to have any adverse effect on the nutritional, toxic, or allergic concerns for humans to date. Neither the American Cancer Society nor the Canadian Cancer Society lists any warnings about GE foods on its website.

- *Approved GE crops (Canada):* Corn, potatoes, soybeans, canola, flax, sunflower, sugar beet, alfalfa, cotton, wheat, rice, papaya, tomato, and squash (yellow crookneck).
- *Additional approved crops (U.S.):* Radicchio, tobacco, and dairy products — some cows in the U.S. are injected with recombinant (genetically modified) bovine growth hormone, or rbGH.

Environmental Risks

GE crops can interbreed with different wild heritage species, reducing biodiversity. Weeds can also become resistant to GE herbicides, resulting in superweeds. There is higher residue of synthetic chemicals on GE foods. Indeed, due to concerns over health and the environment, the European Union had banned all GE products until 2010, when a GE potato was approved. GE foods are not labeled, making it difficult to avoid them. However, products labeled "certified organic" cannot contain GE ingredients. So to avoid GE foods, choose organic versions of GE-approved crops. One main advantage of avoiding GE crops would be lower levels of synthetic chemical residue.

The Nutritional Needs of Palliative Patients

Palliative patients with metastatic disease have a variety of nutritional needs. For those who are nevertheless experiencing a good quality of life, it would be prudent to focus on food, with its beneficial nutrients, to keep fighting their cancer and strengthening the immune system at a cellular level.

When patients with advanced disease are experiencing an overall decline, losing their appetite, feeling unwell more often than not, and no longer responding to their treatment, medical management will become less aggressive. Chemotherapy, radiation, or other forms of treatment may be stopped, especially if the side effects are significant. The medical focus will shift from curing the disease to relief of symptoms and discomfort.

From a nutrition perspective, this might mean that for those with diabetes, blood sugar targets may not be as tight, and for those with heart disease, heart-healthy diet guidelines would not be required. Sodium restrictions may still be necessary, as a buildup of fluid may compromise comfort, but patients can eat what they want and indulge in sweets and higher-fat foods if they wish.

FAQ

Q. *Is it safe to consume flax seeds if I have breast cancer?*

A. Flax seeds are high in the omega-3 fat alpha linolenic acid (ALA) and in plant lignans, which are processed by the bacteria in the colon into compounds that have weak estrogen and anti-estrogen properties. In her studies, researcher Lilian Thompson of the University of Toronto found that flax seeds and flaxseed oil did not interfere with tamoxifen, but rather enhanced its effectiveness in mice with the human version of breast cancer. Most recent reviews suggest that flax-based foods have no adverse effects on breast cancer prognosis. Animal studies have shown that the combination of flax seeds (for their lignans) with soy (for its isoflavones) is more effective than soy alone in reducing the growth of breast tumors.

Part 3

Menu Planning for Side Effect Management

3

Sample Daily Menus

There is no single "cancer diet" for patients to follow during treatment. Rather, the approach to nutrition is based on the goal of minimizing side effects. The meal plans that have been selected for this book are based on the common complaints of cancer patients. These are sample menus and don't need to be followed strictly but rather used as a blueprint. You can substitute foods you prefer as long as they don't contradict the recommendations for your particular symptom. Some of the meals or snacks are recipes that are included in this book. In this case, use the page reference to locate the recipe.

Menu 1
Antidiarrhea Plan
The dietary recommendations to help manage diarrhea are the same whatever the cause. Use this as a temporary meal plan until your bowels return to normal, because it limits many healthy foods (whole grains and many fruits and vegetables) and is not recommended once diarrhea is resolved. If you have lost weight, the first priority is to get the diarrhea under control, and once that happens, then you can choose foods to assist with weight gain

General Guidelines
- Eat soluble fiber.
- Avoid insoluble fiber.
- Avoid raw fruits and vegetables (except bananas).
- Avoid greasy, fatty, or spicy foods.
- Eat foods that will help to bind excess fluid and help make a formed stool.
- Avoid milk and lactose-containing foods if you think you are temporarily lactose intolerant.
- Choose foods with sodium and potassium to help replenish lost electrolytes.
- Try to ingest enough fluid to maintain your hydration.
- Avoid coffee, sweets, and sorbitol (in sugar-free foods).

Meal	Food	Substitutions	Why This Recipe?
Breakfast	• Breakfast Rice (page 159)	• Use short-grain white rice instead of brown rice • Serve with applesauce instead of dried fruit	• Short-grain white rice and applesauce are part of the BRAT diet (bananas, rice, applesauce, toast)
Morning snack	• Oat bran bread with smooth peanut butter	• Use white bread if you can't find oat bran	• Oat bran provides soluble fiber • Smooth peanut butter may help make formed stool
Lunch	• French Toast (page 162)	• Use white bread or oat bran bread instead of whole-grain bread	• Low-fat proteins, such as eggs, are generally well tolerated • White flour is well tolerated, and oat bran provides soluble fiber
Afternoon snack	• Probiotic yogurt and a banana	• Use unsweetened yogurt, if available	• Probiotic bacteria may help with diarrhea • Bananas provide prebiotic fiber
Dinner	• Oven-Fried Fish (page 200) • Creamy Mashed Potato Casserole (page 246)	• Sprinkle the fish with salt for added electrolytes • Use lactose-free milk if you're sensitive to lactose	• Low-fat proteins, such as fish, are generally well tolerated • Peeled potatoes are generally well tolerated • Cheese can be constipating, which can help to control diarrhea
Evening snack	• Salted saltine crackers and sharp (old) Cheddar cheese	• Substitute another type of aged cheese, if desired	• The salt in the crackers and cheese provides electrolytes • The white flour in saltines is well tolerated • Cheese can be constipating, which can help to control diarrhea

Menu 2
Liquid and Soft Foods Plan

This meal plan is recommended if you are experiencing nausea, mouth or throat sores, poor appetite, or dehydration. There are several reasons why this liquid/soft foods meal plan is recommended. Most patients find taking liquids less off-putting than solid foods, and caregivers do not need to worry that they're not getting meat and potatoes into their patient once they see that sufficient calories and protein can be achieved with liquid and soft foods. It has the dual role of providing nutrition and fluid at the same time. No chewing is required, so it is easy if there are mouth sores. The liquid spends less time in the mouth than solid foods, and therefore those with taste alterations are not as put off.

General Guidelines

❶ Avoid dehydration. If you become dehydrated:
• Your nausea will get worse.
• You will become constipated.
• Your body will not be excreting the byproducts of the medications you are taking as quickly as it should.
• Starting an IV will be more difficult.
• Your blood pressure will drop.

❷ Serve foods cold or at room temperature. Foods at this temperature are better tolerated when you are nauseous.

> **Survivor Wisdom**
>
> *After chemo, drink lots of fluids to help flush out the toxins, and keep doing it for a long time — like 3 months after treatment.*

> **Survivor Wisdom**
>
> *I liked all my usual foods — my appetite didn't change. But during chemo, when I had nausea, my favorite food was nutritional drinks.*

Meal	Food	Calories	Protein
Breakfast	Creamy Morning Millet with Apples (page 158)	441	20 g
	8-oz (250 mL) glass of milk	130	9 g
Morning snack	Homemade Chocolate Pudding (page 279)	242*	6 g
Lunch	Green Power Smoothie (page 297)	316**	32 g
Afternoon snack	Sunny Orange Shake (page 294)	199**	10 g
Dinner	Broccoli and Cheddar Cheese Soup (page 171)	339	19 g
	Easy Vanilla Pudding (page 278)	165*	7 g
Evening snack	Island Smoothie (page 299)	274**	5 g
Total		**2106**	**108 g**

* The calories will be higher if you use the higher-calorie options suggested below the recipe.

** Choose the highest-fat yogurt to achieve this calorie level.

Menu 3
High-Energy, High-Protein Plan

This diet is used to promote weight gain and wound healing. Although the body can use protein, carbohydrate, and fat for calories, the goal of a high-energy, high-protein diet is to provide sufficient calories from carbohydrate and fat so that the body can use the protein you consume for building muscle and repairing cells. At times, it can appear to be unhealthy because there is a focus on adding fat to foods, but this diet has a very specific goal of getting these calories into your body.

General Guidelines

- Eat three meals and two to three snacks per day.
- Keep a regular eating schedule.
- Consume protein at every meal and snack.
- Track your protein intake by referring to food labels and the table on page 88.
- Aim for a minimum of 0.45 g of protein per pound of body weight (1 g of protein per kg of body weight) each day. Ask for a referral to a registered dietitian at your cancer center if you need help.

Survivor Wisdom

A food diary can be motivational. See what is helpful. This could be a project for caregivers, since they always want something to do. They can ask you, "Have you had a protein today? A vegetable?"

Meal	Food	Calories	Protein
Breakfast	Overnight Oven French Toast (page 163)	522	20 g
Morning snack	Apple Cranberry Bread (page 258)	310	6 g
Lunch	Tuna Cheddar Melt (page 195)	572	42 g
Afternoon snack	Easy White Bean Purée (page 263) 4 to 6 crackers (not low-fat)	175 180*	8 g 4 g*
Dinner	Italian Chicken Meatloaf (page 210) Turnip Gratin (page 225)	424 301	28 g 18 g
Evening snack	Cinnamon Raison Bread Pudding (page 288)	291	11 g
Throughout the day	Green Power Smoothie (page 297)	316	32 g
Total		**3091**	**169 g**

* These numbers are estimates; for more accurate information, check the Nutrition Facts table on your crackers.

Shopping List

Tips

To promote weight gain, choose higher-fat products and add butter, margarine and/or mayonnaise to your food.

Look for "probiotic" on labels.

Slice fresh ginger to make ginger tea.

Cut up a fresh lemon and hold it to your nose: the scent may help alleviate nausea.

Use broth to moisten meats and other foods if you have dry mouth, to blenderize foods if you have difficulty chewing, as a hydrating fluid, or as a cooking liquid for rice.

Choose a high-iron cereal if you have low iron levels, a high-fiber cereal if you have constipation, and a cereal containing psyllium if you have diarrhea.

Select white or oat bread if you have diarrhea; choose whole-grain if you have constipation or want to increase your nutrient intake.

During your cancer treatment, you may not feel much like cooking. Some days, you may be too busy with medical appointments to put together even simple meals. This shopping list is designed to give you ideas for quick, easy, nourishing foods to have on hand in the event that you don't have the time, energy, or inclination to prepare a meal. You may also want to bring some of these items with you when you go to appointments, which invariably overlap at least one meal or snack time.

Dairy Case
- Yogurt, yogurt drinks
- Cheese, cottage cheese
- Omega-3 eggs
- Non-hydrogenated margarine or butter

Produce
- Fresh gingerroot
- Citrus fruits
- Cut-up fresh fruits
- Fresh juices

Grocery Aisles
- Broth, ready-made soups or stews
- Canned salmon or tuna (light, not white)
- Peanut and other nut butters
- Protein bars, nutrition beverages
- Dried fruit, nuts, trail mix, dried fruit and/or veggie bars
- Pretzels, crackers
- Ginger ale, flavored waters, sports drinks
- Baking soda (for mouth rinses)
- Cereal, fiber biscuits
- Bread
- Skim milk powder, whey powder
- Ready-made puddings
- Mayonnaise

Frozen Foods
- Popsicles or other frozen treats
- Ice cream or frozen yogurt
- Frozen fruit and vegetables
- Individual frozen meals

Food Safety and Storage

Food safety is important for everyone, but the need for safe kitchen practices increases for anyone with a compromised immune system. Following the best practices when shopping, preparing, storing and toting food will limit your exposure to food-borne illnesses and the complications they cause. Follow these guidelines to keep food safe.

When Grocery Shopping

- Pick up packaged goods and non-perishables first, then produce, then refrigerated and frozen foods.
- Place packaged meats, poultry and fish in a clean bag before adding them to the cart, and keep them separate from other foods in the cart.
- Choose only packages that are well sealed and clean on the outside.
- Keep a cooler in the car and place all refrigerated goods directly inside for the ride home. Clean the cooler after you unpack it.
- Plan your errands so grocery shopping is last, and get groceries home promptly.
- Unpack refrigerated and frozen goods first.
- Wash reusable grocery bags and containers with hot water and a sanitizing detergent.

When Cooking

- Thoroughly wash your hands often and sanitize equipment, utensils and surfaces.
- Never thaw perishable foods at room temperature. Thaw in the refrigerator or microwave, and cook the food promptly once thawed.
- Designate separate cutting boards for meat, poultry, fish and produce, and keep them in separate bowls before cooking.
- Never partially cook meats or poultry, then hold them; always cook thoroughly and refrigerate promptly.
- Use an instant-read thermometer to ensure foods are cooked thoroughly; when reheating, heat to 165°F (74°C).
- All hot foods should be served immediately; divide leftovers into smaller portions, place in shallow containers and refrigerate within 30 minutes.

> ### Survivor Wisdom
>
> *Put the date on foods you store in the freezer, or write it on a piece of paper. I had "chemo brain" and would forget, especially when five different people brought over meals within four days.*

To Store Food

- Store all prepared foods in airtight containers in the refrigerator or freezer unless the recipe states otherwise. Label containers with the contents and the date.
- Do not keep foods longer than recommended. If a recipe doesn't specify, 3 days or less in the fridge is a good general rule (freeze within 3 days for longer storage).
- If family and friends bring food, ask when it was prepared. If you're not positive it was prepared or stored safely, do not eat it.
- Check your fridge and freezer frequently and use up foods in the order they were stored. Keep a list of your inventory so you don't forget about something delicious until after it's spoiled.

For Food on the Go

- Always pack food in an insulated bag with an ice pack (even when you think it'll be a short trip), and don't forget eating utensils.
- Sanitize containers, the insulated bag and ice packs after use and let them air-dry thoroughly so they're ready for the next use (keep extra ice packs in the freezer so you always have some frozen).

For more food safety information, visit the USDA's Be Food Safe program (www.fsis.usda.gov/Be_FoodSafe/index.asp) or the Canadian Partnership for Consumer Food Safety Education's website (www.canfightbac.org).

Part 4

Recipes for Cancer Treatment and Beyond

4

Introduction to the Recipes

Knowledge is power, but action is key. The first half of *The Essential Cancer Treatment Nutrition Guide & Cookbook* provides you with the most current information so you can manage your treatment's side effects and be aware of the changes you could make to your diet to increase your chances of remaining cancer-free. But putting that knowledge into daily practice is what will provide you with the peace of mind that you're doing what you can to assist in your fight against cancer. That is why I've provided 150 recipes that incorporate the suggestions from the previous chapters.

Each of the recipes focuses on at least one of three main criteria:

❶ Management of side effects (noted in the "Recommended for" box at the top left of the recipe).

❷ Cancer risk reduction (noted under "Bonus features")

❸ Tasty, easy-to-prepare recipes that are suitable for people who may not be feeling their best.

In addition, many recipes include adjustments you can make, based on your symptoms, to make the dish more suitable for you. These small, easy changes can make all the difference. You'll also find storage and reheating instructions and information on how to prepare certain recipes ahead of time, so they're ready when you are.

There are some classic comfort foods — yes, chicken noodle soup is here — along with some new and interesting dishes so you can try one without a memory of how it "should" taste.

I know that for many of you, eating was once a source of pleasure. You enjoyed the process of choosing your food, the anticipation of the meal, the eating experience, and the look, smell, taste and texture of your food. During cancer treatment, all of this pleasure can be replaced by a sense of duty and obligation to eat, along with stress as mealtimes approach. To those in this situation, I want to say, just do your best. Before the meal, take a couple of deep breaths to relieve some of the tension you hold in your body. Eating in a relaxed manner is

helpful. Make the meal as visually appealing as possible —
don't forget, we eat with our eyes. If fluids are easier, don't be
afraid to follow the liquid and soft foods meal plan (page 138),
knowing that the nutrition from this plan really is sufficient.
Your joy and pleasure in eating will return, and you will
appreciate your robust appetite like you never have in the past.
I hope that day comes soon for you; in the meantime, know
that this too shall pass.

My hope is that these recipes allow you to nourish yourself
throughout your treatment and into your recovery, and that
the book proves to be an understanding companion in this
challenging time of your life.

Bon appétit!
— Jean

About the Nutritional Analyses

Computer-assisted nutrient analysis of the recipes was
prepared by Kimberly Zammit, HBSc (the project supervisor
was Len Piché, PhD, RD, Division of Food & Nutritional
Sciences, Brescia University College, London, ON), using Food
Processor® SQL, version 10.9, ESHA Research Inc., Salem OR
(this software contains over 35,000 food items based largely
on the latest USDA data and the entire Canadian Nutrient
File, 2007b). The database was supplemented when necessary
with data from the Canadian Nutrient File (version 2010) and
documented data from other reliable sources.

The analysis was based on:

- imperial weights and measures (except for foods typically
  packaged and used in metric quantities);
- the smaller ingredient quantity when there was a range;
- the first ingredient listed when there was a choice of
  ingredients.

Calculations involving meat and poultry use lean portions
without skin and with visible fat trimmed. A pinch of salt
was calculated as $1/8$ tsp (0.5 mL). All recipes were analyzed
prior to cooking. Optional ingredients and garnishes, and
ingredients that are not quantified, were not included in
the calculations.

> **Survivor Wisdom**
>
> *People with cancer need to know that sometimes you just may not be hungry and that's okay.*

> **Survivor Wisdom**
>
> *If you are invited over to someone's place for dinner, give yourself permission to approach the host or hostess and say, "If I'm not eating, don't be disturbed by it — I'm just having an off day." Not everyone thinks to ask you ahead of time if there are things you can't tolerate anymore.*

No Ordinary Cookbook

The "Recommended for" and "Bonus features" boxes are designed to help you select the best recipe for you. This chart will help you understand these tools.

Recommended For	Recipe Criteria
Anemia	Is high in iron, B_{12} and/or folate
Constipation	Has ≥ 4 g of fiber and/or contains ingredients with a laxative effect and no constipating ingredients
Dehydration	Has ≥600 mg of sodium* and/or is moist or liquid
Diarrhea	Is a source of soluble fiber or is low in insoluble fiber; contains no raw vegetables and no raw fruits except bananas; contains minimal spices; is low in fat; and is low in sugar
Dry mouth	Has ≤140 mg of sodium* and/or is moist or liquid
Heartburn	Has ≤2 g fat* and is non-spicy
Low appetite	May appeal to those with low appetite
Nausea	Contains ginger; has a mild aroma; is liquid or frozen; and/or is served cold or at room temperature (to reduce aromas)
Sore mouth or throat	Is soft, moist, non-acidic and non-spicy
Taste aversions or reduced sensitivity	Has a strong flavor or interesting texture that will appeal to those with reduced taste sensitivity and/or flavor adjustments are provided to compensate for common taste aversions
Weight gain promotion	*Soups, light meals, main dishes:* has ≥400 calories*; *Grains, potatoes, snacks, desserts, beverages or frozen pops:* has ≥300 calories*; *Vegetable side dishes:* has ≥200 calories*; *Sauces:* has ≥100 calories*
Weight management	*Main dishes:* has ≤200 calories*; *All others:* has ≤150 calories*
Vomiting	Is liquid and is high in sodium and/or potassium

Bonus Feature	Recipe Criteria
Easy prep	Can be prepared by novice cooks or those low on energy
High fiber	Has ≥4 g of fiber*
High protein	*Main dishes:* has ≥21 g of protein*; *Breakfasts, soups, light meals, desserts, beverages or frozen pops:* has ≥7 g of protein*; *Vegetable side dishes, sauces, grains, potatoes, snacks:* has ≥4 g of protein*
Low fat	Has ≤2 g of fat*
Portability	Can be taken to go and eaten away from home
Prepare ahead	Includes make ahead instructions
Risk reduction	The majority of the ingredients have cancer-fighting potential

* Based on 1 serving

Reviving Breakfasts

Breakfast is the most important meal of the day. This adage has never been more true than when you are eating to live. Don't put off eating breakfast. If you don't have an appetite, you may delay and delay eating until suddenly the morning is over and it's lunchtime. If you can only eat a couple of mouthfuls, do that. But eating at regular times will help you regain your appetite as your body learns to develop hunger in anticipation of a scheduled meal.

I have tried to provide comfort foods that will still appeal even if your appetite is off, as well as higher-calorie protein options to give you a head start on your daily requirements. Use the included recipe adjustments to tweak the recipes to meet your needs. If you are experiencing nausea, you may want to eat the hot breakfasts after they have cooled down. Some of these recipes can be made the night before, and that may be just the ticket if you are low on energy in the mornings. And don't restrict these meals to just the morning — they can be eaten any time of day.

**Makes
14 servings**

*Muesli was originally
created by Swiss
physician Maximilian
Bircher-Benner for
hospital patients as part
of their recovery. This
version makes a large
batch to keep on hand,
allowing you to mix each
serving with probiotic
yogurt, milk or soy,
almond or rice beverage
and fresh fruit for a
nutritious cereal that's
ready in seconds.*

Tips

Store flax seeds and wheat germ in the refrigerator.

To add even more fiber and nutrients to this high-fiber cereal, try serving it with peaches and blueberries, topped with probiotic yogurt.

Rolled oats are whole-grain whether they are quick-cooking or large-flake (old-fashioned). The difference is the size of the flake, but all three components that make up a whole grain — the germ, bran and endosperm are present.

Muesli Mix

4 cups	quick-cooking rolled oats	1 L
½ cup	ground flax seeds	125 mL
½ cup	wheat germ	125 mL
½ cup	oat bran	125 mL
½ cup	wheat bran	125 mL
1 cup	dried cranberries	250 mL

1. Mix together all ingredients and pour into an airtight container. Store in a cool, dry place.

This recipe courtesy of dietitian Stefa Katamay.

Nutritional Analysis per Serving

Calories..........164	Sodium..........1 mg	Fiber ....6 g
Fat ....4 g	Carbohydrate .....29 g	Protein ....6 g

Makes 2 servings

This complete breakfast works well for days you have to attend morning appointments, as it is best if made the night before.

Tips

For variety, try serving this muesli with different types of yogurt and fresh fruit in season. If using vanilla or fruit-flavored yogurt, you can omit the honey or reduce the amount you use.

Agave syrup has a glycemic index of 10–19, honey is 35–58 and pure maple syrup is 54. The lower glycemic index of the agave syrup is helping to increase its popularity as a sweetening ingredient.

Variation

To increase the omega-3 and fiber content, add ¼ cup (60 mL) chopped walnuts or 2 tbsp (30 mL) ground flax seeds.

1 cup	large-flake (old-fashioned) or quick-cooking rolled oats (not instant)	250 mL
1 cup	lower-fat plain probiotic yogurt	250 mL
½ cup	2% milk	125 mL
2 tbsp	liquid honey, maple syrup or agave syrup	30 mL
1 cup	assorted berries (fresh or frozen)	250 mL
1	large banana, sliced	1

1. In a plastic container, combine oats, yogurt, milk and honey; gently fold in berries. Cover and refrigerate for at least 4 hours or overnight.

2. Add banana before serving or add to sealable container before taking muesli on the go.

This recipe courtesy of dietitian Renée Crompton.

This recipe should be adjusted based on your symptoms. Follow this symptom guide:

To encourage weight gain:
- Use higher-fat yogurt. Read the label and choose one with a higher % M.F; and/or
- Use whole milk or half-and-half (10%) cream instead of 2%; and/or
- Add ½ cup (125 mL) unflavored whey protein powder or skim milk powder with the oats.

To assist with constipation:
- Add ¼ cup (60 mL) natural wheat bran with the oats; and/or
- Follow this meal with a hot drink, then a cold beverage.

For diarrhea:
- Leave out the fresh fruit.

For lactose intolerance:
- Replace the milk with a lactose-free beverage, such as plain soy milk or lactose-reduced milk.

Nutritional Analysis per Serving

Calories...........416	Sodium....... 112 mg	Fiber .... 8 g
Fat............... 6 g	Carbohydrate..... 78 g	Protein .... 14 g

Recommended for:
- Low appetite
- Nausea
- Sore mouth or throat

Bonus features:
- High protein
- Portability
- Prepare ahead
- Risk reduction

Makes 6 to 8 servings

Three different food groups in this traditional Swiss breakfast cereal combine to make a balanced meal.

Tips

If you're using frozen berries, thaw them in the fridge overnight and drain liquid before adding to the yogurt mixture or microwave on High for 30 seconds.

For added flavor and to increase nutraceutical intake and reduce insulin resistance, try adding 1 tsp (5 mL) ground cinnamon with the oats.

To increase the omega-3 and fiber content, add 1/4 cup (60 mL) chopped walnuts or ground flax seeds, or a combination of the two.

Apple Berry Muesli

2 cups	quick-cooking rolled oats	500 mL
2 cups	low-fat plain probiotic yogurt	500 mL
1 cup	milk	250 mL
3 tbsp	granulated sugar, liquid honey or agave syrup	45 mL
2	large apples, cored	2
	Juice of 1/2 lemon	
1 cup	chopped berries	250 mL
	Raisins and nuts (optional)	

1. In a medium bowl, combine oats, yogurt, milk and sugar. Set aside.
2. Grate apples, leaving the skin on. Sprinkle with lemon juice to prevent browning. Add apples and berries to yogurt mixture. Gently mix together. Cover and refrigerate overnight. Serve topped with raisins and/or nuts, if desired.

This recipe courtesy of dietitian Sandra Gabriele.

This recipe should be adjusted based on your symptoms. Follow this symptom guide:

To encourage weight gain:
- Use higher-fat yogurt. Read the label and choose one with a higher % M.F.; and/or
- Use whole milk or half-and-half (10%) cream in place of the milk; and/or
- Add 1/2 cup (125 mL) unflavored whey protein powder or skim milk powder.

For lactose intolerance:
- Replace the milk with a lactose-free beverage, such as lactose-reduced milk or non-dairy milk such as soy, almond or rice milk.

For sore mouth or throat:
- Peel the apples; and/or
- Omit the lemon juice.
- Do not use the optional nuts.

Nutritional Analysis per Serving

Calories..........201	Sodium........ 58 mg	Fiber .... 4 g
Fat.............. 3 g	Carbohydrate..... 36 g	Protein .... 8 g

Makes 6 to 8 servings

A steaming bowl of this tasty cereal gets you off to a good start in the morning by providing a portion of the nutrients you'll need to remain energized and productive throughout the day.

Tips

Some millet may contain bits of dirt or discolored grains. Rinse it thoroughly in a pot of water before using.

This cereal may get dry and brown around the edges if cooked for longer than 8 hours. If you need to cook it for longer, add an additional $1/2$ cup (125 mL) of water.

Make Ahead

Cooked cereal can be portioned into airtight containers, cooled, covered and refrigerated for up to 2 days. Reheat in the microwave on Medium-High (70%) power for 2 to 3 minutes or until steaming. Stir in additional water or milk to thin to desired consistency.

Multigrain Cereal with Fruit

- **Small (3$1/2$ quart) slow cooker (see tip, page 154)**
- **Greased slow cooker stoneware**

$1/2$ cup	brown rice	125 mL
$1/2$ cup	millet (see tip, at left)	125 mL
$1/2$ cup	wheat berries	125 mL
2	apples, peeled, cored and thinly sliced	2
4 cups	water (see tip, at left)	1 L
$1/2$ tsp	vanilla extract	2 mL
$1/4$ tsp	salt (optional)	1 mL
$1/2$ cup	chopped pitted soft dates, preferably Medjool (see tip, at left)	125 mL
	Chopped toasted nuts (optional)	
	Wheat germ (optional)	

1. In prepared slow cooker stoneware, combine rice, millet, wheat berries and apples. Add water, vanilla and salt, if using. Cover and cook on Low for up to 8 hours or overnight. Add dates and stir well. Serve sprinkled with toasted nuts and/or wheat germ, if using.

This recipe should be adjusted based on your symptoms. Follow this symptom guide:

To assist with constipation:
- Include the optional nuts and wheat germ, using 1 to 2 tbsp (15 to 30 mL) of each.

Nutritional Analysis per Serving

Calories..........249	Sodium..........2 mg	Fiber.............6 g
Fat..............2 g	Carbohydrate.....55 g	Protein..........6 g

Recommended for:
- Low appetite
- Sore mouth or throat

Bonus features:
- High protein
- Prepare ahead
- Risk reduction

Makes 4 servings

Comfort foods are particularly sought after when you aren't feeling well. This version of oatmeal has lots of extras to give you added nutrition.

Tip

To toast wheat germ, heat a skillet over medium heat, add wheat germ and toast gently, shaking occasionally to ensure even toasting, for about 4 minutes or until fragrant.

Make Ahead

Cooked cereal can be portioned into airtight containers, cooled, covered and refrigerated for up to 3 days. Reheat in the microwave on Medium-High (70%) power for 2 to 3 minutes or until steaming. Stir in additional milk or water to thin to desired consistency.

Better-Than-Instant Oatmeal

3 cups	milk or soy milk (approx.)	750 mL
1 cup	quick-cooking rolled oats	250 mL
2 tbsp	packed brown sugar or pure maple syrup	30 mL
1 tbsp	ground flax seeds	15 mL
2 tsp	wheat germ, toasted (see tip, at left)	10 mL
1 tsp	non-hydrogenated margarine or butter	5 mL
½ tsp	ground cinnamon (optional)	2 mL
Pinch	salt	Pinch
⅓ cup	raisins or dried cranberries (optional)	75 mL
	Toasted chopped almonds, walnuts or pecans (optional)	

1. In a large saucepan, over medium-low heat, combine milk, oats, brown sugar, flax seeds, wheat germ, margarine, cinnamon (if using) and salt. Cook, stirring often, for 10 to 15 minutes or until thick and bubbly. Remove from heat and add raisins (if using); let stand for 2 minutes. Stir in additional milk if a thinner texture is desired. Serve topped with nuts, if desired.

This recipe courtesy of dietitian Lisa Diamond.

Nutritional Analysis per Serving

Calories...........230	Sodium....... 165 mg	Fiber .... 3 g
Fat.............. 7 g	Carbohydrate..... 32 g	Protein .... 10 g

Makes 1 serving

Low glycemic index oatmeal combined with the protein of milk and the blood-sugar-stabilizing effect of cinnamon result in a meal with some staying power that you can eat any time of the day.

Tip

This recipe is easily multiplied to make 2, 3 or 4 servings. Increase the cooking time as necessary.

Survivor Wisdom

Things other than treatment can affect your appetite.

Creamy Microwave Oatmeal

½ cup	water	125 mL
½ cup	milk or soy milk (approx.)	125 mL
⅛ tsp	salt	0.5 mL
2 tbsp	raisins	30 mL
1 tsp	wheat bran	5 mL
½ cup	quick-cooking rolled oats	125 mL
¼ tsp	ground cinnamon	1 mL
	Brown sugar or pure maple syrup	

1. In a 4-cup (1 L) microwave-safe bowl, combine water, milk, salt, raisins and bran. Microwave on High for 2 minutes. Stir in oats and cinnamon; microwave on High for 3 to 4 minutes, stirring at 1-minute intervals, or until oatmeal has thickened. Cover and let stand for 1 minute. Serve with brown sugar and additional milk, if desired.

This recipe courtesy of dietitian Bev Callaghan.

This recipe should be adjusted based on your symptoms. Follow this symptom guide:

To encourage weight gain:
- Use whole milk or table cream; and/or
- Add 2 tbsp (30 mL) unflavored whey protein powder or skim milk powder; and/or
- Add 1 to 2 tsp (5 to 10 mL) non-hydrogenated margarine or butter.

To assist with constipation:
- Increase the wheat bran to 1 tbsp (15 mL); and/or
- Add 1 or 2 chopped prunes with the raisins; and/or
- Drink a hot beverage followed by a cold one after eating this cereal.

Nutritional Analysis per Serving

Calories..........294	Sodium.......291 mg	Fiber.............6 g
Fat...............6 g	Carbohydrate.....51 g	Protein..........11 g

Makes 4 servings

Although rolled oats are very popular, the traditional way to eat oatmeal is steel-cut oats, which are often sold under the name Irish oatmeal. They have more flavor than rolled oats and an appealing crunchy texture.

Tip

If you only have a large oval slow cooker, reduce the cooking time by half or double all of the ingredients.

Make Ahead

Cooked cereal can be portioned into airtight containers, cooled, covered and refrigerated for up to 3 days. Reheat in the microwave on Medium-High (70%) power for 2 to 3 minutes or until steaming. Stir in additional milk or water to thin to desired consistency.

Irish Oatmeal

- **Small (3½ quart) slow cooker (see tip, at left)**
- **Greased slow cooker stoneware**

1 cup	steel-cut oats	250 mL
½ tsp	salt	2 mL
4 cups	water	1 L
	Raisins, chopped bananas or pitted dates (optional)	
	Toasted nuts, seeds and milk (optional)	

1. In prepared slow cooker, combine oats and salt. Add water. Cover and cook on High for 4 hours or on Low for 8 hours or overnight. Stir well. Stir in fruit to taste, or garnish with nuts, if using, or add milk, if desired.

This recipe should be adjusted based on your symptoms. Follow this symptom guide:

To encourage weight gain:
- Use half full-fat evaporated milk and half water; and/or
- Add ½ cup (125 mL) unflavored whey protein powder or skim milk powder; and/or
- Add 1 to 2 tsp (5 to 10 mL) non-hydrogenated margarine or butter to each serving; and/or
- Use the optional nut garnish.

To assist with constipation:
- Add 1 to 2 tbsp (15 to 30 mL) wheat bran to each serving; and/or
- Add 1 or 2 chopped prunes to each serving; and/or
- Drink a hot beverage followed by a cold one after eating this cereal.

Nutritional Analysis per Serving

Calories..........140	Sodium....... 291 mg	Fiber............. 4 g
Fat.............. 3 g	Carbohydrate..... 27 g	Protein .... 6 g

Makes 6 servings

This flavorful cereal is an adaptation of a recipe that appeared in Eat, Drink and Be Healthy: The Harvard Medical School Guide to Healthy Eating. *Wheat berries are the kernels of the wheat plant. They are sold in either hard or soft varieties; either will work in this recipe.*

Tips

Wheat berries and brown rice are sources of selenium, a mineral that may have cancer-protective properties.

Magnesium, which is found in whole grains, ranks highest on the anti-inflammatory food index. It is also part of the DASH diet to control high blood pressure.

Make Ahead

Cooked cereal can be portioned into airtight containers, cooled, covered and refrigerated for up to 3 days. Reheat in the microwave on Medium-High (70%) power for 2 to 3 minutes or until steaming. Stir in additional milk or water to thin to desired consistency.

Apple Oatmeal with Wheat Berries

- **Small (3$\frac{1}{2}$ quart) slow cooker (see tip, page 154)**
- **Greased slow cooker stoneware**

1$\frac{1}{2}$ cups	steel-cut oats	375 mL
$\frac{1}{2}$ cup	wheat berries	125 mL
2	apples, peeled, cored and chopped	2
$\frac{1}{2}$ tsp	ground cinnamon	2 mL
$\frac{1}{2}$ tsp	vanilla extract	2 mL
3$\frac{1}{2}$ cups	water	875 mL
1 cup	cranberry or apple juice (see tip, at left)	250 mL
	Sugar, toasted walnuts and wheat germ (optional)	

1. In prepared slow cooker, combine steel-cut oats, wheat berries, apples, cinnamon and vanilla. Add water and cranberry juice. Cover and cook on High for 4 hours or on Low for 8 hours or overnight. Stir well. Top with sugar, walnuts and/or wheat germ, if using.

This recipe should be adjusted based on your symptoms. Follow this symptom guide:

To assist with constipation:
- Replace $\frac{1}{2}$ cup (125 mL) of the cranberry juice with prune juice; and/or
- Drink a hot beverage followed by a cold one after eating this cereal.

Nutritional Analysis per Serving

Calories...........249	Sodium..........2 mg	Fiber ....8 g
Fat...............3 g	Carbohydrate.....52 g	Protein ....8 g

Makes 7 servings

This breakfast cereal combines the goodness of oats and oat bran with high-fiber grains like cracked wheat.

Tips

To vary this recipe, try altering the proportion and types of grains.

This fiber-packed cereal is a new twist on traditional oatmeal. Serve with milk and fresh fruit, and this breakfast will set you up for the day.

Survivor Wisdom

Make a happy face in your oatmeal.

Not Your Same Old Oats

1 cup	large-flake (old-fashioned) rolled oats	250 mL
2/3 cup	5-grain hot cereal	150 mL
1/2 cup	oat bran	125 mL
1/3 cup	medium bulgur (cracked wheat)	75 mL

1. In a large bowl, combine oats, cereal, oat bran and bulgur. Store in airtight container.
2. To prepare 1 serving, place $^1/_3$ cup (75 mL) of the oat mixture in a deep bowl. Add $^3/_4$ cup (175 mL) water and a pinch of salt. Microwave on High for 2 minutes; stir. Microwave for 1 to 2 minutes longer. Or cook in a small saucepan on top of stove for about 5 minutes.

This recipe courtesy of Michael G. Baylis.

Nutritional Analysis per Serving

Calories..........114	Sodium..........1 mg	Fiber .... 4 g
Fat.............. 2 g	Carbohydrate..... 24 g	Protein .... 5 g

**Makes
18 servings**

*Whole grains, dried fruit
and sunflower seeds
combine to make this a
super-nutritious porridge.*

Tips

Look for 9-grain cereal
in the bulk food store or
the bulk food section or
in boxes or bags at your
grocery store.

Add brown sugar and
warmed milk; also
delicious with a handful
of blueberries.

To increase the omega-3
content, add 1½ cups
(375 mL) chopped walnuts
to the dry mix or add 1 tbsp
(15 mL) per serving; add
1 cup (250 mL) ground flax
seeds to the dry mix or add
2 tsp (10 mL) per serving.

Survivor
Wisdom

*If I get five spoonfuls
of cereal in, I need
to say, "That's okay."
Be aware of your
tolerance.*

Big-Batch Power Porridge

6 cups	large-flake (old-fashioned) rolled oats	1.5 L
1 cup	9-grain hot cereal (such as Red River or Bob's Red Mill)	250 mL
¾ cup	wheat germ, toasted (see tip, page 152)	175 mL
½ cup	oat bran	125 mL
½ cup	raisins or dried cranberries	125 mL
½ cup	sunflower seeds	125 mL

1. In a large bowl, combine oats, 9-grain cereal, wheat germ, oat bran, raisins and sunflower seeds. Store in a large covered container at room temperature for up to 1 week or in the refrigerator for up to 3 months.

2. To prepare 1 serving, bring 1 cup (250 mL) water to a boil in a small saucepan. Add ½ cup (125 mL) porridge mixture; stir and reduce heat to low. Cook, stirring occasionally, for about 5 minutes or until thickened.

This recipe courtesy of Konnie Kranenburg.

Nutritional Analysis per Serving

Calories...........201	Sodium..........4 mg	Fiber ....5 g
Fat...............5 g	Carbohydrate.....33 g	Protein ....9 g

Makes 4 to 6 servings

Millet is a nutritious whole-grain, gluten-free seed that is high in fiber and relatively high in protein. It also contains an assortment of beneficial phytochemicals. To boot, millet is particularly easy to digest.

Tip

Regular cow's milk does not work in the slow cooker, as the long exposure to the heat will cause it to curdle.

Make Ahead

Cooked cereal can be portioned into airtight containers, cooled, covered and refrigerated for up to 2 days. Reheat in the microwave on Medium-High (70%) power for 2 to 3 minutes or until steaming. Stir in additional milk or water to thin to desired consistency.

Creamy Morning Millet with Apples

- **Small (3½ quart) slow cooker (see tip, page 154)**
- **Greased slow cooker stoneware**

1 cup	millet (see tip, page 151)	250 mL
3 to 4 cups	evaporated milk, enriched rice milk or soy milk or water (or a mixture)	750 mL to 1 L
3	apples, peeled, cored and chopped	3
¼ tsp	salt	1 mL
	Chopped pitted dates, fresh berries and toasted nuts (optional)	

1. In prepared slow cooker stoneware, combine millet, rice milk, apples and salt. Cover and cook on High for 4 hours or on Low for 8 hours or overnight. Stir well, spoon into bowls and sprinkle with fruit and/or nuts, if using.

This recipe should be adjusted based on your symptoms. Follow this symptom guide:

If foods taste too sweet:
- Add a few drops of lemon juice, to taste.

To encourage weight gain:
- Use half full-fat evaporated milk and half water; and/or
- Add ½ cup (125 mL) unflavored whey protein powder or skim milk powder; and/or
- Add 1 to 2 tsp (5 to 10 mL) non-hydrogenated margarine or butter to each serving; and/or
- Use the optional nut garnish.

Nutritional Analysis per Serving

Calories..........441	Sodium....... 329 mg	Fiber .... 6 g
Fat.............. 6 g	Carbohydrate..... 78 g	Protein .... 20 g

Makes 4 servings

Simple yet delicious, this tasty combination couldn't be easier to make.

Tips

Made with this quantity of liquid, the rice will be a bit crunchy around the edges, which is fine if you don't have mouth sores. If you prefer a softer version or will be cooking it longer than 8 hours, add ½ cup (125 mL) of water or rice milk to the recipe.

Cherries (along with cranberries, blueberries and other red, purple and blue fruits) contain anthocyanins, a flavonoid with anti-inflammatory properties.

Make Ahead

Cooked cereal can be portioned into airtight containers, cooled, covered and refrigerated for up to 2 days. Reheat in the microwave on Medium-High (70%) power for 2 to 3 minutes or until steaming. Stir in additional milk or water to thin to desired consistency.

Breakfast Rice

- Small (3½ quart) slow cooker (see tip, page 154)
- Greased slow cooker stoneware

1 cup	brown rice	250 mL
4 cups	vanilla-flavored enriched rice milk, soy milk or evaporated milk	1 L
½ cup	dried cherries or cranberries	125 mL

1. In prepared slow cooker stoneware, combine rice, rice milk and cherries. Place a clean tea towel folded in half (so you will have two layers) over top of stoneware to absorb moisture. Cover and cook on High for 4 hours or on Low for up to 8 hours or overnight. Stir well and serve.

This recipe should be adjusted based on your symptoms. Follow this symptom guide:

To assist with constipation:
- Use half brown rice and half wheat berries; and/or
- Drink a hot beverage followed by a cold one after eating this cereal.

For diarrhea:
- Use short-grain white rice; and/or
- Omit the dried fruit and serve with applesauce and/or probiotic yogurt.

Nutritional Analysis per Serving

Calories..........326	Sodium........ 90 mg	Fiber .... 2 g
Fat.............. 3 g	Carbohydrate..... 73 g	Protein .... 4 g

Makes about 12 pancakes

These tasty pancakes are so easy to make. Maple syrup or mixed berries on the side will allow you to adjust the flavor to suit your taste buds. The egg white and cottage cheese provide protein.

Tip

These pancakes taste great topped with fresh berries and a dollop of your favorite yogurt.

Make Ahead

Let extra pancakes cool on a wire rack. Wrap in plastic wrap, layering with waxed or parchment paper, then place in a freezer bag or airtight container. Refrigerate for up to 3 days or freeze for up to 1 month. Reheat in toaster or toaster oven.

Oatmeal Pancakes

6	egg whites	6
1 cup	large-flake (old-fashioned) rolled oats	250 mL
1 cup	fat-free or regular cottage cheese	250 mL
2 tsp	granulated sugar	10 mL
1 tsp	ground cinnamon (optional)	5 mL
1 tsp	vanilla extract	5 mL
	Vegetable cooking spray	

1. In a blender, on medium speed, blend egg whites, oats, cottage cheese, sugar, cinnamon (if using) and vanilla until smooth.

2. Heat a griddle or large nonstick skillet over medium-low heat. Spray lightly with vegetable cooking spray. For each pancake, pour $1/4$ cup (60 mL) batter onto griddle and cook until bubbly around the edges, about 2 minutes. Flip and cook until golden brown, about 2 minutes. Transfer to a plate and keep warm in a low oven. Repeat with remaining batter, spraying griddle with vegetable cooking spray and adjusting heat between batches as needed.

This recipe courtesy of Jorie Janzen.

Nutritional Analysis per Pancake

Calories............58	Sodium........ 62 mg	Fiber ....1 g
Fat...............1 g	Carbohydrate......7 g	Protein ....6 g

Makes 4 servings

You can have this impressive oven pancake assembled and in the oven in very short order. Serve with a drizzle of maple syrup and vanilla yogurt.

Tips

The brown sugar you use in recipes is totally your preference. Brown sugar comes in both light and dark brown. Dark brown sugar is noticeably darker in color and has a stronger molasses taste.

In place of the cake pans, you could use 9-inch (23 cm) glass pie plates.

Survivor Wisdom

So many people will tell you what you should be doing. Advice is generous.

Apple Puff Pancake

- Preheat oven to 400°F (200°C)
- Two 8- or 9-inch (20 or 23 cm) cake pans

1 cup	all-purpose flour	250 mL
1 cup	milk	250 mL
4	eggs	4
2 tbsp	granulated sugar	30 mL
¼ tsp	salt	1 mL
4 tbsp	butter or non-hydrogenated margarine divided	60 mL
3	apples, peeled and thinly sliced (about 4 cups/1 L)	3
¼ cup	packed brown sugar	60 mL
1½ tsp	ground cinnamon	7 mL

1. In a blender or food processor, blend flour, milk, eggs, granulated sugar and salt to make a smooth batter. Let stand while cooking apples.

2. In a large nonstick skillet, melt 2 tbsp (30 mL) butter over medium heat. Add apple slices, brown sugar and cinnamon. Cook, stirring often, for 5 minutes or until apples are softened.

3. Add 1 tbsp (15 mL) butter to each baking pan and place in preheated oven until melted. Swirl to coat bottom and sides. Pour batter into pans, dividing evenly, and top each with an even layer of warm apple mixture.

4. Bake for 20 to 25 minutes or until puffed and golden.

This recipe should be adjusted based on your symptoms. Follow this symptom guide:

For risk reduction:
- Use whole wheat flour instead of all-purpose; and/or
- Use omega-3 fortified eggs; and/or
- Leave the peel on the apples; and/or
- Reduce the brown sugar to 2 tbsp (30 mL).

Nutritional Analysis per Serving

Calories..........463	Sodium.......624 mg	Fiber.............4 g
Fat..............17 g	Carbohydrate.....69 g	Protein..........12 g

Makes 6 servings

Here's a lower-fat, higher-fiber version of an old favorite. This version will be more suited to those with difficulty tolerating fat or those who are concerned with unwanted weight gain during treatment.

Tips

Both the whites and the yolks of eggs provide such valuable nutrients as vitamin A, magnesium, iron and riboflavin, in addition to protein.

Sprinkle with fresh berries and serve with probiotic yogurt. This will add calcium, vitamin C and other beneficial nutrients to this breakfast favorite.

If you have an aversion to meat, then make sure to use non-meat sources of protein to supply this important nutrient. Eggs and milk both provide protein. Each large egg provides 7 g of protein and every ounce (30 mL) of milk provides 1 g of protein.

French Toast

4	egg whites	4
2 tbsp	skim milk	30 mL
½ tsp	vanilla extract	2 mL
Pinch	ground nutmeg and/or cinnamon	Pinch
6	slices whole-grain bread	6

1. Beat together egg whites, milk, vanilla and nutmeg until frothy. Pour into a large flat dish; dip both sides of bread slices into mixture.

2. In a large nonstick or lightly buttered skillet, cook bread over medium heat until brown on one side. Flip and cook other side. Serve immediately.

This recipe courtesy of Lise Parisien.

This recipe should be adjusted based on your symptoms. Follow this symptom guide:

For diarrhea:
- Use white or oat bread instead of whole-grain bread.

Nutritional Analysis per Serving

Calories............79	Sodium........ 165 mg	Fiber .... 2 g
Fat............... 1 g	Carbohydrate..... 13 g	Protein .... 5 g

Makes 4 servings

Energy low in the mornings? Here's a great breakfast dish that can be assembled a day ahead or frozen. When ready to serve, arrange the toasts on greased baking sheets and pop in the oven. This version, which uses whole eggs and regular milk, is more appropriate for those who need to maintain or gain weight during treatment, as opposed to the lower-fat version.

Tip

The sugar in this recipe will be welcome if you have a bitter, metallic or bland taste in your mouth.

Make Ahead

Freeze unbaked slices in a single layer on a baking sheet lined with plastic wrap; when frozen, transfer to plastic storage bags and freeze. No need to defrost before baking; bake as directed in recipe, increasing baking time by about 5 minutes.

Overnight Oven French Toast

- **Preheat oven to 425°F (220°C)**
- **13- by 9-inch (33 by 23 cm) baking dish**
- **Baking sheet, well greased or lined with parchment paper**

4	eggs	4
1 cup	milk	250 mL
1 tbsp	granulated sugar	15 mL
1 tsp	vanilla extract	5 mL
12	slices day-old French bread, cut $\frac{3}{4}$ inch (2 cm) thick	12
3 tbsp	melted butter	45 mL

1. In a bowl, whisk together eggs, milk, sugar and vanilla. Arrange bread slices in a single layer in baking dish. Pour egg mixture over. Turn slices over and let stand until egg mixture is absorbed. Cover and refrigerate until ready to bake. (Recipe can be prepared up to this point the night before.)

2. Arrange toasts in a single layer on prepared baking sheet and brush tops with half of melted butter.

3. Bake in preheated oven for 10 minutes. Turn slices over; brush tops with remaining melted butter. Bake for 8 minutes longer or until puffed and golden.

This recipe should be adjusted based on your symptoms. Follow this symptom guide:

For risk reduction:
- Use whole-grain bread; and/or
- Use omega-3 fortified eggs; and/or
- Use canola oil instead of butter; and/or
- Add $\frac{1}{2}$ tsp (2 mL) ground cinnamon and/or nutmeg with the milk; and/or
- Reduce or omit the sugar.

Nutritional Analysis per Serving

Calories............522	Sodium........846 mg	Fiber.............3 g
Fat..............14 g	Carbohydrate.....76 g	Protein..........20 g

Restorative Soups and Uplifting Light Meals

Soup is a great food when you are unwell, providing a full serving of fluids, as well as three to four food groups. Follow the freeze-thaw instructions so that you can cook when you have the energy and use your stockpile (no pun intended) when you don't. Be sure to label what you freeze, since "chemo brain" can challenge your ability to remember details.

If you have a sore mouth, blend the soup or cook it until the ingredients are extra-soft — all of the nutrients will still be captured in the broth. If you need extra calories, choose the recipes recommended for weight gain promotion. In addition, with any recipe, you can melt a spoonful of butter into your soup, drizzle with vegetable oil or sprinkle with grated cheese. For more protein (and to thicken a soup), add puréed meat; every ounce (30 g) adds 7 g of protein.

These recipes use reduced-sodium broth; however, not everyone with cancer needs to reduce their sodium. If your blood pressure is low or you are dehydrated, don't be afraid to add salt or use high-sodium ingredients — your body needs sodium to retain fluid and expand the blood supply.

The light meals in this chapter avoid the use of red meat, a common food aversion. Eggs, cheese, fish, seafood and legumes provide the protein you need, without a heavy meat component. These meals will see you through times of altered eating and may become favorites for years to come.

Basic Vegetable Stock

Makes about 12 cups (3 L)

Stock, often called broth, can be used in many circumstances: as a clear fluid when you're recovering from surgery, as a light first meal after vomiting or diarrhea, as a warm rehydrating beverage, or as a base for homemade recipes.

Tips

Adding 1 tsp (5 mL) salt to this stock increases the sodium quantity to 215 mg per 1-cup (250 mL) serving.

To freeze stock, transfer to airtight containers in measured portions (2 cups/500 mL or 4 cups/ 1 L are handy), leaving at least 1 inch (2.5 cm) headspace for expansion. Refrigerate until chilled, then freeze for up to 3 months. Thaw in the refrigerator or microwave before use.

- Large (minimum 6 quart) slow cooker (optional)

8	carrots, coarsely chopped	8
6	stalks celery, coarsely chopped	6
3	onions, coarsely chopped	3
3	cloves garlic, coarsely chopped	3
6	sprigs parsley	6
3	bay leaves	3
10	black peppercorns	10
1 tsp	dried thyme leaves	5 mL
	Salt (optional)	
12 cups	water	3 L

Slow Cooker Method

1. In slow cooker stoneware, combine carrots, celery, onions, garlic, parsley, bay leaves, peppercorns, thyme, salt to taste, if using, and water. Cover and cook on Low for 8 hours or on High for 4 hours.

2. Strain and discard solids. Cover and refrigerate for up to 5 days or freeze in an airtight container.

Stovetop Method

1. In a large pot, combine carrots, celery, onions, garlic, parsley, bay leaves, peppercorns, thyme, salt to taste, if using, and water. Bring to a boil over high heat. Reduce heat to low, cover and simmer gently for about 1 hour or until liquid is flavorful.

2. Strain and discard solids. Cover and refrigerate for up to 5 days or freeze in an airtight container.

Nutritional Analysis per 1 cup (250 mL)

Calories............18	Sodium........ 23 mg	Fiber .... 1 g
Fat............... 0 g	Carbohydrate...... 4 g	Protein .... 1 g

Makes about 8 cups (2 L)

It's easy to make homemade stock instead of resorting to commercial stock cubes and powders, which are loaded with salt.

Tips

Adding 1 tsp (5 mL) salt to this stock increases the sodium to 289 mg per 1-cup (250 mL) serving.

To freeze stock, see page 166.

Celery can test high in synthetic pesticide residue. To reduce your exposure, you may want to buy organic celery. Onions, on the other hand, test very low in residue.

Variation

Turkey Stock: Substitute raw turkey wings for the chicken bones, or use the cooked carcass of a roasted turkey (cleaned of meat, skin and fat).

Chicken Stock

3 lbs	chicken bones (such as neck, backbones and wing tips)	1.5 kg
2	carrots, coarsely chopped	2
2	stalks celery, including leaves, chopped	1
1	large onion, chopped	1
½ tsp	dried thyme leaves	2 mL
1	bay leaf	1
	Freshly ground black pepper	

1. Place chicken bones in a large stockpot. Add water to cover (about 10 cups/2.5 L). Add carrots, celery, onion, thyme and bay leaf. Bring to a boil over high heat and skim. Reduce heat to low and simmer, covered, for 2 hours.

2. Strain through a fine sieve. Season with pepper to taste. Cover and refrigerate for up to 2 days or freeze in an airtight container.

Nutritional Analysis per 1 cup (250 mL)

Calories 8	Sodium . . . . 11 mg	Fiber . . . . 1 g
Fat . . . . 0 g	Carbohydrate . . . . . . 2 g	Protein . . . . 0 g

Makes 8 servings

Often called "Jewish penicillin," chicken soup is the perfect antidote to an off day.

Tip

You don't have to slave over the stove to make this soul-satisfying soup. Adding the chicken and the vegetables to the pot at the same time streamlines the process. The results are every bit as restorative.

Make Ahead

Prepare the soup through step 4, cover tightly and refrigerate for up to 3 days, or transfer individual portions to airtight containers, leaving at least 1 inch (2.5 cm) headspace for expansion, and freeze for up to 3 months. Thaw in the refrigerator or microwave. Reheat individual portions in the microwave on Medium-High (70%) for 1 to 2 minutes, or in a saucepan over medium heat, stirring often, for 4 to 5 minutes, until steaming. (The noodles will get very soft after freezing, so you may prefer to leave them out, then cook them separately and stir them into the reheated soup.)

Chicken Noodle Soup

3 lbs	whole chicken or chicken pieces, such as legs and breasts	1.5 kg
10 cups	water (approx.)	2.5 L
1	large onion, finely chopped	1
3	carrots, peeled and chopped	3
2	stalks celery, including leaves, chopped	2
2 tbsp	chopped fresh parsley	30 mL
1/2 tsp	dried thyme leaves	2 mL
2 tsp	salt	10 mL
1/4 tsp	freshly ground black pepper	1 mL
1	bay leaf	1
2 cups	medium or broad egg noodles	500 mL
1 cup	finely diced zucchini or small cauliflower florets	250 mL
2 tbsp	chopped fresh dill or parsley	30 mL

1. Rinse chicken; remove as much skin and excess fat as possible. Place in a large stockpot; add water to cover. Bring to a boil over high heat; using a slotted spoon, skim off foam as it rises to the surface.

2. Add onion, carrots, celery, parsley, thyme, salt, pepper and bay leaf. Reduce heat to medium-low; cover and simmer for about $1\frac{1}{4}$ hours or until chicken is tender.

3. Remove chicken with a slotted spoon and place in a large bowl; let cool slightly. Pull chicken meat off the bones, discarding skin and bones. Cut meat into bite-size pieces. Reserve 2 cups (500 mL) for soup. (Use remainder for casseroles and sandwiches.)

4. Skim fat from surface of soup; bring to a boil. Add cubed chicken, noodles, zucchini and dill; cook for 10 minutes or until noodles and vegetables are tender. Remove bay leaf. Adjust seasoning with salt and pepper to taste.

Nutritional Analysis per Serving

Calories..........159	Sodium....... 643 mg	Fiber .... 1 g
Fat.............. 3 g	Carbohydrate..... 13 g	Protein .... 20 g

Borscht

1 tbsp	vegetable oil	15 mL
1 cup	diced onion	250 mL
1 tbsp	minced garlic	15 mL
1	can (14 oz/398 mL) beets, including juice	1
2 cups	reduced-sodium ready-to-use beef or chicken broth	500 mL
$\frac{1}{2}$	bag (10 oz/300 g) baby spinach or 2 cups (500 mL) tightly packed baby spinach	$\frac{1}{2}$
2 tbsp	freshly squeezed lemon juice	30 mL
	Salt and freshly ground black pepper	

Makes 4 servings

Beets owe their color to a family of pigments called betalains. They are high in lutein and zeaxanthin, two antioxidants from the carotenoid family, and are a good source of folacin, vitamin C and potassium.

Tips

You can also use homemade beef stock, Chicken Stock (page 167) or Basic Vegetable Stock (page 166) in this recipe.

If you are dehydrated, make sure to add salt to this soup.

Make Ahead

Cover soup tightly and refrigerate for up to 3 days, or transfer individual portions to airtight containers, leaving at least 1 inch (2.5 cm) headspace for expansion, and freeze for up to 3 months. Thaw in the refrigerator or microwave. Serve cold or reheat individual portions in the microwave on Medium-High (70%) for 1 to 2 minutes, or in a saucepan over medium-high heat, stirring often, for 4 to 5 minutes, until steaming.

1. In a large saucepan, heat oil over medium heat. Add onion and cook, stirring, until softened, about 3 minutes. Add garlic and cook, stirring, for 1 minute.
2. Add beets with juice and broth. Bring to a boil. Reduce heat to low and simmer for 10 minutes to combine flavors. Add spinach and cook, stirring, just until wilted. Stir in lemon juice. Season with salt and pepper to taste.
3. Using a slotted spoon, transfer solids plus $\frac{1}{2}$ cup (125 mL) of the liquid to a food processor or blender. Process until smooth. (You can also do this in the saucepan, using a hand-held immersion blender.)
4. Return mixture to saucepan and stir to blend. Serve hot or chill thoroughly.

Nutritional Analysis per Serving

Calories............95	Sodium.......263 mg	Fiber.............3 g
Fat..............4 g	Carbohydrate.....14 g	Protein...........3 g

Makes 6 to 8 servings

This soup is good hot or cold. It provides fluid, cancer-fighting nutrients and a burst of flavor for those whose taste buds need an extra hit of pizzazz.

Tips

If you prefer, use Basic Vegetable Stock (page 166) in place of the ready-to-use broth. If your stock is unsalted, add ½ tsp (2 mL) salt, or to taste, just before serving.

Cranberries are beneficial for the treatment and prevention of urinary tract infections, because they prevent bacteria from attaching to the urethra and bladder. They are being investigated for their cancer-fighting ability thanks to their beneficial phytochemicals.

Make Ahead

Cover soup tightly and refrigerate for up to 3 days. Reheat individual portions in the microwave on Medium-High (70%) for 1 to 2 minutes, or in a saucepan over medium-high heat, stirring often, for about 5 minutes or until steaming.

Cranberry Borscht

6	beets, peeled and quartered	6
	Leaves from the beets, coarsely chopped and set aside in refrigerator	
4	cloves garlic, chopped	4
5 cups	reduced-sodium ready-to-use beef or vegetable broth	1.25 L
1 tsp	salt	5 mL
½ tsp	freshly ground black pepper	2 mL
1 cup	cranberries	250 mL
2 tbsp	granulated sugar or liquid honey	30 mL
	Grated zest and juice of 1 orange	
	Sour cream	

1. In a large saucepan or stockpot over medium heat, combine beets, garlic, broth, salt and pepper. Bring to a boil. Cover, reduce heat to low and simmer until beets are tender, about 45 minutes. Add cranberries, sugar, orange zest and juice and beet leaves. Cover and cook until cranberries are popping from their skins, about 10 minutes.

2. Place a strainer over a large bowl and strain soup. Transfer solids to work bowl fitted with metal blade and add 1 cup (250 mL) of the liquid. Purée until smooth. If serving hot, return puréed solids to saucepan, stir in remaining liquid and reheat. If serving cold, add puréed solids to bowl, cover and chill thoroughly, for at least 3 hours.

3. When ready to serve, ladle into individual bowls and top with a dollop of sour cream.

Nutritional Analysis per Serving

Calories............77	Sodium....... 569 mg	Fiber .... 4 g
Fat.............. 0 g	Carbohydrate..... 18 g	Protein .... 2 g

---

Makes 4 servings

There is a rich Cheddar taste in this hearty soup, a suitable choice for those who want more than just clear soup but aren't yet ready for a solid meal.

Tips

If you prefer, use Chicken Stock (page 167) or Basic Vegetable Stock (page 166) in place of the ready-to-use broth. If don't have broth or stock, use 3 cups (750 mL) water instead.

Taste before serving and add salt if needed.

For a hit of heat, add hot pepper sauce to taste just before serving.

Make Ahead

Cover soup tightly and refrigerate for up to 3 days. Reheat individual portions in the microwave on Medium (50%) for 2 to 3 minutes, or in a saucepan over medium heat, stirring often, for about 5 minutes or until steaming (do not let boil).

Broccoli and Cheddar Cheese Soup

1 tbsp	vegetable oil	15 mL
1 cup	diced onion	250 mL
1 tbsp	minced garlic	15 mL
Pinch	cayenne pepper	Pinch
	Freshly ground black pepper	
1	can (10 oz/284 mL) condensed Cheddar cheese soup, undiluted	1
1 tbsp	Dijon mustard	15 mL
3 cups	reduced-sodium ready-to-use vegetable or chicken broth	750 mL
4 cups	broccoli florets	1 L
2 cups	shredded Cheddar cheese	500 mL

1. In a large saucepan, heat oil over medium heat. Add onion and cook, stirring, until softened, about 3 minutes. Add garlic, cayenne and black pepper to taste. Cook, stirring, for 1 minute.

2. Add soup and mustard, stirring until smooth. Gradually stir in stock. Add broccoli and bring to a boil. Reduce heat to low and simmer until broccoli is tender, about 10 minutes.

3. Using a slotted spoon, transfer solids to a food processor or blender. Add $1/2$ cup (125 mL) of the cooking liquid and process until smooth. (You can also do this in the saucepan, using a hand-held blender.)

4. Return mixture to saucepan over low heat. Add Cheddar cheese and stir until smooth, being careful not to let the mixture boil. Serve piping hot.

Nutritional Analysis per Serving

Calories..........339	Sodium.......659 mg	Fiber.............4 g
Fat..............23 g	Carbohydrate.....16 g	Protein..........19 g

Makes 6 servings

Ginger has a long tradition as a treatment for nausea. Depending on what appeals to you, you may want to leave out the curry powder.

Tip

Gingerroot keeps well in the freezer for up to 3 months and can be grated from frozen.

Make Ahead

Cover soup tightly and refrigerate for up to 3 days. Reheat individual portions in the microwave on Medium (50%) for 2 to 3 minutes, or in a saucepan over medium heat, stirring often, for about 5 minutes or until steaming (do not let boil).

To freeze the soup, omit the milk in step 3. Transfer individual portions to airtight containers, leaving at least 1 inch (2.5 cm) headspace for expansion, and freeze for up to 3 months. Thaw in the refrigerator or microwave. Stir in ¼ cup (60 mL) milk per portion. Reheat as directed above.

Carrot and Ginger Soup

3 cups	water	750 mL
2	cloves garlic, crushed	2
4 cups	sliced carrots	1 L
½ cup	chopped onion	125 mL
1 tbsp	vegetable bouillon powder	15 mL
2 tsp	pure maple syrup	10 mL
1 tsp	curry powder	5 mL
½ tsp	grated gingerroot	2 mL
1½ cups	milk	375 mL

1. In a large saucepan, bring water to a boil. Add garlic, carrots, onion, bouillon powder, maple syrup, curry powder and ginger; return to a boil. Reduce heat, cover and simmer for 40 to 45 minutes or until carrots are tender. Remove from heat.

2. Working in batches, transfer soup to blender and purée on high speed until smooth.

3. Return soup to saucepan and add milk. Heat over low heat (do not boil or milk will curdle).

This recipe courtesy of dietitian Karine Gravel.

This recipe should be adjusted based on your symptoms. Follow this symptom guide:

To encourage weight gain:
- Use any type of cream or evaporated milk instead of milk.

For lactose intolerance:
- Replace the milk with a lactose-free beverage, such as lactose-reduced milk, or a non-dairy milk, such as soy, almond or rice milk or a 14-oz (400 mL) can of coconut milk.

Nutritional Analysis per Serving

Calories...........66	Sodium.......319 mg	Fiber.............2 g
Fat..............2 g	Carbohydrate.....11 g	Protein..........3 g

Makes 6 servings

Oranges and carrots make a delicious flavor combination and make this soup a powerhouse of beta carotene.

Make Ahead

Cover soup tightly and refrigerate for up to 3 days. Reheat individual portions in the microwave on Medium (50%) for 2 to 3 minutes, or in a saucepan over medium heat, stirring often, for about 5 minutes or until steaming (do not let boil).

To freeze the soup, omit the milk in step 3. Transfer individual portions to airtight containers, leaving at least 1 inch (2.5 cm) headspace for expansion, and freeze for up to 3 months. Thaw in the refrigerator or microwave. Stir in 1/4 cup (60 mL) milk per portion. Reheat as directed above.

Carrot Orange Soup

2 tbsp	butter, non-hydrogenated margarine or canola oil	30 mL
1/2 cup	chopped onion	125 mL
4 cups	sliced carrots	1 L
4 cups	reduced-sodium ready-to-use chicken or vegetable broth	1 L
1/2 cup	orange juice	125 mL
1/2 tsp	ground nutmeg	2 mL
1/4 tsp	ground white or black pepper	1 mL
1 cup	milk	250 mL

1. In a large saucepan, heat butter over medium-high heat; add onions and cook for 4 to 5 minutes or until softened. Add carrots and broth; bring to a boil. Reduce heat and simmer for 15 to 20 minutes or until carrots are very soft. Stir in orange juice, nutmeg and pepper.

2. In a food processor or blender, purée carrot mixture in batches until smooth.

3. Return soup to pan; stir in milk. Simmer over very low heat for 2 to 3 minutes or until heated through.

This recipe courtesy of Mary Persi.

This recipe should be adjusted based on your symptoms. Follow this symptom guide:

To encourage weight gain:
- Use any type of cream or evaporated milk instead of milk.

For lactose intolerance:
- Replace the milk with a lactose-free beverage, such as lactose-reduced milk, or non-dairy milk, such as soy, almond, rice or coconut milk.

Nutritional Analysis per Serving

Calories..........113	Sodium.......129 mg	Fiber.............3 g
Fat...............5 g	Carbohydrate.....15 g	Protein...........4 g

Makes 8 servings

This chicken, leek and barley soup, full of cancer-fighting ingredients, is an old Scottish favorite. The prunes deepen the flavor and add a pleasant note of sweetness.

Make Ahead

Cover soup tightly and refrigerate for up to 3 days. Reheat individual portions in the microwave on Medium (50%) for 2 to 3 minutes, or in a saucepan over medium heat, stirring often, for about 5 minutes or until steaming (thin as necessary with more stock or water).

Variation

To make this soup in a slow cooker, complete steps 1 and 2, reducing the quantity of water in step 2 to 1 cup (250 mL). Transfer to slow cooker stoneware. Cover and cook on Low for 8 hours or on High for 4 hours, until barley is tender. Add prunes and soaking water, if using. Cover and cook on High for 15 minutes, until heated through.

Traditional Cockaleekie Soup

10	pitted prunes, finely chopped (about $\frac{1}{2}$ cup/125 mL whole pitted prunes)	10
3 cups	water, divided	750 mL
1 tbsp	olive oil	15 mL
4	large leeks, white part with just a bit of green, thinly sliced	4
4	stalks celery, diced	4
4	carrots, peeled and diced	4
1 tsp	dried thyme leaves, crumbled	5 mL
$\frac{1}{2}$ tsp	cracked black peppercorns	2 mL
4	whole cloves	4
1	piece cinnamon, about 1 inch (2.5 cm) long	1
$1\frac{1}{4}$ cups	whole (hulled) barley, rinsed and drained	300 mL
2 lbs	skinless boneless chicken thighs, coarsely chopped	1 kg
4 cups	reduced-sodium ready-to-use chicken broth	1 L
$\frac{1}{2}$ cup	finely chopped parsley	125 mL

1. In a small bowl, combine prunes and 1 cup (250 mL) of the water. Stir well. Cover and set aside.

2. In a large saucepan, stockpot or Dutch oven, heat oil over medium heat for 30 seconds. Add leeks, celery and carrots and cook, stirring, until softened, about 7 minutes. Add thyme, peppercorns, cloves and cinnamon stick and cook, stirring, for 1 minute. Add barley and toss until well coated with mixture. Add chicken, broth and 2 cups (500 mL) of water and bring to a boil.

3. Reduce heat to low. Cover and simmer until chicken is falling apart and barley is tender, about 1 hour. Discard cloves and cinnamon stick.

4. Add prunes and soaking water, if using. Stir well. Cover and cook to allow flavors to meld, about 15 minutes. Ladle into bowls and garnish with parsley.

Nutritional Analysis per Serving

Calories...........285		Sodium........607 mg		Fiber.............6 g	
Fat...............5 g		Carbohydrate.....30 g		Protein..........30 g	

Recommended for:
- Sore mouth or throat

Bonus features:
- High protein
- Prepare ahead
- Risk reduction

Makes 8 servings

This soup goes together quickly, and the smooth texture is very soothing.

Tip

If you prefer, use Chicken Stock (page 167) or Basic Vegetable Stock (page 166) in place of the ready-to-use broth. If your stock is unsalted, add ¾ tsp (3 mL) salt, or to taste, with the stock.

Make Ahead

Cover soup tightly and refrigerate for up to 3 days, or transfer individual portions to airtight containers, leaving at least 1 inch (2.5 cm) headspace for expansion, and freeze for up to 3 months. Thaw in the refrigerator or microwave. Reheat individual portions in the microwave on Medium (50%) for 2 to 3 minutes, or in a saucepan over medium heat, stirring often, for about 5 minutes, until steaming (do not let boil).

Variation

Replace the sweet potatoes with butternut squash and the leeks with yellow onions.

Leek and Sweet Potato Soup

2 tbsp	vegetable oil	30 mL
4 cups	chopped leeks (white and light green parts only)	1 L
4 cups	diced peeled large sweet potatoes	1 L
4 cups	reduced-sodium ready-to-use chicken or vegetable broth	1 L
1	can (12 oz or 370 mL) evaporated milk	1
1 tsp	dried dillweed	5 mL
	Salt and freshly ground black pepper	

1. In a large saucepan, heat oil over medium heat. Sauté leeks for 10 minutes or until lightly browned. Add potatoes and broth; bring to a boil. Reduce heat, cover and simmer for 30 minutes or until potatoes are soft. Remove from heat.

2. Working in batches, transfer soup to blender and purée until smooth.

3. Return soup to saucepan and add evaporated milk and dill. Heat over low heat (do not let boil). Season to taste with salt and pepper.

This recipe courtesy of Eileen Campbell.

This recipe should be adjusted based on your symptoms. Follow this symptom guide:

To encourage weight gain:
- Use any type of cream instead of evaporated milk; and/or
- Increase the vegetable oil to ¼ cup (60 mL).

For lactose intolerance:
- Replace the milk with a lactose-free beverage, such as lactose-reduced milk, or non-dairy milk, such as unsweetened soy, almond or rice milk.

Nutritional Analysis per Serving

Calories..........164	Sodium.......402 mg	Fiber.............2 g
Fat...............5 g	Carbohydrate.....22 g	Protein...........8 g

Recommended for:
- Nausea
- Taste aversions
- Weight management

Bonus features:
- Prepare ahead
- Risk reduction

Makes 6 servings

To pamper your patient and increase the visual appeal of this soup, cut the tofu into stars with cookie cutters.

Tips

If you prefer, use Chicken Stock (page 167) in place of the ready-to-use broth. If your stock is unsalted, add 1 tsp (5 mL) salt, or to taste, with the stock.

Be sure to use firm tofu in this soup. Otherwise, it won't retain its shape.

Mushrooms are the only plant source of vitamin D; in addition, mushrooms demonstrate cancer-fighting activity when added to cancer cells in laboratory studies.

Make Ahead

Cover soup tightly and refrigerate for up to 3 days. Reheat individual portions in the microwave on Medium-High (70%) for 1 to 2 minutes, or in a saucepan over medium-high heat, stirring often, for about 5 minutes or until steaming.

Ginger Soy Mushroom Soup

5 cups	reduced-sodium ready-to-use chicken broth	1.25 L
4 tsp	finely chopped gingerroot	20 mL
8 oz	sliced mushrooms (shiitake, oyster, portobello or a combination), about 2 cups (500 mL)	250 g
2 tbsp	reduced-sodium soy sauce	30 mL
1 tsp	sesame oil	5 mL
8 oz	firm tofu, cut into small cubes	250 g
1	green onion, thinly sliced	1

1. In a saucepan, combine broth, ginger and mushrooms; bring to a boil. Reduce heat and simmer, uncovered, for 15 minutes. Stir in soy sauce and sesame oil.

2. Place tofu and green onion in individual soup bowls or a tureen. Add soup and serve.

This recipe courtesy of chef Samuel Glass and dietitian Rosie Schwartz.

This recipe should be adjusted based on your symptoms. Follow this symptom guide:

For dehydration or low blood pressure:
- Use regular-sodium broth and soy sauce.

Nutritional Analysis per Serving

Calories............70	Sodium....... 239 mg	Fiber............. 1 g
Fat............... 3 g	Carbohydrate...... 5 g	Protein .... 7 g

Cheese-Smothered Onion Soup

Makes 6 servings

A good melting cheese with a nice nutty flavor, such as Gruyère or raclette, works very well in this savory soup that will warm you when you have a chill. The assertive flavor of onions mellows and sweetens when they're cooked until golden. This classic comfort food might be just what you need on a day when your appetite is wavering.

Make Ahead

The onion soup base can be made ahead through step 1. Cover and refrigerate for up to 3 days, or transfer individual portions to airtight containers, leaving 1 inch (2.5 cm) headspace for expansion, and freeze for up to 3 months. Thaw in the refrigerator or microwave. Reheat individual portions in the microwave on Medium-High (70%) for 1 to 2 minutes, or in a saucepan over medium-high heat, stirring often, for about 5 minutes or until steaming. Proceed with step 2.

- Large, shallow baking pan

3 tbsp	butter	45 mL
8 cups	thinly sliced Spanish onions (about 2 to 3)	2 L
¼ tsp	dried thyme leaves	1 mL
¼ tsp	freshly ground black pepper	1 mL
2 tbsp	all-purpose flour	30 mL
6 cups	reduced-sodium ready-to-use beef broth	1.5 L
1 tbsp	olive oil	15 mL
1	large clove garlic, minced	1
6	slices French bread, about ¾ inch (2 cm) thick	6
2 cups	shredded Gruyère cheese	500 mL

1. In a Dutch oven or large heavy saucepan, melt butter over medium heat. Add onions, thyme and pepper; cook, stirring often, for 15 minutes or until onions are tender and a rich golden color. Blend in flour; stir in broth. Bring to a boil, stirring, until thickened. Reduce heat to medium-low, cover and simmer for 15 minutes.

2. Meanwhile, position oven rack 6 inches (15 cm) from broiler; preheat broiler.

3. In a small bowl, combine olive oil and garlic; lightly brush oil mixture over both sides of bread. Arrange on baking sheet; place under broiler and toast on both sides.

4. Place toasts in deep ovenproof soup bowls; sprinkle with half the cheese. Arrange bowls in baking pan. Ladle hot soup into bowls. Sprinkle with remaining cheese. Place under broiler for 3 minutes or until cheese melts and is lightly browned. Serve immediately.

Nutritional Analysis per Serving

Calories..........464	Sodium.......487 mg	Fiber.............5 g
Fat.............21 g	Carbohydrate.....46 g	Protein..........22 g

Makes 4 servings

This soup contains vegetables, protein and grains, making it a balanced meal.

Tips

If you prefer, use Chicken Stock (page 167) in place of the ready-to-use broth. If your stock is unsalted, add ½ tsp (2 mL) salt, or to taste, with the stock.

Instead of frozen vegetables, add the same quantity of fresh vegetables, such as chopped carrots, celery, zucchini and cauliflower, when the pasta goes into the pot. Some frozen Italian vegetable mixes include fava beans, which provide additional protein.

Make Ahead

Cover soup tightly and refrigerate for up to 3 days. Reheat individual portions in the microwave on Medium-High (70%) for 1 to 2 minutes, or in a saucepan over medium-high heat, stirring often, for about 5 minutes or until steaming (thin with more stock or water if desired).

Vegetable Tortellini Soup

2 tsp	olive oil	10 mL
1	small onion, finely chopped	1
2	cloves garlic, finely chopped	2
½ tsp	dried basil leaves	2 mL
3 cups	reduced-sodium ready-to-use chicken broth	750 mL
1	can (19 oz/540 mL) Italian stewed tomatoes	1
2 cups	fresh or frozen cheese- or meat-filled tortellini	500 mL
2 cups	frozen mixed Italian vegetables	500 mL
	Salt and freshly ground black pepper	
	Freshly grated Parmesan cheese	

1. In large saucepan, heat oil over medium heat. Cook onion, garlic and basil, stirring, for 3 minutes or until softened. Add chicken broth and tomatoes; bring to a boil. Add tortellini. Reduce heat, cover and simmer, stirring occasionally, for 5 minutes.

2. Add frozen vegetables. Cover and simmer for 8 minutes more or until pasta and vegetables are just tender. Season with salt and pepper to taste. Ladle into soup bowls; sprinkle generously with Parmesan cheese.

This recipe should be adjusted based on your symptoms. Follow this symptom guide:

For meat aversion:
- Use cheese tortellini, and use vegetable broth instead of chicken broth.

Nutritional Analysis per Serving

Calories..........268	Sodium....... 705 mg	Fiber .... 6 g
Fat............... 5 g	Carbohydrate..... 44 g	Protein .... 11 g

Makes 6 servings

The combination of vegetables and lentils makes a balanced meal.

Tips

If you prefer, use Basic Vegetable Stock (page 167) in place of the ready-to-use broth. If your stock is unsalted, add 1/4 tsp (1 mL) salt, or to taste, with the stock.

Lentils come in many colors, but the most common are red, brown or green. A member of the legume family, lentils are rich in protein and other nutrients.

Make Ahead

Cover soup tightly and refrigerate for up to 3 days, or transfer individual portions to airtight containers, leaving at least 1 inch (2.5 cm) headspace for expansion, and freeze for up to 3 months. Thaw in the refrigerator or microwave. Reheat individual portions in the microwave on Medium-High (70%) for 1 to 2 minutes, or in a saucepan over medium heat, stirring often, for 4 to 5 minutes, until steaming.

Chunky Vegetable Lentil Soup

2 cups	reduced-sodium ready-to-use vegetable broth	500 mL
1 cup	chopped carrots	250 mL
1	can (28 oz/796 mL) diced tomatoes	1
1	can (19 oz/540 mL) lentils, drained and rinsed	1
2 tsp	minced garlic	10 mL
1 tsp	dried basil	5 mL
1/2 tsp	ground thyme	2 mL
1/2 tsp	ground cumin	2 mL

1. In a large saucepan, bring vegetable broth to a boil over high heat.

2. Add carrots; reduce heat to medium and cook, covered, for 10 minutes.

3. Add tomatoes, lentils, garlic, basil, thyme and cumin; reduce heat to medium-low and cook, stirring often, for 10 minutes or until carrots are tender.

This recipe courtesy of dietitian Lynn Roblin.

Nutritional Analysis per Serving

Calories 126	Sodium . . . . 501 mg	Fiber . . . . 9 g
Fat . . . . 0 g	Carbohydrate . . . . . 23 g	Protein . . . . 8 g

Recommended for:
- Constipation

Bonus features:
- High fiber
- High protein
- Low fat
- Prepare ahead
- Risk reduction

Makes 6 servings

Lentils make a valuable contribution to your daily protein intake.

Tip

If you prefer, use Chicken Stock (page 167) or Basic Vegetable Stock (page 166) in place of the ready-to-use broth. If your stock is unsalted, add 1½ tsp (7 mL) salt, or to taste, with the stock.

Variation

Lentil-Rice Soup: Reduce the lentils to ⅔ cup (150 mL) and add ⅓ cup (75 mL) long-grain white or brown rice with the lentils.

Make Ahead

See page 179.

Suppertime Lentil Soup

8 cups	reduced-sodium ready-to-use chicken or vegetable broth	2 L
1 cup	dried green lentils, rinsed and sorted	250 mL
8 oz	mushrooms, chopped	250 g
3	carrots, peeled and chopped	3
2	stalks celery, including leaves, chopped	2
1	large onion, chopped	1
2	cloves garlic, finely chopped	2
1 tsp	dried thyme or marjoram leaves	5 mL
¼ cup	chopped fresh dill or parsley	60 mL
	Salt and freshly ground black pepper	

1. In a large Dutch oven or stockpot, combine broth, lentils, mushrooms, carrots, celery, onion, garlic and thyme.
2. Bring to a boil; reduce heat, cover and simmer for 35 to 40 minutes or until lentils are tender. Stir in dill or parsley. Adjust seasoning with salt and pepper to taste.

Nutritional Analysis per Serving

Calories...........154	Sodium.......262 mg	Fiber.............8 g
Fat...............1 g	Carbohydrate.....30 g	Protein...........9 g

---

Makes 4 servings

This soup is so light and refreshing, it's hard to believe that it's also packed with nutrition.

Tips

You can use cooked dried lentils instead of canned. Thoroughly rinse 1 cup (250 mL) dried brown lentils under cold running water, then place in a large saucepan. Cover with 3 cups (750 mL) cold water. Bring to a boil over medium heat. Reduce heat to low and simmer until tender, about 25 minutes. Drain.

If you prefer, use Chicken Stock (page 167) or Basic Vegetable Stock (page 166) in place of the ready-to-use broth. If your stock is unsalted, add 1 tsp (5 mL) salt, or to taste, with the stock.

Variation

Curried Lentil and Spinach Soup: Add 1 to 3 tsp (5 to 15 mL) curry powder, depending upon the degree of spice you prefer, with the garlic.

Make Ahead

See page 179.

Lemony Lentil Soup with Spinach

1 tbsp	vegetable oil	15 mL
1 cup	diced onion	250 mL
1 tbsp	minced garlic	15 mL
Pinch	cayenne pepper	Pinch
	Freshly ground black pepper	
1	package (10 oz/300 g) frozen chopped spinach or 1 bag (10 oz/300 g) fresh spinach, stems removed and chopped	1
1	can (19 oz/540 mL) lentils, drained and rinsed	1
5 cups	reduced-sodium ready-to-use vegetable or chicken broth	1.25 L
¼ cup	freshly squeezed lemon juice	60 mL
	Salt	

1. In a large saucepan, heat oil over medium heat. Add onion and cook, stirring, until softened, about 3 minutes. Add garlic, cayenne and black pepper to taste. Cook, stirring, for 1 minute.

2. Add spinach and cook, stirring and breaking up with spoon, until thawed (if frozen) or wilted (if fresh). Add lentils and broth. Bring to a boil. Reduce heat to low and simmer for 15 minutes to cook spinach and combine flavors. Stir in lemon juice, and salt to taste. Serve immediately.

Nutritional Analysis per Serving

Calories...........215	Sodium....... 526 mg	Fiber .... 16 g
Fat.............. 4 g	Carbohydrate..... 36 g	Protein .... 12 g

Makes 6 servings

This light soup is perfect when your appetite is weak. It is good hot or cold.

Tip

If you prefer, use Chicken Stock (page 167) or Basic Vegetable Stock (page 166) in place of the ready-to-use broth. If your stock is unsalted, add ¾ tsp (3 mL) salt, or to taste, with the stock.

Make Ahead

Do not reserve whole peas for garnish. Cover soup tightly and refrigerate for up to 3 days, or transfer individual portions to airtight containers, leaving at least 1 inch (2.5 cm) headspace for expansion, and freeze for up to 3 months. Thaw in the refrigerator or microwave. Reheat individual portions in the microwave on Medium-High (70%) for 1 to 2 minutes, or in a saucepan over medium heat, stirring often, for 4 to 5 minutes, until steaming.

Sweet Green Pea Soup

2 tbsp	butter	30 mL
1 cup	diced onion	250 mL
½ tsp	dried tarragon, thyme or mint	2 mL
½ tsp	salt	2 mL
	Freshly ground black pepper	
10	Boston or romaine lettuce leaves, shredded (optional)	10
4 cups	reduced-sodium ready-to-use vegetable or chicken broth	1 L
1	package (12 oz/375 g) frozen sweet green peas	1
Pinch	granulated sugar	Pinch
	Finely chopped parsley or chives	

1. In a large saucepan, melt butter over medium heat. Add onion and cook, stirring, until softened, about 3 minutes. Add tarragon, salt and pepper to taste and cook, stirring, for 1 minute. Add lettuce, if using, and stir until wilted.

2. Add chicken broth, green peas and sugar. Bring to a boil. Reduce heat to low and simmer until peas are tender, about 7 minutes.

3. Using a slotted spoon, remove about ¼ cup (60 mL) of the whole peas from the saucepan and set aside. Using a slotted spoon, transfer remaining solids to a food processor or blender. Add ½ cup (125 mL) of the cooking liquid and process until smooth. (You can also do this in the saucepan, using a hand-held blender.) Ladle into bowls and garnish with reserved peas and parsley.

Nutritional Analysis per Serving

Calories..........104	Sodium.......334 mg	Fiber.............5 g
Fat..............4 g	Carbohydrate.....14 g	Protein..........4 g

Makes 8 servings

Here's a homey, satisfying soup that's perfect to serve as the main dish when you need a meal that feels like a warm blanket.

Tip

This soup thickens as it cools, so you may want to thin it with additional stock before serving if you've made it ahead.

Make Ahead

Prepare the soup through step 2, cover tightly and refrigerate for up to 3 days, or transfer individual portions to airtight containers, leaving at least 1 inch (2.5 cm) headspace for expansion, and freeze for up to 3 months. Thaw in the refrigerator or microwave. Reheat individual portions in the microwave on Medium-High (70%) for 1 to 2 minutes, or in a saucepan over medium heat, stirring often, for 4 to 5 minutes, until steaming.

Curried Split Pea Soup

1 tbsp	vegetable oil	15 mL
2	onions, chopped	2
4	cloves garlic, finely chopped	4
1 tbsp	mild curry paste, or to taste	15 mL
1 tsp	ground cumin	5 mL
1 tsp	paprika	5 mL
1/4 tsp	cayenne pepper	1 mL
3	large carrots, peeled and chopped	3
2	large stalks celery, including leaves, chopped	2
2 cups	dried yellow or green split peas, rinsed and sorted	500 mL
1/4 cup	tomato paste	60 mL
10 cups	Basic Vegetable Stock (page 166) or Chicken Stock (page 167) or no-salt-added ready-to-use chicken broth	2.5 L
1/3 cup	chopped fresh cilantro or parsley	75 mL
	Salt and freshly ground black pepper	
	Plain yogurt (optional)	

1. In a large Dutch oven or stockpot, heat oil over medium heat. Add onions, garlic, curry paste, cumin, paprika and cayenne pepper; cook, stirring, for 3 minutes or until softened.

2. Add carrots, celery, split peas, tomato paste and stock. Bring to a boil; reduce heat, cover and simmer for about 1 to 1½ hours or until peas are tender.

3. Stir in cilantro; season with up to ½ tsp (2 mL) salt and pepper to taste. Ladle into bowls; top with a dollop of yogurt, if desired.

Nutritional Analysis per Serving

Calories..........230	Sodium.......227 mg	Fiber...........15 g
Fat..............3 g	Carbohydrate.....39 g	Protein..........13 g

---

Makes 4 servings

This tasty soup can be made in less time than it takes to order from a restaurant.

Tips

If you have fresh basil or parsley, use 1 tbsp (15 mL) or more of each instead of the dried.

Limit nitrate intake by using beans in tomato sauce and not "beans with pork."

Make Ahead

Prepare the soup through step 1, cover tightly and refrigerate for up to 3 days, or transfer individual portions to airtight containers, leaving at least 1 inch (2.5 cm) headspace for expansion, and freeze for up to 3 months. Thaw in the refrigerator or microwave. Reheat individual portions in the microwave on Medium-High (70%) for 1 to 2 minutes, or in a saucepan over medium heat, stirring often, for 4 to 5 minutes, until steaming.

Tomato and Bean Soup

1	can (19 oz/540 mL) stewed tomatoes	1
1	can (14 oz/398 mL) baked beans in tomato sauce	1
1 cup	water	250 mL
½ cup	chopped onions	125 mL
½ tsp	dried basil	2 mL
½ tsp	dried parsley	2 mL
1 cup	shredded Cheddar cheese	250 mL

1. In a saucepan over medium heat, combine tomatoes, beans in sauce, water, onion, basil and parsley; bring to a boil. Reduce heat and simmer, uncovered and stirring occasionally, for 10 to 15 minutes or until onions are softened.

2. Top each serving with ¼ cup (60 mL) Cheddar cheese.

This recipe courtesy of Marylin Cook.

This recipe should be adjusted based on your symptoms. Follow this symptom guide:

If foods taste too sweet:
- Choose baked beans with lower sugar content by reading the label; and/or
- Add 1 to 2 tbsp (15 mL) cider vinegar or lemon juice at the end of cooking; and/or
- Choose sharp (old) Cheddar cheese.

Nutritional Analysis per Serving

Calories..........274	Sodium.......913 mg	Fiber.............7 g
Fat..............10 g	Carbohydrate.....36 g	Protein..........14 g

Makes 6 servings

Chances are you'll have the basic items on hand to make this hearty soup — the most famous soup in Italy, where it's known as pasta e fagioli.

Make Ahead

Omit the fresh basil or use dried basil (see tip, above). Cover soup tightly and refrigerate for up to 3 days, or transfer individual portions to airtight containers, leaving at least 1 inch (2.5 cm) headspace for expansion, and freeze for up to 3 months. Thaw in the refrigerator or microwave. Reheat individual portions in the microwave on Medium-High (70%) for 1 to 2 minutes, or in a saucepan over medium heat, stirring often, for 4 to 5 minutes, until steaming. Add fresh basil just before serving.

Variation

Bean, Pasta and Swiss Chard Soup: Increase the broth to 6 cups (1.5 L) and stir in 4 cups (1 L) shredded Swiss chard or spinach with the pasta.

Pasta and Bean Soup

1 tbsp	olive oil	15 mL
1	onion, chopped	1
2	cloves garlic, finely chopped	2
1 cup	chopped drained canned plum tomatoes	250 mL
5 cups	reduced-sodium ready-to-use chicken or vegetable broth (approx.)	1.25 L
1	can (19 oz/540 mL) white kidney beans, drained and rinsed, divided	1
¾ cup	small pasta shapes, such as ditali or shells	175 mL
2 tbsp	chopped fresh basil or parsley	30 mL
	Salt and freshly ground black pepper	
	Freshly grated Parmesan cheese	

1. In a large saucepan, heat oil over medium heat. Cook onion and garlic, stirring, for 3 minutes or until softened. Add tomatoes and cook, stirring occasionally, for 5 minutes or until sauce-like.

2. Add broth; bring to a boil over high heat. In a bowl, using a fork, mash half of the beans. Stir into stock along with pasta; reduce heat to medium, partially cover and cook, stirring occasionally, for 8 to 10 minutes or until pasta is just tender.

3. Add remaining whole beans and basil; heat until piping hot. Season with salt and pepper to taste. Thin with additional stock, if necessary. Ladle soup into bowls; sprinkle generously with Parmesan cheese.

Nutritional Analysis per Serving

Calories..........155	Sodium.......513 mg	Fiber.............7 g
Fat..............3 g	Carbohydrate.....26 g	Protein..........8 g

---

Makes 4 servings

This chilled, fruity soup is perfect when you need something cool and fresh to restore you. It can be eaten with a spoon as a cool lunch or poured into a tall glass for a nutrient-packed elixir. For an appealing presentation, garnish with fresh mint.

Tips

Although this soup does not freeze well, it will keep for up to 3 days in the refrigerator.

Chilled soups travel well in a Thermos, so consider taking this to an appointment.

Survivor Wisdom

I ate anything with a creamy texture — custard, puréed soups. They felt like comfort.

Chilled Melon Soup with Mango

2 cups	cubed cantaloupe	500 mL
1 cup	diced mango	250 mL
¾ cup	orange juice	175 mL
½ cup	lower-fat plain yogurt	125 mL
2 tbsp	freshly squeezed lime juice	30 mL
2 tbsp	liquid honey	30 mL
	Chopped fresh mint (optional)	

1. In a food processor or blender, combine fruit; purée until smooth. Add orange juice, yogurt, lime juice and honey. Blend until combined. Chill. Serve sprinkled with mint, if desired.

This recipe courtesy of dietitian Bev Callaghan.

This recipe should be adjusted based on your symptoms. Follow this symptom guide:

For sore mouth or throat:
- Replace the orange juice and lime juice with unsweetened mango juice or peach nectar.

Nutritional Analysis per Serving

Calories..........130	Sodium........ 36 mg	Fiber .... 2 g
Fat.............. 1 g	Carbohydrate..... 29 g	Protein .... 3 g

Makes 6 servings

The flavors of grape juice, lime, honey, ginger and melon blend to make a fruity, layered soup that will be appreciated by anyone whose taste buds need a pick-me-up.

Tips

Patients should check with their doctor before consuming alcohol. Even when simmered in this recipe, some alcohol may remain, so if you need to avoid alcohol, use the white grape juice or a dealcoholized wine instead.

Purée melon in a food processor or blender to make about 4 cups (1 L) for this recipe.

Although this soup does not freeze well, it will keep for up to 3 days in the refrigerator.

Chilled soups travel well in a Thermos, so consider taking this to an appointment.

Chilled Melon Soup with Ginger and Lime

2 cups	white wine or white grape juice (see tip, at left)	500 mL
¼ cup	grated lime zest	60 mL
2 tbsp	freshly squeezed lime juice	30 mL
2 tbsp	liquid honey	30 mL
3 tbsp	grated gingerroot	45 mL
1	large honeydew melon, peeled, seeded, cut into chunks and puréed	1

1. In a saucepan, combine wine, lime zest and juice, honey and ginger; bring to a boil. Reduce heat and simmer, uncovered, until reduced by half. Cool to room temperature. Strain through a fine sieve.

2. Add melon purée to wine mixture. Chill thoroughly.

This recipe courtesy of chef Kenneth Peace and dietitian Maye Musk.

Nutritional Analysis per Serving

Calories...........197	Sodium........ 39 mg	Fiber .... 2 g
Fat.............. 0 g	Carbohydrate..... 38 g	Protein .... 1 g

Makes 4 servings

This classic soup is a meal in itself. It features clams, which are a good source of iron and vitamin B$_{12}$.

Tip

Clams provide 2 mg of iron and 75 mcg of vitamin B$_{12}$ per 2$^1/_2$ oz (75 g).

Make Ahead

Cover soup tightly and refrigerate for up to 2 days. Reheat individual portions in the microwave on Medium-High (70%) for 1 to 2 minutes, or in a saucepan over medium heat, stirring often, for 4 to 5 minutes, until steaming.

Survivor Wisdom

I never ate steak and baked potato.

New England Clam Chowder

2 tbsp	butter or canola oil	30 mL
1 cup	diced onion	250 mL
1 cup	diced celery	250 mL
1 tsp	paprika	5 mL
	Freshly ground black pepper	
2	cans (each 5 oz/142 g) clams, including juice	2
1	can (19 oz/540 mL) whole potatoes, drained and cut into $^1/_2$-inch (1 cm) cubes, or 2 cups (500 mL) cubed cooked potatoes	2
1	bottle (8 oz/240 mL) clam juice	1
1 cup	water	250 mL
1 cup	whipping (35%) cream	250 mL

1. In a large saucepan, melt butter over medium heat. Add onion and celery and cook, stirring, until softened, about 3 minutes. Add paprika and pepper to taste. Cook, stirring, for 1 minute.

2. Add clams with juice, potatoes, bottled clam juice and water. Bring to a boil. Reduce heat to low and simmer for at least 10 minutes to combine flavors. Stir in cream, remove from heat and serve.

Nutritional Analysis per Serving

Calories..........387	Sodium.......978 mg	Fiber.............4 g
Fat.............27 g	Carbohydrate.....29 g	Protein...........9 g

---

Recommended for:
- Constipation
- Dehydration
- Nausea

Bonus features:
- High fiber
- High protein
- Prepare ahead
- Risk reduction

Makes 4 servings

There are many variations of this dish, most of which can be found in Mediterranean or Indian cooking.

Tips

If you don't have fresh parsley on hand, garnish with finely chopped red or green onion instead.

Chickpeas, like other legumes, contain valuable phytonutrients and provide soluble fiber, which helps control blood sugar levels.

Make Ahead

Cover tightly and refrigerate for up to 3 days, or transfer individual portions to airtight containers, leaving at least 1 inch (2.5 cm) headspace for expansion, cover and freeze for up to 3 months. Thaw in the refrigerator or microwave. Reheat individual portions in the microwave on Medium-High (70%) for 1 to 2 minutes, or in a saucepan over medium heat, stirring often, for 4 to 5 minutes, until steaming.

Chickpeas in Tomato Sauce

1	large onion, cut into thin wedges	1
2	cloves garlic, minced	2
1 tbsp	olive oil	15 mL
1	can (28 oz/796 mL) chickpeas, drained and rinsed	1
1½ cups	canned crushed tomatoes	375 mL
½ tsp	salt	2 mL
½ tsp	freshly ground black pepper	2 mL
½ tsp	dried thyme	2 mL
¼ tsp	cayenne pepper	1 mL
1	bay leaf	1
	Chopped fresh parsley	

1. In a large saucepan over medium-high heat, cook onion and garlic in oil for about 5 minutes or until tender. Add chickpeas; cook for 3 to 4 minutes. Add tomatoes and seasonings except parsley; cook over low heat for about 25 minutes. Remove bay leaf before serving; garnish with chopped parsley.

This recipe courtesy of Chantal Haddad.

This recipe should be adjusted based on your symptoms. Follow this symptom guide:

To assist with nausea:
- Add 1 tbsp (15 mL) minced gingerroot with the garlic.

Nutritional Analysis per Serving

Calories...........241	Sodium........882 mg	Fiber.............9 g
Fat................6 g	Carbohydrate.....38 g	Protein..........10 g

Overnight Broccoli and Cheese Strata

This is a comforting meal to make ahead and serve for breakfast, lunch or dinner.

Tips

This is a great way to use up stale bread, which actually works better than fresh in this recipe — it absorbs more of the egg and milk mixture, making the strata taste creamier.

Frozen broccoli can be used in place of fresh. Place frozen broccoli in a microwave-safe bowl, cover and microwave on High for 2 minutes. Drain, pat dry and proceed with the recipe.

Survivor Wisdom

My energy was depleted throughout my entire treatment.

- **Preheat oven to 350°F (180°C)**
- **9-inch (23 cm) casserole, greased**

2 cups	chopped fresh broccoli or asparagus	500 mL
4 cups	cubed whole wheat bread (preferably stale)	1 L
2 cups	shredded Swiss or Cheddar cheese	500 mL
4	eggs	4
2 cups	milk	500 mL
½ to 1 tsp	dry mustard	2 to 5 mL
	Cayenne pepper to taste (optional)	

1. In a pot of boiling water, cook broccoli just until tender-crisp; drain and pat dry. Set aside.
2. Place bread cubes in casserole dish. Add cheese and broccoli; gently toss together.
3. In a bowl, beat together eggs, milk, mustard and, if using, cayenne; pour evenly over bread mixture. Cover and refrigerate for 2 hours or overnight.
4. Bake in preheated oven for 50 to 60 minutes or until golden brown and just set in center. Let stand for 3 to 4 minutes before serving.

This recipe courtesy of the Canadian Egg Marketing Agency.

This recipe should be adjusted based on your symptoms. Follow this symptom guide:

To encourage weight gain:
- Replace the milk with half-and-half (10%) or table (18%) cream; and/or
- Spread butter or non-hydrogenated margarine on slices of bread before cutting them into cubes.

Nutritional Analysis per Serving

Calories..........523	Sodium....... 709 mg	Fiber .... 12 g
Fat.............. 28 g	Carbohydrate..... 44 g	Protein .... 33 g

Makes 2 servings

Here's a hearty, no-nonsense dish that is very easy to make. With pre-shredded cheese, it can be completed in less than 15 minutes.

Tips

If your immune system is compromised, be sure to cook the eggs thoroughly.

If the handle of your skillet is not ovenproof, wrap it in foil.

Survivor Wisdom

It's nice when a host or hostess asks, "Do you have any food issues?" or "I was thinking of making X — would this work for you?"

Cheese and Hash Brown Omelet

- Ovenproof skillet (see tip, at left)

6	eggs	6
¼ tsp	salt	1 mL
2 tbsp	vegetable oil, divided	30 mL
1 cup	frozen hash brown potatoes	250 mL
	Freshly ground black pepper	
1 cup	shredded Cheddar or Swiss cheese	250 mL

1. In a bowl, lightly beat eggs and salt. Set aside.
2. In an ovenproof skillet, heat 1 tbsp (15 mL) of the oil over medium heat. Add potatoes and season with black pepper to taste. Cook, stirring, until potatoes are crisp and browned, 7 to 8 minutes. Transfer to a paper towel–lined plate to drain and wipe skillet clean.
3. Add remaining oil to skillet and return to heat. Add egg mixture and cook until mixture begins to form a crust on the bottom, about 2 minutes.
4. Sprinkle cheese evenly over top and arrange potatoes evenly over cheese. Bake in preheated oven until eggs are set and cheese is melted, 2 to 3 minutes.

This recipe should be adjusted based on your symptoms. Follow this symptom guide:

To encourage weight gain:
- Serve topped with sour cream.

Nutritional Analysis per Serving

Calories...........624	Sodium.......833 mg	Fiber.............1 g
Fat..............44 g	Carbohydrate.....17 g	Protein..........34 g

Makes 1 to 2 servings

This delicious and unusual omelet is reminiscent of potato pancakes. Your tummy will be smiling!

Tips

To flip the omelet, put a plate over the skillet and turn it out. Flip it over into the skillet to cook the other side.

Substitute sliced green beans, chopped bean sprouts, finely chopped bell pepper, diced mushrooms or any combination of your favorite vegetables for the sweet potatoes, then serve with bread or toast for a balanced meal.

Sweet Potato Omelet

2	eggs	2
1 cup	shredded peeled sweet potatoes	250 mL
½ cup	chopped onion	125 mL
1	clove garlic, chopped	1
¼ tsp	salt (or 1 tsp/5 mL soy sauce)	1 mL
1 tbsp	vegetable oil	15 mL

1. In a small bowl, beat eggs with a fork. Stir in sweet potatoes, onion, garlic and salt until well combined.

2. Heat a medium skillet over medium-high heat. Add oil and swirl to coat the pan. Pour in egg mixture; cook, turning once, until lightly browned on both sides, about 2 minutes per side.

This recipe courtesy of dietitian Nena Wirth.

This recipe should be adjusted based on your symptoms. Follow this symptom guide:

To encourage weight gain:
- Serve topped with sour cream; and/or
- Sprinkle each serving with ¼ cup (60 mL) shredded cheese.

Nutritional Analysis per Serving

Calories...........223	Sodium........391 mg	Fiber.............3 g
Fat..............11 g	Carbohydrate.....22 g	Protein...........8 g

Makes 6 servings

When it comes to a no-fuss dinner, this salmon loaf has it all: protein, vegetables, whole grains and dairy.

Tip

Salmon is a great source of beneficial omega-3 fatty acids. You can increase your intake even further by choosing eggs fortified with omega-3s.

Survivor Wisdom

Be aware of your surroundings. People, places and situations will affect your mood and your ability to eat.

Cheesy Salmon Loaf

- **Preheat oven to 350°F (180°C)**
- **9- by 5-inch (23 by 12.5 cm) loaf pan, lightly greased**

2	eggs	2
1 cup	quick-cooking rolled oats	250 mL
2	cans (each 7½ oz/213 g) salmon, skin removed	2
1 cup	shredded part-skim mozzarella cheese	250 mL
¼ cup	chopped onion	60 mL
1	stalk celery, chopped	1
1	large carrot, grated	1
2 tbsp	freshly squeezed lemon juice	30 mL

1. In a large bowl, beat eggs. Stir in rolled oats, salmon, cheese, onion, celery, carrot and lemon juice until well combined. Turn salmon mixture into prepared loaf pan. Bake in preheated oven for about 35 minutes. Let stand for 5 minutes before slicing.

This recipe courtesy of dietitian Clair Lightfoot.

This recipe should be adjusted based on your symptoms. Follow this symptom guide:

If you are low on energy:
- Purchase skinless canned salmon to save some prep time and buy pre-shredded cheese.

To encourage weight gain:
- Use full-fat mozzarella cheese rather than part-skim; and/or
- Serve the loaf topped with tartar sauce or mayonnaise mixed with green relish or sliced pickles.

Nutritional Analysis per Serving

Calories..........220	Sodium.......725 mg	Fiber.............2 g
Fat..............10 g	Carbohydrate.....11 g	Protein..........21 g

Makes 4 servings

For those whose taste buds register bland, this perky meal has a variety of flavor and texture elements that will wake up the mouth. Combined with simple preparation and cancer-fighting ingredients, the result is a memorable meal.

Tip

Salmon and yellow curry powder are two anti-inflammatory ingredients.

Variation

To boost the vitamin B_{12} content, replace the salmon with 2 cans (each $3\frac{3}{4}$ oz/106 g) sardines, drained and rinsed.

Salmon Oasis

- Preheat broiler
- Baking sheet, ungreased

4	whole wheat English muffins	4
1	can (7½ oz/213 g) salmon, drained, skin removed	1
¼ cup	light mayonnaise	60 mL
2 tbsp	finely chopped green onion	30 mL
2 tsp	freshly squeezed lemon juice	10 mL
½ tsp	curry powder	2 mL
¼ tsp	freshly ground black pepper	1 mL
8	green bell pepper strips	8
¾ cup	shredded part-skim mozzarella cheese	175 mL
	Paprika	

1. Split muffins in half and toast.
2. Combine salmon, mayonnaise, onion, lemon juice, curry powder and pepper. Spread on muffin halves; top with green pepper and cheese. Sprinkle with paprika to taste. Place on ungreased baking sheet. Broil for about 3 minutes or just until cheese melts.

This recipe courtesy of Ellen Craig.

This recipe should be adjusted based on your symptoms. Follow this symptom guide:

If you are low on energy:
- Choose skinless canned salmon to save some prep time and buy pre-shredded cheese.

To encourage weight gain:
- Use full-fat mayonnaise and mozzarella cheese.

Nutritional Analysis per Serving

Calories..........349	Sodium....... 707 mg	Fiber .... 5 g
Fat.............. 14 g	Carbohydrate..... 36 g	Protein .... 22 g

Makes 2 servings

The protein from the tuna and the whole-grain bread combine to make a meal that will help sustain your energy.

Tip

To reduce your exposure to environmental pollutants, always try to choose smaller fish. Select yellowfin, skipjack or tongol (often labeled "light") tuna and limit your intake of albacore tuna (often labeled "white").

Survivor Wisdom

I would walk around the block before a meal to help with my appetite.

Tuna Cheddar Melt

- Preheat broiler
- Baking sheet

1	can (6 oz/170 g) tuna, drained and flaked	1
¼ cup	light mayonnaise	60 mL
¼ cup	finely chopped celery	60 mL
1	green onion, finely chopped	1
1 tsp	fresh lemon juice	5 mL
4	slices whole-grain bread	4
8	thin tomato slices	8
	Salt and freshly ground black pepper	
4	slices Cheddar cheese	4

1. In a bowl, combine tuna, mayonnaise, celery, green onion and lemon juice.
2. Spread bread slices with tuna mixture. Layer with tomato slices; season with salt and pepper. Top with Cheddar cheese slices.
3. Arrange on baking sheet; place under broiler for about 3 minutes or until cheese is melted. Serve immediately.

This recipe should be adjusted based on your symptoms. Follow this symptom guide:

To encourage weight gain:
- Use full-fat mayonnaise; and/or
- Spread butter or non-hydrogenated margarine on bread before adding tuna mixture; and/or
- Use full-fat cheese and add 2 slices to each serving.

Nutritional Analysis per Serving

Calories...........572	Sodium......1,016 mg	Fiber ....5 g
Fat..............31 g	Carbohydrate.....31 g	Protein ....42 g

**Makes
4 sandwiches**

This sandwich is a favorite with cancer survivors at the Wellspring Support Center in Toronto, Ontario.

Tips

If your taste buds are not strong, you will appreciate the mix of textures in this sandwich.

While turmeric does have cancer-fighting properties, it can add a bitter note, so you may wish to replace it with an additional $\frac{1}{2}$ tsp (10 mL) curry powder.

Curcumin, the cancer-fighting compound in turmeric, is best absorbed when eaten along with black pepper, so add some pepper to the mayonnaise mixture if your curry powder does not already include it.

Curry Chickpea and Avocado Sandwich

$1\frac{1}{2}$ tsp	curry powder	7 mL
$\frac{1}{2}$ tsp	ground turmeric (see tip, at left)	2 mL
$\frac{1}{4}$ cup	mayonnaise	60 mL
1	can (19 oz/540 mL) chickpeas, rinsed and drained (or 2 cups/500 mL cooked)	1
$\frac{1}{4}$ cup	chopped walnuts, toasted	60 mL
$\frac{1}{4}$ cup	dried cranberries	60 mL
2 tbsp	chopped fresh cilantro or parsley	30 mL
1	avocado, diced	1
Pinch	salt (optional)	Pinch
8	slices whole-grain bread	8

1. In a small bowl, combine curry powder, turmeric and mayonnaise.

2. In a medium bowl, using a fork, mash the chickpeas until broken apart, but not puréed. Stir in walnuts, cranberries, cilantro and curry mayonnaise, stirring until evenly blended. Gently stir in avocado. Stir in salt, if desired.

3. Spoon chickpea mixture onto 4 slices of the bread, then top with remaining bread to sandwich.

Nutritional Analysis per Serving

Calories..........457	Sodium.......682 mg	Fiber............13 g
Fat..............21 g	Carbohydrate.....59 g	Protein..........14 g

---

Encouraging Main Dishes

The recipes in this chapter range from simple dishes with short ingredient lists, such as Simple Grilled Fish, to the more complex Moroccan Chicken with Couscous and Cinnamon-Spiked Prunes. Some people, when sick, want simple flavors and easy, straightforward preparation — this is likely the case if your energy is low and you don't have much of an appetite. Others want layered flavors and detest anything bland and flavorless — likely the case if your cancer (or its treatment) has numbed your taste buds and you crave excitement and diversity in your meals. I have tried to include recipes from both ends of this continuum, as well as those in between. As your needs change, so can your recipes. As with the previous chapters, the recipe adjustments will help you get the most from the meals.

Makes 6 servings

This meatless dish, with its combination of rice, cheese and sour cream, is the epitome of comfort food.

Survivor Wisdom

One piece of advice I would give to caregivers is that if you bug cancer patients too much about eating, it will turn them off.

California Casserole

- **Preheat oven to 350°F (180°C)**
- **6-cup (1.5 L) baking dish, lightly greased**

2 cups	water	500 mL
¾ cup	long-grain white rice	175 mL
1 cup	light sour cream	250 mL
1 cup	shredded medium Cheddar cheese	250 mL
½ cup	lower-fat cottage cheese	125 mL
½ cup	chopped onion	125 mL
¼ cup	chopped mushrooms	60 mL
¼ cup	chopped green bell pepper	60 mL
½ tsp	salt	2 mL
¼ tsp	freshly ground black pepper	1 mL

1. In a large saucepan, bring water to a boil; add rice. Cover and cook on low for about 20 minutes or until rice is tender and water is absorbed. Let stand for 5 minutes.

2. Combine hot rice, sour cream, Cheddar and cottage cheese, onion, mushrooms, green pepper and seasonings. Pour into prepared baking dish. Bake, uncovered, in preheated oven for about 25 minutes.

This recipe courtesy of Lauren Forsyth.

This recipe should be adjusted based on your symptoms. Follow this symptom guide:

To encourage weight gain:
- Use full-fat sour cream, cottage cheese and cheese.

For dehydration and low blood pressure:
- Cook the rice in chicken or vegetable broth (not reduced-sodium) to increase electrolytes.

To reduce gas and bloating:
- Omit the green bell pepper.

Nutritional Analysis per Serving

Calories..........243	Sodium....... 430 mg	Fiber .... 1 g
Fat.............. 10 g	Carbohydrate..... 25 g	Protein .... 12 g

Makes 4 servings

The most appealing food sometimes comes from simple ingredients and an easy preparation. This lovely fish dish provides protein, as well as fresh ingredients that contain important nutraceuticals.

Tips

Refrigerate any leftovers in an airtight container for up to 2 days. Flake the fish and mix it with mayonnaise and sliced pickles or tartar sauce to make a sandwich filling.

White fish has a mild flavor and aroma. While pink fish, such as trout, is stronger, it is also higher in beneficial omega-3 fats.

Variation

Substitute tilapia, sole, haddock or halibut for the orange roughy.

Simple Grilled Fish

- Preheat broiler
- Rimmed baking sheet, lightly greased

1 tbsp	chopped fresh parsley	15 mL
1 tbsp	butter, melted, or olive oil	15 mL
	Juice of 1 lemon	
4	orange roughy or rainbow trout fillets (about 1¾ lbs/875 g total)	4

1. In a small bowl, combine parsley, butter and lemon juice.
2. Place fish fillets on prepared baking sheet and baste both sides with butter mixture.
3. Broil for 5 to 10 minutes or until fish is opaque and flakes easily with a fork.

This recipe courtesy of Eileen Campbell.

This recipe should be adjusted based on your symptoms. Follow this symptom guide:

To assist with a bitter or metallic taste:
- Reduce lemon juice to 1 tbsp (15 mL) and add 1 tbsp (15 mL) pure maple syrup to the parsley mixture.

Nutritional Analysis per Serving

Calories 170	Sodium . . . . 150 mg	Fiber . . . . 0 g
Fat . . . . 4 g	Carbohydrate . . . . . . 1 g	Protein . . . . 30 g

Makes 4 servings

With its mild taste and soft texture, fish makes an excellent protein for those who are struggling to eat. Preparing the fish in the oven helps to reduce cooking odors, so it is less likely to trigger nausea.

Tips

For the fish fillets, try tilapia, sole, haddock or orange roughy.

Create seasoned bread crumbs by combining regular dry bread crumbs with a little salt, lemon pepper and dried parsley, or ½ tsp (2 mL) ground turmeric and 2 tbsp (30 mL) chopped fresh parsley.

Variations

For more texture and flavor in the coating and to increase the fiber, replace 2 tbsp (30 mL) of the bread crumbs with an equal quantity of wheat germ, ground nuts, ground flax seeds or stone-ground cornmeal.

For an exotic flavor and to boost the antioxidants, add 1 tbsp (15 mL) finely crushed green tea leaves to the crumbs.

Oven-Fried Fish

- **Preheat oven to 350°F (180°C)**
- **Baking sheet, greased**

1	egg	1
½ cup	milk	125 mL
½ cup	all-purpose flour	125 mL
1	pouch (2 oz/57 g) seasoned bread crumbs for fish (see tip, at left)	1
4	thin white fish fillets (about 1½ lbs/ 750 g total)	4
	Vegetable cooking spray	

1. In a shallow bowl, whisk egg and milk. Place flour on one plate and bread crumbs on another.

2. Dip both sides of fish in flour, then in egg mixture. Coat well with crumbs. Place on prepared baking sheet and spray top lightly with vegetable cooking spray. Discard any excess flour, egg and crumb mixtures.

3. Bake in preheated oven for 10 minutes or until fish is opaque and flakes easily with a fork.

This recipe courtesy of Eileen Campbell.

Nutritional Analysis per Serving

Calories...........262	Sodium.......368 mg	Fiber.............1 g
Fat...............4 g	Carbohydrate.....19 g	Protein..........34 g

Makes 6 servings

Broiling the fish on only one side keeps it moist, delicious and full of flavor. The use of fresh herbs and lemon juice will be appreciated by those with metallic, bitter or reduced taste.

Tips

To eliminate cooking odors in the house, cook the fish on a barbecue with two or more burners. Preheat one side to medium, place the salmon on the other side and close the lid. This indirect cooking method is great for delicate proteins like fish. There will be enough heat to cook the salmon without burning it or drying it out.

The ginger in this recipe may be a welcome flavor for those with nausea.

Refrigerate any extra salmon in an airtight container for up to 2 days, then serve cold.

Broiled Cilantro Ginger Salmon

- **Rimmed baking sheet, greased**

3	cloves garlic, roughly chopped	3
2 tbsp	grated gingerroot	30 mL
½ tsp	salt	2 mL
½ cup	chopped fresh cilantro	125 mL
2 tbsp	olive oil	30 mL
½ tsp	freshly ground black pepper	2 mL
	Grated zest of 2 limes	
6	salmon fillets (about 2¼ lbs/1.125 kg total)	6

1. Using a mortar and pestle (or a food processor), crush garlic, ginger and salt to form a paste. Stir in cilantro, olive oil, pepper and lime zest.

2. Place salmon on a plate and coat top evenly with paste. Cover and refrigerate for at least 30 minutes or for up to 2 hours. Preheat broiler, with rack set 4 inches (10 cm) from the top.

3. Transfer salmon to prepared baking sheet and broil for 7 to 10 minutes or until salmon is opaque and flakes easily with a fork.

This recipe courtesy of Eileen Campbell.

Nutritional Analysis per Serving

Calories..........327	Sodium.......276 mg	Fiber.............0 g
Fat..............21 g	Carbohydrate......1 g	Protein..........30 g

Makes 8 servings

In this elegant recipe, salmon is smothered with seasonings, green onion and minced garlic, then poached in the oven on spinach leaves. Served with rice, this delicious dish makes a nourishing meal.

Tips

When buying spinach, look for crisp, unblemished and fresh-smelling leaves. Spinach that has passed its peak has an acrid and unpleasant taste. Spinach that hasn't been prewashed is very sandy, so wash loose spinach leaves well in a container of tepid water, then rinse thoroughly in a colander before using.

Refrigerate any leftovers in an airtight container for up to 2 days. Flake the fish and mix it with mayonnaise and sliced pickles or tartar sauce to make a sandwich filling, or serve chilled on top of a green salad.

Smothered Salmon with Spinach

- **Preheat oven to 325°F (160°C)**
- **13- by 9-inch (33 by 23 cm) baking dish**

12	large spinach leaves	12
2 lb	whole salmon	1 kg
1 tbsp	chopped fresh dill (or 1 tsp/5 mL dried dillweed)	15 mL
½ tsp	salt	2 mL
½ tsp	freshly ground black pepper	2 mL
1 cup	cold water	250 mL
1½ tsp	olive oil	7 mL
1	bunch green onions, sliced (about ⅔ cup/150 mL)	1
1	clove garlic, minced	1

1. Arrange spinach leaves on bottom of baking dish. Top with salmon; sprinkle with dill, salt and pepper. Pour water and oil over salmon. Top with green onions and garlic. Cover tightly with foil.

2. Bake in preheated oven for 25 to 30 minutes or until salmon flakes easily when tested with a fork, basting twice. Arrange salmon with spinach on serving platter with pan juices.

This recipe courtesy of chef Yvonne Levert and dietitian Nanette Porter-MacDonald.

Nutritional Analysis per Serving

Calories...........214	Sodium....... 204 mg	Fiber .... 0 g
Fat.............. 13 g	Carbohydrate...... 1 g	Protein .... 23 g

Makes 6 servings

This moist protein dish will be welcomed by those with a dry mouth. To make this a balanced meal, serve with brown rice and a colorful vegetable, such as broccoli.

Tips

Replace the sole fillets with halibut, haddock or turbot, if desired.

Add the grapes just before serving — otherwise, the color will disappear and you won't notice them in the sauce.

The combination of sweet from the orange juice, grapes and honey, sour from the Dijon mustard and bitter from the orange zest provides interest for your taste buds.

Sole with Fresh Fruit Sauce

Fish

1½ lbs	sole fillets	750 g
1½ cups	boiling water	375 mL
⅓ cup	finely chopped onion	75 mL
2 tbsp	freshly squeezed lemon juice	30 mL
¾ tsp	salt	4 mL

Sauce

1 cup	orange juice	250 mL
¼ cup	water	60 mL
2 tbsp	cornstarch	30 mL
2 tbsp	liquid honey	30 mL
1 tsp	grated orange zest	5 mL
1 tsp	grated lemon zest	5 mL
1 tsp	Dijon mustard	5 mL
1 cup	fresh orange sections	250 mL
1 cup	seedless green grapes, halved	250 mL
	Fresh mint leaves	

1. *Fish:* Roll fish fillets and secure with toothpicks. Arrange in shallow skillet. Add boiling water, onion, lemon juice and salt. Poach, covered, over low heat for about 8 minutes. To microwave, place fish in casserole; omit water but sprinkle fish with onion, lemon juice and salt. Cover and microwave on High for 5 to 7 minutes or until fish flakes easily when tested with a fork.

2. *Sauce:* Meanwhile, in a small saucepan, combine orange juice, water, cornstarch, honey, orange zest, lemon zest and mustard. Cook over low heat, stirring constantly. Add orange sections and green grapes. Spoon sauce over drained fish fillets and garnish with mint leaves.

This recipe courtesy of Fran J. Maki.

Nutritional Analysis per Serving

Calories..........166	Sodium.......626 mg	Fiber.............1 g
Fat..............2 g	Carbohydrate.....23 g	Protein..........14 g

Makes 4 to 6 servings

This meatless comfort food will provide you with nourishment when you crave something warm, soft and inviting.

Tip

Transfer leftover casserole portions to individual airtight containers and refrigerate for up to 2 days. Reheat in the microwave on Medium-High (70%) for 4 to 5 minutes or until steaming.

Make Ahead

Cook noodles, rinse under cold water to chill, then drain. Combine cold noodles and cold sauce, spoon into casserole dish, cover and refrigerate for up to 2 days. Add crumb topping just before baking to prevent it from getting soggy.

Tuna Noodle Bake

- Preheat oven to 350°F (180°C)
- 13- by 9-inch (33 by 23 cm) casserole dish, lightly greased

1 tbsp	butter	15 mL
8 oz	mushrooms, sliced	250 g
3/4 cup	chopped green onions	175 mL
2 tbsp	all-purpose flour	30 mL
1	can (10 oz/284 mL) chicken broth, undiluted	1
1 cup	milk	250 mL
4 oz	cream cheese, softened	125 g
1	can (6 oz/170 g) chunk light tuna, drained and flaked	1
1 cup	frozen peas	250 mL
8 oz	broad egg noodles	250 g

Cheddar Crumb Topping

1/2 cup	dry bread crumbs	125 mL
2 tbsp	melted butter	30 mL
1 cup	shredded Cheddar cheese	250 mL

1. In a saucepan, melt butter over medium heat. Add mushrooms and green onions; cook, stirring, for 3 minutes or until softened.

2. Blend in flour; pour in broth and milk. Bring to a boil, stirring constantly, until slightly thickened. Stir in cream cheese until melted. Add tuna and peas; cook 2 minutes more or until heated through. Remove from heat.

3. Cook noodles in a large pot of boiling water until tender but still firm. Drain well. Stir noodles into sauce. Spoon into prepared casserole dish.

4. *Topping:* In a bowl, toss bread crumbs with melted butter; add Cheddar cheese. Just before baking, sprinkle topping over noodles.

5. Bake in preheated oven for about 30 minutes (10 minutes longer if refrigerated) or until top is golden.

Nutrients per serving

Calories..........489	Sodium.......536 mg	Fiber.............3 g
Fat.............23 g	Carbohydrate.....47 g	Protein..........25 g

Makes 8 servings

Roast chicken that is crispy on the outside and juicy on the inside is hard to beat. As a bonus, the seasonings all contain beneficial cancer-fighting compounds.

Tip

Using a V-shaped rack is an excellent and healthy way to roast chicken. The open cavity of the chicken is placed over the rack, allowing the chicken to roast upright. If you don't have a V-shaped rack, you can place the chicken on a flat rack or directly in the roasting pan. However, the overall result is better with the rack — the chicken skin crisps all around, and any excess fat drips off into the pan.

Make Ahead

Roast the chicken and remove the meat from the bones while it's still warm. Let cool for 15 minutes, then refrigerate in an airtight container for up to 3 days. Use the cooked chicken to prepare chicken sandwiches to take to your appointments, add it on top of salads or stir it into soups or other dishes that could use a protein boost.

Lemon-Thyme Roast Chicken

- **Roasting pan with rack (preferably V-shaped)**

1	whole roasting chicken (5 to 6 lbs/2.5 to 3 kg)	1
4	cloves garlic, minced	4
1/4 cup	olive oil	60 mL
2 tbsp	chopped fresh thyme	30 mL
1 tsp	freshly ground black pepper	5 mL
	Grated zest and juice of 1 lemon	
	Salt	

1. Prepare chicken by trimming excess fat from body or cavity. Rinse inside and out under cold running water and pat dry.

2. In a bowl large enough to hold the chicken, whisk together garlic, olive oil, thyme, pepper, lemon zest, lemon juice and salt to taste. Place chicken in bowl and turn to coat completely, inside and out. Cover and refrigerate for at least 1 hour or overnight. Preheat oven to 450°F (230°C) and remove top rack.

3. Place chicken on rack in roasting pan and baste with marinade. Roast for 15 to 20 minutes. Reduce heat to 375°F (190°C) and roast for 1 1/2 to 2 hours (depending on the size of the chicken) or until skin is dark golden and crispy, drumsticks wiggle when touched, and a meat thermometer inserted into the thickest part of a thigh registers 180°F (82°C). Remove from oven and let rest, tented with foil, for 10 to 15 minutes before carving. (This allows the juices to redistribute and provides a much moister chicken.)

This recipe courtesy of Eileen Campbell.

Nutrients per serving

Calories..........231	Sodium........ 74 mg	Fiber .... 0 g
Fat.............. 15 g	Carbohydrate...... 1 g	Protein .... 24 g

Makes 6 servings

This is a wonderfully warming dish, a mélange of spirited flavors such as cinnamon, ginger, saffron and lemon. These ingredients make for a comforting, healthy meal.

Tip

Let the minced garlic stand for 10 minutes before cooking to maximize its cancer-fighting properties.

Survivor Wisdom

My favorite foods when I was sick were tuna casserole, soy desserts and stews with small amounts of meat and a lot of vegetables. I couldn't handle a large hunk of meat. In my family, when we were sick, we had junket. I really liked the flavored soy desserts; they reminded me of junket.

Moroccan Chicken with Couscous and Cinnamon-Spiked Prunes

1 cup	pitted prunes	250 mL
1 tsp	ground cinnamon	5 mL
1 tbsp	olive oil	15 mL
2 lbs	skin-on bone-in chicken breasts, cut into serving-size pieces, rinsed and patted dry	1 kg
3	onions, halved and thinly sliced on the vertical	3
2	cloves garlic, minced	2
2 tbsp	minced gingerroot	30 mL
1 tsp	ground cumin	5 mL
1 tsp	salt	5 mL
1 tsp	finely grated lemon zest	5 mL
1/4 tsp	cayenne pepper	1 mL
	Freshly ground black pepper	
2 tbsp	freshly squeezed lemon juice	30 mL
3 cups	reduced-sodium ready-to-use chicken broth, divided	750 mL
1/4 tsp	crumbled saffron threads, dissolved in 2 tbsp (30 mL) boiling water	1 mL
1 tbsp	liquid honey	15 mL
1 cup	whole wheat couscous	250 mL
	Toasted sliced almonds	

1. In a saucepan, combine prunes and cinnamon with cold water to cover. Bring to a boil over medium-high heat. Reduce heat and simmer until prunes are tender and water has been absorbed, about 30 minutes. Set aside.

2. In a skillet, heat oil over medium heat for 30 seconds. Add chicken, in batches, and cook, turning once, until nicely browned, about 6 minutes per batch. Transfer to a plate.

Tightly cover the chicken
and sauce and refrigerate
for up to 3 days, or transfer
individual portions
to airtight containers,
leaving at least 1 inch
(2.5 cm) headspace for
expansion, and freeze for
up to 3 months. Thaw in the
refrigerator or microwave.
Reheat in a saucepan over
medium heat, stirring
often, for 5 to 10 minutes or
until the chicken is heated
through (the microwave
can make chicken tough
and rubbery). For the
best texture, prepare
the couscous just
before serving.

3. Add onions and cook, stirring, until they begin to brown, about 10 minutes. Add garlic, ginger, cumin, salt, lemon zest, cayenne and black pepper to taste and cook, stirring, for 1 minute. Add lemon juice, $1\frac{1}{2}$ cups (375 mL) of the broth and saffron liquid and bring to a boil. Return chicken to pan, skin side up. Reduce heat to low. Cover and simmer until chicken is no longer pink inside, 25 to 40 minutes. Remove chicken from pan and keep warm.

4. Increase heat to medium and cook, stirring frequently, until mixture is reduced by one-third, about 10 minutes. Add honey and stir well. Stir in reserved prunes and cook, stirring, until heated through. Return chicken to pan, cover and heat through.

5. Meanwhile, in a saucepan over medium heat, bring remaining $1\frac{1}{2}$ cups (375 mL) of stock to a boil. Add couscous in a steady stream, stirring constantly. Remove from heat. Cover and let stand until tender and liquid is absorbed, about 15 minutes. Fluff with a fork and use your hands to break up any lumps.

6. Spoon couscous in a ring around the edge of shallow serving bowls or plates, leaving the center hollow. Arrange chicken mixture in hollow and garnish with almonds.

Nutritional Analysis per Serving

Calories...........372	Sodium....... 482 mg	Fiber .... 7 g
Fat............... 5 g	Carbohydrate..... 52 g	Protein .... 29 g

Makes 4 servings

This classic chicken casserole is easy to make and a balanced meal. For ease of cleanup and to speed preparation time, you can make it in the microwave, using only one dish.

Tip

If desired, use 1 cup (250 mL) fresh mushrooms, sliced. Cook them with the onion and celery if using the oven method. Increase the water to 2½ cups (625 mL).

Make Ahead

Transfer cooked casserole portions to individual airtight containers and refrigerate for up to 2 days. Reheat in the microwave on Medium-High (70%) for 4 to 5 minutes or until steaming.

Easy Chicken 'n' Rice Casserole

- **Preheat oven to 350°F (180°C)**
- **8-cup (2 L) baking dish (microwave-safe, if necessary)**

½ cup	chopped onion	125 mL
½ cup	chopped celery	125 mL
2 tbsp	butter, non-hydrogenated margarine or canola oil	30 mL
2 cups	cooked bite-size chicken pieces	500 mL
1¾ cups	hot water	425 mL
⅔ cup	long-grain white rice	150 mL
1	can (10 oz/284 mL) mushrooms, with liquid	1
1 cup	frozen peas and carrots	250 mL
½ tsp	dried thyme	2 mL
½ tsp	dried rosemary	2 mL

Microwave Method

1. Combine onion, celery and butter in microwave-safe baking dish. Microwave, covered, on High for 5 minutes. Stir in chicken, water, rice, mushrooms, peas, carrots, thyme and rosemary. Microwave on High for 6 minutes, then microwave on Medium (50%) for 10 to 12 minutes or until rice is tender and most of the water has been absorbed. Let stand for 10 minutes before serving.

Oven Method

1. In a skillet, cook onion and celery in butter over medium heat until soft. Stir in chicken, water, rice, mushrooms, peas, carrots, thyme and rosemary. Transfer to baking dish and bake in preheated oven for about 30 minutes or until rice is tender.

This recipe courtesy of Karen Quinn.

Nutritional Analysis per Serving

Calories...........151	Sodium.......347 mg	Fiber.............3 g
Fat...............7 g	Carbohydrate.....16 g	Protein...........8 g

Makes 4 servings

Herbs and spices add not just flavor, but also powerful cancer-fighting nutraceuticals in this balanced meal that provides protein, grains and vegetables.

Tips

If you prefer, use Chicken Stock (page 167) in place of the ready-to-use broth. If your stock is unsalted, add up to $\frac{1}{4}$ tsp (1 mL) salt, or to taste, with the rice.

Of the protein options for this recipe, mussels (see variation, below) are the highest in iron, followed by beef, then turkey, then chicken.

Variation

To boost the iron and vitamin B_{12} content, add 1 lb (500 g) scrubbed mussels in step 4 after 5 minutes of simmering. Cover pan and simmer for 5 to 8 minutes or until mussels have opened. Discard any that do not open.

Spanish Chicken and Rice

2 cups	reduced-sodium ready-to-use chicken broth	500 mL
1 cup	long-grain white rice	250 mL
1 lb	lean ground chicken, turkey or beef	500 g
1 tbsp	canola oil	15 mL
2	cloves garlic, finely chopped	2
1	small onion, finely chopped	1
1	green bell pepper, diced	1
1	large stalk celery, finely chopped	1
$1\frac{1}{2}$ tsp	chili powder	7 mL
1 tsp	dried oregano	5 mL
1 tsp	paprika	5 mL
$\frac{1}{2}$ tsp	salt	2 mL
$\frac{1}{4}$ tsp	freshly ground black pepper	1 mL
1	can (14 oz/398 mL) diced tomatoes, including juice	1

1. In a medium saucepan, bring broth to a boil. Add rice, reduce heat to low, cover and simmer for 20 minutes or until liquid is absorbed and rice is tender.

2. In a large saucepan over medium-high heat, cook chicken, breaking up with a wooden spoon, for 5 minutes or until no longer pink. Transfer to a bowl.

3. Add oil to pan. Cook garlic, onion, green pepper, celery, chili powder, oregano, paprika, salt and pepper, stirring often, for 4 minutes or until vegetables are softened.

4. Return chicken to pan, along with tomatoes and their juice; bring to a boil. Reduce heat to medium-low, cover and simmer for 10 minutes or until vegetables are tender.

5. Stir in cooked rice. Cover and let stand for 5 minutes to blend the flavors.

Nutritional Analysis per Serving

Calories..........354	Sodium.......650 mg	Fiber.............2 g
Fat..............19 g	Carbohydrate.....21 g	Protein..........23 g

Makes 6 servings

This moist, Italian-inspired meatloaf is flavored with a winning combination of sausage, mozzarella and basil pesto. It's an appealing way for someone with dry mouth to consume meat.

Tip

Because of increased awareness about the risk of consuming nitrates, many meat processors are making nitrate-free versions of cold cuts, sausage and other processed meats. Look for these products in specialty stores or health food stores.

Make Ahead

See page 211.

Italian Chicken Meatloaf

- **Preheat oven to 375°F (190°C)**
- **9- by 5-inch (23 by 12.5 cm) loaf pan, greased**

1 lb	lean ground chicken, turkey or beef	500 g
8 oz	mild Italian pork, beef or chicken sausage, casings removed (see tip, at left)	250 g
1 cup	shredded mozzarella or provolone cheese	250 mL
1 cup	soft fresh Italian bread crumbs	250 mL
1	egg	1
1 cup	tomato pasta sauce, divided	250 mL
2 tbsp	basil pesto	30 mL
1	small onion, finely chopped	1
1	clove garlic, finely chopped	1
½ tsp	salt	2 mL
½ tsp	freshly ground black pepper	2 mL

1. In a bowl, combine chicken, sausage meat, cheese and bread crumbs.

2. In another bowl, beat egg. Stir in ½ cup (125 mL) pasta sauce, pesto, onion, garlic, salt and pepper. Pour over chicken mixture and gently mix until evenly combined.

3. Press meat mixture into prepared loaf pan. Spread remaining ½ cup (125 mL) pasta sauce over top. Bake in preheated oven for 55 to 60 minutes or until a meat thermometer inserted into center registers 170°F (77°C). Let stand for 5 minutes. Drain pan juices; turn out onto a plate and cut into slices.

Nutritional Analysis per Serving

Calories..........424	Sodium......1,178 mg	Fiber.............1 g
Fat.............26 g	Carbohydrate.....18 g	Protein..........28 g

---

Makes 6 servings

Ground turkey is lean and pairs well with the tartness of apple, making for a moist and delicious protein source.

Make Ahead

Wrap cooled slices of meatloaf tightly in plastic wrap, then in foil, or place in an airtight container; refrigerate for up to 3 days or freeze for up to 2 months. Let thaw in the refrigerator or defrost in the microwave, if necessary. Remove plastic wrap and wrap in foil, then reheat in a 350°F (180°C) toaster oven or conventional oven for 10 to 15 minutes or until steaming. To microwave, unwrap, place on a microwave-safe plate, cover loosely and microwave on Medium-High (70%) for 2 to 3 minutes or until steaming.

Variation

Turkey Apple Burgers: This mixture can also be used to make burgers, which can be cooked on a barbecue or grill or in the oven. They're excellent served on a whole wheat bun with sliced tomato and a spoonful of cucumber dressing.

Turkey Apple Meatloaf

- Preheat oven to 350°F (180°C)
- 9- by 5-inch (23 by 12.5 cm) loaf pan, lightly greased

2	cloves garlic, minced	2
1	egg	1
1	tart apple, such as Mutsu or Granny Smith, finely chopped	1
1 lb	lean ground turkey	500 g
½ cup	chopped onion	125 mL
⅓ cup	oat bran	75 mL
⅓ cup	ground flax seeds	75 mL
3 tbsp	prepared yellow mustard	45 mL
1 tbsp	ketchup	15 mL
1 tsp	salt	5 mL

1. In a large bowl, combine garlic, egg, apple, turkey, onion, oat bran, flaxseed, mustard, ketchup and salt. Pack into prepared loaf pan.
2. Bake in preheated oven for 45 to 60 minutes or until a meat thermometer inserted in the center registers an internal temperature of 175°F (80°C).

This recipe courtesy of dietitian Gillian Proctor.

Nutritional Analysis per Serving

Calories..........197	Sodium.......583 mg	Fiber.............3 g
Fat..............10 g	Carbohydrate.....11 g	Protein..........17 g

Makes 2 loaves, 8 servings each

Cinnamon and bulgur give this meatloaf Mediterranean flavor. This change from the expected might be just what you need if your taste buds crave something different.

Tip

Make this big batch and refrigerate and freeze the extras to reheat on those days when you're low on energy.

Make Ahead

See page 211.

Variation

Substitute an equal amount of lean or extra-lean ground beef for the pork.

Survivor Wisdom

I had to eat something that had flavor to get rid of the bad taste in my mouth.

Big-Batch Mediterranean Bulgur Meatloaf

- Preheat oven to 350°F (180°C)
- Two 9- by 5-inch (23 by 12.5 cm) loaf pans, lightly greased

¾ cup	bulgur, rinsed	175 mL
1½ cups	hot water	375 mL
2	eggs	2
1	onion, finely chopped	1
1 lb	lean ground pork	500 g
1 lb	ground chicken	500 g
¼ cup	finely chopped fresh parsley	60 mL
2 tbsp	freshly squeezed lemon juice	30 mL
2 tsp	ground cinnamon	10 mL
1 tsp	ground allspice	5 mL
1 tsp	paprika	5 mL
½ tsp	salt	2 mL
½ tsp	freshly ground black pepper	2 mL
	Olive oil	

1. Place bulgur in a large bowl and pour in hot water. Cover and let stand for 10 minutes or until most of the water is absorbed. Squeeze out excess water. Add eggs, onion, ground pork, ground chicken, parsley, lemon juice, cinnamon, allspice, paprika, salt and pepper; mix ingredients together, using hands, and divide in half. Pack each half into a prepared loaf pan. Brush lightly with olive oil.

2. Bake in preheated oven for about 45 minutes or until a meat thermometer inserted in the center of a loaf registers an internal temperature of 175°F (80°C).

This recipe courtesy of dietitian Marketa Graham.

Nutritional Analysis per Serving

Calories..........202	Sodium....... 152 mg	Fiber .... 1 g
Fat.............. 11 g	Carbohydrate...... 8 g	Protein .... 17 g

Makes 8 servings

Here's a chili you can have ready in about half an hour.

Tip

Transform leftovers into a chili baked potato. Scrub a medium potato and pierce with a fork. Microwave on High for 3 to 4 minutes. Let stand for 2 minutes. Cut an X in the top of potato and squeeze open. Top with hot chili and shredded cheese.

Make Ahead

Cover chili tightly and refrigerate for up to 3 days, or transfer individual portions to airtight containers, leaving at least 1 inch (2.5 cm) headspace for expansion, and freeze for up to 3 months. Thaw in the refrigerator or microwave. Reheat individual portions in the microwave on Medium-High (70%) for 3 to 4 minutes, or in a saucepan over medium heat, stirring often, for 4 to 5 minutes or until steaming.

Fast Chili

1 lb	lean ground beef	500 g
1	can (19 oz/540 mL) stewed tomatoes	1
2	cans (each 14 oz/398 mL) beans in tomato sauce	2
2	cans (each 19 oz/540 mL) kidney beans, drained and rinsed	2
1 cup	sliced white or red onions	250 mL
2 cups	diced green bell peppers	500 mL
1 tbsp	chili powder	15 mL

1. In a large saucepan or Dutch oven over medium-high heat, brown meat, breaking up with a wooden spoon, for about 8 minutes or until no longer pink inside. Drain off fat.
2. Add tomatoes, beans in tomato sauce, kidney beans, onions, green peppers and chili powder. Reduce heat and simmer, covered and stirring occasionally, for 20 to 30 minutes or until vegetables are tender and flavors are blended.

This recipe courtesy of Barbara McGillivary.

This recipe should be adjusted based on your symptoms. Follow this symptom guide:

For meat aversion:
- Omit the ground beef and skip step 1. The beans still provide plenty of protein.

Nutritional Analysis per Serving

Calories...........400	Sodium......1,047 mg	Fiber .... 14 g
Fat.............. 6 g	Carbohydrate..... 59 g	Protein .... 28 g

Makes 4 servings

Comfort foods save the day when your appetite is low.

Tip

For a speedy meal-in-a-pot, add 3 to 4 cups (750 mL to 1 L) small broccoli florets to the pot of boiling pasta for the last 3 minutes of cooking; remove from heat when broccoli is tender-crisp.

Make Ahead

Cover macaroni tightly and refrigerate for up to 3 days. Reheat individual portions in the microwave on Medium-High (70%) for 2 to 3 minutes, or in a saucepan over medium heat, stirring gently, for 3 to 4 minutes or until steaming. Stir in additional milk until sauce is creamy.

Survivor Wisdom

Foods that appealed to me during my treatment were ice pops, grapes, milkshakes, and macaroni and cheese.

Easy One-Pot Macaroni and Cheese

2 tbsp	all-purpose flour	30 mL
1½ cups	milk	375 mL
1½ cups	shredded Cheddar cheese	375 mL
¼ cup	freshly grated Parmesan cheese	60 mL
1 tsp	Dijon mustard	5 mL
	Salt and cayenne pepper	
2 cups	elbow macaroni	500 mL

1. In a large saucepan, whisk flour with ¼ cup (60 mL) milk to make a smooth paste; stir in remaining milk until smooth. Place over medium heat; cook, stirring, until mixture comes to a boil and thickens. Reduce heat to low; stir in cheeses and mustard. Cook, stirring, until melted. Season with salt and a pinch of cayenne pepper to taste; keep warm.

2. Cook pasta in a large pot of boiling salted water until tender but firm. Drain well; stir into cheese mixture. Cook, stirring gently, for 1 minute or until sauce coats the pasta. Serve immediately.

This recipe should be adjusted based on your symptoms. Follow this symptom guide:

For lactose intolerance:
- Replace the milk with a lactose-free beverage, such as lactose-reduced milk or non-dairy milk (e.g., soy milk or rice milk). Depending on your tolerance level, you can likely use the cheese as is, since aged cheeses, such as Cheddar and Parmesan, are very low in lactose.

Nutritional Analysis per Serving

Calories..........451	Sodium.......551 mg	Fiber.............5 g
Fat..............19 g	Carbohydrate.....48 g	Protein..........24 g

Makes 8 servings

Many people love lasagna but don't have the time or energy to make it even when they are healthy. This uncomplicated version makes this comfort food more accessible.

Make Ahead

Wrap cooled slices of baked lasagna tightly in plastic wrap, then in foil, or place in an airtight container; refrigerate for up to 3 days or freeze for up to 2 months. Let thaw in the refrigerator or defrost in the microwave, if necessary. Remove plastic wrap and wrap in foil, then reheat in a 350°F (180°C) toaster oven or conventional oven for 15 to 20 minutes or until steaming. To microwave, unwrap, place on a microwave-safe plate, cover loosely and microwave on Medium-High (70%) for 4 to 6 minutes or until steaming.

Alternatively, prepare through step 3 (do not bake), cover with plastic wrap, then with foil, and freeze for up to 2 months. Thaw in the refrigerator overnight before baking as directed in step 4.

Easy Lasagna

- **Preheat oven to 350°F (180°C)**
- **13- by 9-inch (33 by 23 cm) glass baking dish, lightly greased**

2 cups	ricotta cheese	500 mL
2	eggs, beaten	2
1/3 cup	freshly grated Parmesan cheese	75 mL
1/4 tsp	freshly ground black pepper	1 mL
1/4 tsp	freshly grated nutmeg	1 mL
3 cups	spaghetti sauce (homemade or store-bought)	750 mL
12	lasagna noodles, cooked	12
2 cups	shredded mozzarella cheese	500 mL

1. In a bowl, combine ricotta, eggs and Parmesan cheese; season with pepper and nutmeg.

2. Depending on thickness of the spaghetti sauce, add about 3/4 cup (175 mL) water to thin sauce. (Sauce should be fairly loose because noodles absorb extra moisture while cooking.)

3. Spoon 1/2 cup (125 mL) sauce in bottom of prepared baking dish. Layer with 3 lasagna noodles. Spread with 3/4 cup (175 mL) of the sauce and then one-third of the ricotta mixture. Repeat with two more layers of noodles, sauce and ricotta cheese. Layer with rest of noodles and top with remaining sauce. Sprinkle with mozzarella cheese.

4. Bake, uncovered, in preheated oven for 45 minutes or until cheese is melted and sauce is bubbly.

This recipe should be adjusted based on your symptoms. Follow this symptom guide:

For risk reduction:
- Use whole wheat lasagna noodles and add 4 cups (1 L) small-cut frozen mixed vegetables, thawed and drained, dividing the vegetables evenly on top of the ricotta mixture when layering the lasagna.

Nutritional Analysis per Serving

Calories..........423	Sodium.......737 mg	Fiber.............5 g
Fat..............20 g	Carbohydrate.....36 g	Protein..........25 g

Makes 4 servings

Pasta with clams is an Italian classic and for good reason — it's as good to eat as it is easy to make. The high iron level in clams makes this recipe a sensible part of a plan to improve iron levels.

Tips

Patients should check with their doctor before consuming alcohol. Even when simmered in this recipe, some alcohol may remain, so if you need to avoid alcohol, use a dealcoholized wine or substitute 1/4 cup (60 mL) additional clam juice or vegetable broth and 1 tbsp (15 mL) white wine vinegar.

Fresh clams are superb in this dish. Substitute 2 cups (500 mL) shucked clams for the canned clams. Instead of the reserved clam juice, use 3/4 cup (175 mL) fish stock or vegetable broth.

For a change of color, try making this with red clam sauce: just add 1 cup (250 mL) chopped tomatoes to the sauce at the end of step 1.

Pasta with White Clam Sauce

1 tbsp	olive oil	15 mL
1/4 cup	chopped onions	60 mL
2 cups	sliced mushrooms	500 mL
2 tsp	all-purpose flour	10 mL
1/3 cup	dry white wine	75 mL
2	cans (each 5 oz/142 g) clams, drained (reserve 3/4 cup/175 mL clam juice)	2
1 tsp	minced garlic	5 mL
2/3 cup	evaporated milk	150 mL
1/8 tsp	ground nutmeg	0.5 mL
8 oz	capellini or vermicelli pasta	250 g
2 tbsp	chopped fresh parsley (or 2 tsp/10 mL dried)	30 mL
	Freshly ground black pepper	

1. In a large nonstick skillet, heat oil over medium-high heat. Add onions and mushrooms; sauté for 5 to 6 minutes or until softened and moisture has evaporated. Sprinkle with flour; blend well. Add wine, reserved clam juice and garlic; bring to a boil. Reduce heat and simmer for 2 to 3 minutes or until thickened. Stir in clams, evaporated milk and nutmeg; simmer for 1 to 2 minutes or until heated through.

2. Just before serving, cook pasta according to package directions or until tender but firm; drain. Toss with sauce. Sprinkle with parsley. Season with pepper to taste.

This recipe courtesy of Mary Anne Pucovsky.

This recipe should be adjusted based on your symptoms. Follow this symptom guide:

For weight gain promotion:
- Replace the evaporated milk with heavy or whipping (35%) cream.

Nutritional Analysis per Serving

Calories..........408	Sodium....... 236 mg	Fiber .... 3 g
Fat.............. 8 g	Carbohydrate..... 57 g	Protein .... 24 g

Recuperative Vegetables and Calming Sauces

One thing cancer researchers seem to agree on is that a plant-based diet — including vegetables, fruits, whole grains, nuts, seeds, legumes, herbs and spices — provides beneficial cancer-fighting nutrients. Cancer patients are often highly motivated to improve their diet, as it makes them feel like they are doing their part to ensure this doesn't happen to them again.

Whether you were already a vegetable lover or are charting new territory, you will enjoy these recipes, which go beyond plain steamed or boiled vegetables, adding pizzazz that will appeal to a palate that has been damaged by treatment. They will also give you ideas when it comes to combining vegetables and other plant-based foods to maximize the cancer-fighting potential of every bite.

If you have a dry or sore mouth, the calming sauces moisten food so that you can enjoy every mouthful without worrying about the food getting stuck in your throat. Some sauces also contribute cancer-fighting ingredients (try Mango Mint Mojo) or additional calories and protein (try Foolproof Hollandaise). Your needs and appetite will dictate which ones are right for you.

Makes 4 to 6 servings

These seasoned carrots are a great way to add flavor when your taste buds need a boost.

Tips

Use the side of a spoon to scrape off the skin before chopping or grating gingerroot. Gingerroot keeps well in the freezer for up to 3 months and can be grated from frozen.

Let the minced garlic stand for 10 minutes before cooking to maximize its cancer-fighting properties.

Survivor Wisdom

Some of your friends will be pickup trucks and some will be bulldozers. The bulldozer will say, "Is that all you're eating? You look pretty anorexic right now." Some people don't know how to be supportive.

Ginger Carrots

4 cups	chopped carrots	1 L
½ cup	reduced-sodium vegetable or chicken broth	125 mL
2 tsp	minced gingerroot	10 mL
1 tsp	minced garlic	5 mL
1 tsp	packed brown sugar	5 mL
¼ tsp	freshly squeezed lemon juice	1 mL

1. In a large saucepan, combine carrots, broth, ginger, garlic, brown sugar and lemon juice. Bring to a boil over high heat. Reduce heat to medium-low, cover and simmer for about 20 minutes or until carrots are tender-crisp and liquid is absorbed.

This recipe courtesy of dietitian Roberta Lowcay.

This recipe should be adjusted based on your symptoms. Follow this symptom guide:

If food tastes too sweet:
- Omit the sugar and add extra lemon juice to taste after cooking.

If food tastes too salty:
- Replace the broth with water or unsalted stock or broth.

If food tastes too bitter or metallic:
- Add more sugar and lemon juice to taste after cooking.

Nutritional Analysis per Serving

Calories............34	Sodium....... 128 mg	Fiber .... 2 g
Fat .... 0 g	Carbohydrate...... 8 g	Protein .... 1 g

Makes 4 servings

Jazz up simple carrots with flavorful, on-hand ingredients when your taste buds need a lift.

Tip

The ginger in this recipe may help with nausea.

Survivor Wisdom

I had neuropathy, so I added two nails to my cutting board so I could cut vegetables with one hand.

Honey-Glazed Carrots

1 lb	carrots, cut into 1-inch (2.5 cm) pieces	500 g
½ tsp	ground ginger	2 mL
1 tbsp	liquid honey, brown sugar or agave nectar	15 mL
½ tsp	grated orange zest (optional)	2 mL
1 tbsp	orange juice	15 mL
2 tsp	butter, non-hydrogenated margarine or olive oil	10 mL

1. In a medium saucepan, combine carrots and cold water to cover. Bring to a boil over high heat. Reduce heat and boil gently for 15 to 20 minutes or until tender-crisp; drain and return to pan over medium-low heat.
2. Add ginger, honey, orange zest (if using), orange juice and butter to pan. Quickly stir for 2 to 3 minutes or until glaze forms.

This recipe courtesy of dietitian Lynn Roblin.

This recipe should be adjusted based on your symptoms. Follow this symptom guide:

If food tastes too sweet:
- Omit the honey and add extra orange zest and/or juice to taste after cooking.

If food tastes too bitter or metallic:
- Omit the orange zest and add salt and extra honey to taste after cooking.

Nutritional Analysis per Serving

Calories............85	Sodium........ 78 mg	Fiber .... 3 g
Fat............... 3 g	Carbohydrate..... 16 g	Protein .... 1 g

Makes 8 servings

The maple syrup in this recipe makes sweet-tasting vegetables, which will be especially welcomed by those with bitter or metallic taste alterations.

Tip

Not only does roasting vegetables add a sweet, smoky taste, more nutrients are preserved than when they are boiled.

Make Ahead

The vegetables can be tightly covered and refrigerated for up to 3 days. Reheat individual portions in the microwave on Medium-High (70%) for 2 to 3 minutes, or place in a saucepan with enough water to moisten and heat over medium heat, stirring often, for 2 to 3 minutes or until steaming.

Roasted Carrots and Parsnips

- **Preheat oven to 400°F (200°C)**
- **13- by 9-inch (33 by 23 cm) glass baking dish, greased**

1 lb	parsnips, cut into 1-inch (2.5 cm) pieces	500 g
1 lb	carrots, cut into 1-inch (2.5 cm) pieces	500 g
1	large onion, cut into wedges	1
2 tbsp	vegetable oil	30 mL
1 tsp	dried thyme	5 mL
2 tbsp	pure maple syrup	30 mL
1 tbsp	Dijon mustard	15 mL

1. Place parsnips, carrots, onions, oil and thyme in prepared baking dish; toss until vegetables are well coated with oil. Roast in preheated oven for 30 minutes.

2. Meanwhile, in a small bowl, combine maple syrup and mustard. Pour over vegetables; toss to coat. Roast for another 20 to 25 minutes or until vegetables are tender and golden, stirring once.

This recipe courtesy of dietitian Bev Callaghan.

This recipe should be adjusted based on your symptoms. Follow this symptom guide:

If food tastes too sweet:
- Reduce or omit the maple syrup and add extra mustard to taste once the vegetables are cooked.

If food tastes too salty:
- Reduce the amount of mustard to 1 tsp (5 mL) and add extra maple syrup to taste once the vegetables are cooked.

If food tastes too bitter or metallic:
- Omit the thyme and mustard.

Nutritional Analysis per Serving

Calories..........116	Sodium.......232 mg	Fiber.............4 g
Fat..............4 g	Carbohydrate.....21 g	Protein...........2 g

Makes 4 servings

This is an easy way to add flavor to spinach. You can substitute Swiss chard, kale, rapini or mustard greens for the spinach and increase the cooking time accordingly. If you don't have pine nuts, try chopped pecans or walnuts.

Tip

Stir-frying vegetables is a great way to preserve nutrients. When boiled, vegetables can lose up to 45% of their vitamin C, compared with a loss of only 5% when stir-fried.

Survivor Wisdom

I eat organic food as much as I can.

Sautéed Spinach with Pine Nuts

2 tsp	olive oil	10 mL
¼ cup	pine nuts	60 mL
1	package (10 oz/300 g) fresh spinach, trimmed	1
1 tsp	minced garlic	5 mL
1 tsp	freshly squeezed lemon juice	5 mL
⅛ tsp	ground nutmeg	0.5 mL
	Freshly ground black pepper	

1. In a large nonstick skillet, heat 1 tsp (5 mL) of the oil over medium heat. Add pine nuts and cook, stirring constantly, for 2 to 3 minutes or until golden. Remove pine nuts from pan and set aside.

2. Add remaining oil to pan. Add spinach in several bunches (it will cook down quickly), stirring constantly. Add garlic and cook, stirring, for 1 to 2 minutes, until fragrant. Stir in lemon juice and nutmeg. Season with pepper to taste. Add reserved pine nuts. Cook until heated through.

This recipe courtesy of dietitian Bev Callaghan.

This recipe should be adjusted based on your symptoms. Follow this symptom guide:

If food tastes too sweet:
- Add more lemon juice to taste.

If food tastes too bitter or metallic:
- Add a bit of sweetness in the form of agave syrup, maple syrup or honey to taste once the spinach is cooked.

Nutritional Analysis per Serving

Calories...........109	Sodium....... 119 mg	Fiber .... 4 g
Fat............... 8 g	Carbohydrate...... 9 g	Protein .... 3 g

Makes 5 servings

Raisins, herbs, lemon and pepper combine to give this healthy vegetable added flavor for those whose taste buds need a little encouraging. This healthy, flavorful side dish is particularly good with fish.

Tips

Use fresh herbs to replace any of the dried herbs in this recipe, but double or triple the amount, as the drying process intensifies the flavor of herbs.

Like all dark, leafy greens, spinach is a source of vitamin A, folate and non-heme iron. When consuming foods that contain iron, avoid drinking caffeinated beverages, such as coffee, tea or cola, for at least an hour, as caffeine can reduce the body's ability to absorb iron. The vitamin C in the lemon juice will help with non-heme iron absorption.

Variation

Replace the spinach with 6 cups (1.5 L) chopped trimmed kale and increase the cooking time in step 2 to 8 to 10 minutes, stirring occasionally.

Spinach Fancy

1 tbsp	butter, olive oil or non-hydrogenated margarine	15 mL
3 tbsp	raisins	45 mL
Pinch	dried mint	Pinch
Pinch	ground fennel	Pinch
Pinch	dried oregano	Pinch
1	package (10 oz/300 g) fresh spinach, stems trimmed, leaves chopped	1
2 tbsp	water	30 mL
1 tsp	freshly squeezed lemon juice	5 mL
½ tsp	salt	2 mL
Pinch	freshly ground black pepper	Pinch
	Lemon slices	

1. In a large skillet, melt butter over medium heat; add raisins, mint, fennel and oregano and cook, stirring, for 1 minute.
2. Add spinach and water; cover and steam for 2 to 3 minutes or until wilted. Drain liquid. Sprinkle with lemon juice, salt and pepper; toss well. Serve with lemon slices.

This recipe courtesy of Martine Lortie.

Nutritional Analysis per Serving

Calories............69	Sodium........329 mg	Fiber.............3 g
Fat...............3 g	Carbohydrate.....11 g	Protein...........2 g

Makes 4 servings

Squash, a favorite fall vegetable, makes a wonderful container for rice, meats or fruit.

Tips

Have you ever wrestled with a squash, trying to cut it into pieces? Here's a technique that simplifies the chore. First, split off the stem. Then, using a large, sharp knife, pierce the skin of the squash where you want to cut it. Insert the knife slightly into the squash and tap it several times with a hammer or meat mallet. The squash should split open. Alternatively, place the squash in the microwave and cook on High for 2 minutes. Then cut.

Squash is rich in beta carotene, a form of vitamin A, which promotes healthy tissues and cells.

Apple-Stuffed Squash

- Preheat oven to 375°F (190°C)
- Shallow baking pan

2	small acorn squash	2
2 cups	unsweetened applesauce	500 mL
1/2 cup	raisins	125 mL
1/4 cup	liquid honey or molasses	60 mL
1/4 cup	chopped walnuts	60 mL
1 tbsp	butter, non-hydrogenated margarine or olive oil	15 mL
1 tbsp	grated lemon zest	15 mL
2 tsp	freshly squeezed lemon juice	10 mL
1/4 tsp	ground cinnamon	1 mL

1. Cut squash in half lengthwise; remove seeds. Combine applesauce, raisins, honey and walnuts. Fill squash with mixture; dot each squash with butter. Sprinkle with lemon zest, juice and cinnamon.

2. Place filled squash in shallow baking pan; pour in hot water to 1/4-inch (0.5 cm) depth. Bake, covered, in preheated oven for 30 minutes; uncover and bake for another 20 minutes or until squash is tender.

This recipe courtesy of Irene Mofina.

This recipe should be adjusted based on your symptoms. Follow this symptom guide:

If food tastes too sweet:
- Reduce or eliminate the honey or molasses; and/or
- Add more lemon juice to taste after baking.

If food tastes too salty:
- Use unsalted butter or margarine or the olive oil.

If food tastes too bitter or metallic:
- Reduce or omit the lemon zest; and/or
- Add more honey or molasses and salt to taste after baking.

Nutritional Analysis per Serving

Calories..........247	Sodium........ 13 mg	Fiber .... 4 g
Fat.............. 8 g	Carbohydrate..... 49 g	Protein .... 3 g

Makes 4 servings

Squash, like other orange-colored vegetables, is a source of the antioxidant beta carotene. The chives and cayenne add even more cancer-fighting potential.

Tip

Substitute butternut or another orange winter squash for the acorn squash.

Make Ahead

Cover purée tightly and refrigerate for up to 3 days, or transfer individual portions to airtight containers, leaving at least 1 inch (2.5 cm) headspace for expansion, and freeze for up to 3 months. Thaw in the refrigerator or microwave. Reheat individual portions in the microwave on Medium-High (70%) for 2 to 3 minutes, or in a saucepan over medium heat, stirring often, for 2 to 3 minutes or until steaming.

Roasted Squash Purée

- **Preheat oven to 400°F (200°C)**
- **Food processor or potato masher**

1	acorn squash (see tip, at left)	1
2 tbsp	butter or olive oil, divided	30 mL
1 tbsp	packed brown sugar, divided	15 mL
¼ cup	coarsely snipped chives	60 mL
½ tsp	salt	2 mL
⅛ tsp	cayenne pepper	0.5 mL
	Freshly ground black pepper	

1. Cut squash in half lengthwise and scoop out seeds. Place half the butter and half the brown sugar in each cavity. Wrap each half tightly in foil. Bake in preheated oven until tender, about 45 minutes.

2. Remove foil, scoop out flesh and transfer to work bowl fitted with metal blade, being careful not to lose the melted butter (or transfer to a bowl). Discard skins. Add chives, salt, cayenne and black pepper to taste and purée until smooth (or use a potato masher in the bowl). Serve hot.

This recipe should be adjusted based on your symptoms. Follow this symptom guide:

If food tastes too sweet:
- Reduce or eliminate the brown sugar; and/or
- Add lemon juice to taste after puréeing.

If food tastes too salty:
- Reduce or eliminate the salt and use unsalted butter or the olive oil.

If food tastes too bitter or metallic:
- Add more brown sugar and lemon to taste after puréeing.

For sore mouth or throat:
- Omit the cayenne pepper.

Nutritional Analysis per Serving

Calories............75	Sodium........ 292 mg	Fiber .... 0 g
Fat............... 7 g	Carbohydrate...... 4 g	Protein .... 0 g

Makes 4 servings

This dish, which smells like the holidays, is a wonderful way to send an enticing aroma through the house, drawing dull but curious palates to the table. If appetite permits, serve with turkey or other hearty fare.

Tips

Make quick work of slicing the turnips by using a mandolin or a food processor fitted with the slicing blade. You can shred the cheese using the shredding blade of a food processor.

Confused about the difference between a turnip and a rutabaga? A rutabaga is a cross between a turnip and a cabbage. Rutabagas are bigger, have a yellow color and become yellow-orange once cooked. They are often sold with a thick wax coating. Turnips are more bitter, while rutabaga are sweeter.

Make Ahead

Cover the gratin tightly and refrigerate for up to 3 days. Reheat individual portions in the microwave on Medium-High (70%) for 3 to 4 minutes or until steaming.

Turnip Gratin

- Preheat oven to 375°F (190°C)
- 6-cup (1.5 L) shallow baking dish, buttered

1½ cups	whole milk, divided (approx.)	375 mL
2 lbs	white turnips, peeled and thinly sliced (about 6 turnips)	1 kg
6 oz	Gruyère cheese, shredded, divided	175 g
¼ tsp	freshly grated nutmeg	1 mL
	Salt and freshly ground black pepper	

1. Pour ½ cup (125 mL) of the milk into prepared baking dish. Layer half the turnips over top, overlapping as necessary. Sprinkle with half each cheese and nutmeg and season with salt and pepper to taste. Repeat. Add remaining milk (more, if necessary to cover turnips).

2. Bake in preheated oven until turnips are tender, about 1½ hours. Let stand for 10 minutes before serving.

This recipe should be adjusted based on your symptoms. Follow this symptom guide:

For lactose intolerance:
- Use lactose-reduced milk or plain soy milk.

To encourage weight gain:
- Add 2 tbsp (30 mL) melted butter or olive oil with the milk; and/or
- Use half-and-half (10%) or table (18%) cream in place of the milk.

If food tastes too bitter or metallic:
- Replace the turnips with 4 cups (1 L) thinly sliced rutabaga (2-inch/5 cm pieces), as it is sweeter. Or use half carrots and half turnips.

Nutritional Analysis per Serving

Calories 301	Sodium . . . . 397 mg	Fiber . . . . 4 g
Fat . . . . 17 g	Carbohydrate . . . . . 19 g	Protein . . . . 18 g

Makes 8 servings

With this recipe, all the chopping (except the potatoes) can be done up to a day ahead, then you can simply pop the pan in the oven 30 to 40 minutes before mealtime.

Tips

For the herbs, try any combination of thyme, oregano, basil, dill, parsley, chives and rosemary — whatever suits your taste!

To save time and energy, you can buy some of these vegetables already cleaned and cut. The oil mixture can also be made a day in advance, covered and stored in the fridge.

Make Ahead

Cover the roasted vegetables tightly and refrigerate for up to 3 days. Reheat individual portions in the microwave on Medium-High (70%) for 2 to 3 minutes, or in a skillet over medium heat, stirring often, for 3 to 4 minutes or until steaming.

Roasted Vegetables

- Preheat oven to 325°F (160°C)
- 13- by 9-inch (33 by 23 cm) roasting pan or shallow casserole dish, lightly greased

2	bell peppers (any color)	2
2	parsnips, peeled	2
2	carrots	2
2	potatoes (unpeeled)	2
1	onion	1
1	zucchini	1
1	bulb fennel	1
3	cloves garlic	3
2 tbsp	vegetable oil	30 mL
2 tbsp	pure maple syrup or liquid honey	30 mL
1 tbsp	Dijon mustard	15 mL
2 tbsp	chopped fresh herbs (or 2 tsp/10 mL dried)	30 mL
	Freshly ground black pepper	

1. Chop peppers, parsnips, carrots, potatoes, onion, zucchini and fennel into bite-size chunks. Spread vegetables and garlic in prepared pan.

2. In a medium bowl, combine oil, maple syrup, mustard and herbs. Pour over vegetables and toss to coat. Sprinkle with pepper to taste.

3. Roast in preheated oven, tossing vegetables once, for 30 to 40 minutes or until fork-tender and golden.

This recipe courtesy of dietitian Dianna Bihun.

This recipe should be adjusted based on your symptoms. Follow this symptom guide:

If food tastes too bitter or metallic:
- Add more maple syrup or honey and lemon juice to taste to each serving.

Nutritional Analysis per Serving

Calories..........150	Sodium........ 62 mg	Fiber .... 5 g
Fat............... 4 g	Carbohydrate..... 28 g	Protein .... 3 g

Makes 6 servings

This soft dish is perfect when a sore mouth or throat have you looking for smooth and creamy food.

Make Ahead

Cover the purée tightly and refrigerate for up to 3 days, or transfer individual portions to airtight containers, leaving at least 1 inch (2.5 cm) headspace for expansion, and freeze for up to 3 months. Thaw in the refrigerator or microwave. Reheat individual portions in the microwave on Medium-High (70%) for 2 to 3 minutes, or in a saucepan over medium heat, stirring often, for 2 to 3 minutes or until steaming.

Fresh Vegetable Purée

- **Food processor**

1 tbsp	butter or olive oil	15 mL
1	onion, chopped	1
3	carrots, chopped	3
3 lbs	butternut squash, peeled and chopped	1.5 kg
1 cup	unsweetened apple juice	250 mL
2 tbsp	pure maple syrup	30 mL
½ tsp	ground nutmeg	2 mL
¼ tsp	ground coriander	1 mL
	Salt and freshly ground white pepper	

1. In a saucepan, melt butter over medium heat. Add onion and cook, stirring, for about 3 minutes or until just tender. Add carrots and squash and cook, stirring, for 6 to 8 minutes or until softened.

2. Pour apple juice over vegetables. Reduce heat to low, cover and simmer for 25 minutes or until vegetables are softened. Stir in maple syrup, nutmeg and coriander.

3. In food processor, working in batches, process vegetable mixture until smooth. Transfer to a bowl and season with salt and pepper to taste.

This recipe should be adjusted based on your symptoms. Follow this symptom guide:

If food tastes too sweet:
- Reduce or eliminate the maple syrup; and/or
- Substitute vegetable broth for the apple juice (choose reduced-sodium broth or unsalted homemade Basic Vegetable Stock, page 166, if you have fluid retention or high blood pressure); and/or
- Add lemon juice to taste with the salt and pepper.

If food tastes too bitter or metallic:
- Add more maple syrup and lemon juice to taste to each serving.

Nutritional Analysis per Serving

Calories...........152	Sodium........ 66 mg	Fiber .... 7 g
Fat............... 3 g	Carbohydrate..... 34 g	Protein .... 2 g

This pretty, light green dressing contains beneficial monounsaturated fat. Use it on any salad, as a dip for carrot and celery sticks, or to moisten cooked poultry, fish or vegetables.

Make Ahead

Cover the dressing tightly and refrigerate for up to 3 days.

The sweetness of mango and the freshness of lime juice and mint make a dynamite combination. This sauce will wake up sleeping taste buds and put some joy back into eating. Serve over chicken or fish.

Avocado Dressing

- Food processor or blender

½ cup	cottage cheese	125 mL
½ cup	buttermilk	125 mL
½ cup	mayonnaise	125 mL
1	ripe avocado	1
2 tsp	chopped fresh dill	10 mL
1 tsp	freshly squeezed lemon juice	5 mL

1. In food processor, combine cottage cheese, buttermilk, mayonnaise, avocado, dill and lemon juice and process until smooth, about 2 minutes.

Nutritional Analysis per 2 tbsp (30 mL)

Calories............57	Sodium........ 90 mg	Fiber .... 1 g
Fat............... 5 g	Carbohydrate...... 4 g	Protein .... 2 g

Mango Mint Mojo

- Blender or food processor

12	fresh mint leaves	12
1	ripe mango, peeled, pitted and chopped	1
½ cup	freshly squeezed lime juice	125 mL

1. In blender, combine mint, mango and lime juice and purée until smooth. Use immediately, or for best results, cover and refrigerate for at least 4 hours to allow the flavors to develop. Store in the refrigerator for up to 2 days.

This recipe courtesy of Eileen Campbell.

Nutritional Analysis per 2 tbsp (30 mL)

Calories............21	Sodium..........1 mg	Fiber .... 1 g
Fat............... 0 g	Carbohydrate...... 6 g	Protein .... 0 g

**Makes about
2 cups (500 mL)**

*Adding a fruity gravy
to lean protein, such as
chicken, turkey or pork,
helps moisten it for those
with dry mouth, as well as
boosting the flavor.*

Tips

If you prefer a sauce with a
bit more tartness, increase
the cider vinegar to 2 tbsp
(30 mL).

If you prefer a bit of spice,
add as much as $\frac{1}{4}$ tsp
(1 mL) cayenne pepper with
the brown sugar.

Make Ahead

Transfer gravy to an airtight
container and refrigerate
for up to 3 days. Reheat in
a saucepan over medium
heat, stirring often, or
microwave on Medium-
High (70%), until steaming.

Savory Cranberry Gravy

1 tbsp	vegetable oil	15 mL
1 tbsp	all-purpose flour	15 mL
$\frac{1}{2}$ cup	reduced-sodium chicken or vegetable broth	125 mL
1 tbsp	cider vinegar	15 mL
2 tbsp	packed brown sugar	30 mL
1 tbsp	Dijon mustard	15 mL
1	can (14 oz/398 mL) cranberry sauce, preferably whole berry	1
	Salt and freshly ground pepper to taste	

1. In a saucepan, heat oil over medium heat. Sprinkle with flour and cook, stirring, for 1 minute (do not let brown). Gradually whisk in broth and cider vinegar and bring to a boil. Boil, whisking, for about 2 minutes or until liquid is reduced by half, about 2 minutes.

2. Stir in brown sugar and mustard until blended. Stir in cranberry sauce and bring to a boil, stirring often. Season to taste with salt and pepper.

Nutritional Analysis per $\frac{1}{4}$ cup (60 mL)

Calories............64	Sodium........ 55 mg	Fiber .... 0 g
Fat............... 1 g	Carbohydrate..... 14 g	Protein .... 0 g

---

Makes about 1 cup (250 mL)

When your mouth is dry, a smooth sauce makes fish, eggs, vegetables, potatoes, rice or anything that appeals to you easier to swallow. In addition, because it's made with eggs, this sauce adds 1 g of protein per serving.

Tip

When making hollandaise, keep a small quantity of boiling water at the side of the stove. If your eggs start to curdle during the final whisking, add 1 tbsp (15 mL) boiling water to the mixture. Whisk until smooth and thickened, then transfer to the blender.

Variations

Chive Hollandaise: Add ¼ cup (60 mL) coarsely chopped chives with the salt and blend until smooth.

Dill Hollandaise: Add ¼ cup (60 mL) coarsely chopped fresh dill with the salt and blend until smooth.

Foolproof Hollandaise

- **Blender or small food processor**

3	egg yolks	3
3 tbsp	water	45 mL
1 tbsp	freshly squeezed lemon juice	15 mL
½ cup	butter, melted	125 mL
½ tsp	salt	2 mL
	Cayenne pepper	

1. In a small saucepan over low heat, combine egg yolks, water and lemon juice. Cook, whisking constantly, until eggs begin to thicken, about 1 minute. Whisk rapidly for about 5 seconds longer to ensure the yolks are cooked, then immediately transfer to blender.

2. With motor running, slowly add butter through the hole in the lid or through the feed tube, in a thin stream, blending until mixture is smooth and creamy. Add salt and cayenne and blend until smooth. Serve immediately.

This recipe should be adjusted based on your symptoms. Follow this symptom guide:

For dry mouth:
- Reduce the salt.

Nutritional Analysis per 2 tbsp (30 mL)

Calories..........120	Sodium.......150 mg	Fiber.............0 g
Fat..............13 g	Carbohydrate......0 g	Protein.............1

**Makes about
1 cup (250 mL)**

A simple cheese sauce can dress up broccoli or cauliflower, a broiled fish fillet or, of course, cooked macaroni, and makes everything go down that much easier. You not only get a boost in flavor, but also in added protein, calcium and energy.

Tips

For extra cheese flavor, use a sharp (old) or extra-sharp (extra-old) Cheddar cheese and/or add 2 tbsp (30 mL) freshly grated Parmesan cheese with the Cheddar.

Once it has chilled and thickened, you can use this sauce as a cheese spread on toast, crackers, apple slices or celery sticks.

Make Ahead

Transfer sauce to an airtight container and refrigerate for up to 3 days. Reheat in a saucepan over medium-low heat, stirring often, or microwave on Medium (50%), until steaming (do not let boil).

Easy Cheese Sauce

2 tbsp	all-purpose flour	30 mL
1 cup	milk	250 mL
½ tsp	dry mustard or Dijon mustard	2 mL
Pinch	ground nutmeg (optional)	Pinch
1 cup	shredded Cheddar cheese, preferably sharp (old)	250 mL
	Freshly ground black pepper	

1. Place flour in a small saucepan. Gradually whisk in milk. Whisk in mustard and nutmeg (if using). Bring to a boil over medium heat, whisking often.
2. Reduce heat and boil gently, whisking constantly, for about 3 minutes or until thick. Remove from heat and stir in cheese until melted. Season to taste with pepper.

Nutritional Analysis per ¼ cup (60 mL)

Calories..........160	Sodium.......326 mg	Fiber.............0 g
Fat.............11 g	Carbohydrate......7 g	Protein..........10 g

Makes about 3½ cups (875 mL)

This is my favorite all-purpose tomato sauce, and it's terrific to have on hand for a last-minute pasta dinner, to use as a base for spaghetti sauce or to pour over cooked meats, fish or grains to moisten them. Alternatively, you could use canned crushed (ground) tomatoes for a sauce.

Tip

Let the minced garlic stand for 10 minutes before cooking to maximize its cancer-fighting properties.

Make Ahead

Cover the sauce tightly and refrigerate for up to 3 days, or transfer individual portions to airtight containers, leaving at least 1 inch (2.5 cm) headspace for expansion, and freeze for up to 3 months. Thaw in the refrigerator or microwave. Reheat individual portions in the microwave on Medium-High (70%) for 2 to 3 minutes, or in a saucepan over medium heat, stirring often, for 2 to 3 minutes or until steaming.

Jean's Tomato Sauce

1 tbsp	olive oil	15 mL
2 to 3	cloves garlic, minced	2 to 3
1	small onion, chopped	1
1	can (28 oz/796 mL) diced tomatoes, with juice	1
1½ tbsp	basil pesto	22 mL

1. In a deep saucepan, heat oil over medium heat. Add garlic to taste and onion and cook, stirring, for about 5 minutes or until softened.

2. Add tomatoes with juice and bring to a boil, stirring often. Reduce heat and simmer, stirring occasionally, for about 10 minutes or until slightly thickened. Stir in pesto and simmer, stirring often, for about 5 minutes to blend the flavors.

3. If desired, purée sauce with an immersion blender for a finer texture.

Nutritional Analysis per ¼ cup (60 mL)

Calories............32	Sodium....... 159 mg	Fiber .... 1 g
Fat.............. 2 g	Carbohydrate...... 4 g	Protein .... 1 g

Comforting Grains and Potatoes

Whole grains are becoming more popular and more available as they are recognized for their health benefits. Your choice of whole grains or refined grains will largely depend on your bowel status. If you are regular or constipated, opt for the higher fiber and beneficial nutrition of whole grains. If you are just starting solid food or are experiencing diarrhea or bowel obstruction, then refined, lower-fiber grains are a better choice. To address the varying needs of cancer patients, some of the recipes in this chapter use whole grains, others refined. Either way, these traditional comfort foods will provide that hug-in-a-bowl you may need right now.

If plain rice tastes like cardboard because of reduced taste sensitivity, this recipe should hold some appeal for your damaged taste buds.

Tip

Rice can harbor a bacteria, *Bacillus cereus*, that can grow rapidly if rice is not cooled promptly and/or stored too long.

Make Ahead

Transfer cooked rice to individual shallow airtight containers and refrigerate for up to 2 days or freeze for up to 2 months. If frozen, thaw in the microwave or refrigerator. Reheat individual portions in the microwave on Medium-High (70%) for 2 to 3 minutes, or in a saucepan over medium heat, stirring often and adding a little water as necessary to moisten, for 3 to 4 minutes or until very hot.

Variation

To boost the fiber content and increase the cancer-fighting properties of this recipe, use brown basmati rice, increase the water to 3¾ cups (925 mL) and increase the cooking time to 30 minutes.

Basmati Rice with Ginger

1½ cups	basmati rice	375 mL
1 tbsp	butter or olive oil	15 mL
1	small onion, finely chopped	1
1 tbsp	minced gingerroot	15 mL
1	stick cinnamon, about 4 inches (10 cm) long, broken in half	1
1	large bay leaf, broken in half	1
1 tsp	salt	5 mL
2¼ cups	water	550 mL
¼ cup	chopped fresh cilantro (or 2 tbsp/30 mL chives or green onions)	60 mL

1. Place rice in sieve and rinse. Transfer to a bowl and add water to cover. Let soak for 15 minutes. Drain.

2. In a medium saucepan, melt butter over medium heat. Add onion, ginger, cinnamon and bay leaf; cook, stirring, for 2 minutes or until onion is softened.

3. Add rice, salt and water; bring to a boil. Reduce heat to low, cover and simmer for 10 minutes or until water is absorbed. Let stand, covered, for 5 minutes.

4. Fluff rice with a fork and remove and discard cinnamon stick and bay leaf. Serve sprinkled with cilantro.

Nutritional Analysis per Serving

Calories..........167	Sodium.......388 mg	Fiber.............2 g
Fat..............4 g	Carbohydrate.....33 g	Protein...........3 g

Makes 4 servings

Saffron seems exotic and is expensive, but a little goes a long way in adding a deep flavor and vibrant color to a simple rice pilaf. Plus, the valuable cancer-fighting properties of saffron justify the cost.

Tip

To toast whole almonds, place them in a dry skillet over medium heat. Toast, stirring constantly, for about 5 minutes or until golden and fragrant. Immediately transfer to a bowl and let cool, then chop.

Make Ahead

Transfer cooked rice to individual shallow airtight containers and refrigerate for up to 2 days or freeze for up to 2 months. If frozen, thaw in the microwave or refrigerator. Reheat individual portions in the microwave on Medium-High (70%) for 2 to 3 minutes, or in a saucepan over medium heat, stirring often and adding a little water as necessary to moisten, for 3 to 4 minutes or until very hot.

Saffron Basmati Rice with Almonds

1½ cups	reduced-sodium ready-to-use vegetable or chicken broth	375 mL
¼ tsp	saffron threads, crumbled	1 mL
1 cup	brown basmati rice	250 mL
1 tbsp	olive oil	15 mL
2	cloves garlic, minced	2
½ cup	sliced green onions	125 mL
¼ tsp	salt	1 mL
1 cup	water	250 mL
¼ cup	almonds, toasted and chopped	60 mL

1. In a glass measuring cup, combine broth and saffron threads; heat in microwave on High power for 1 to 2 minutes or until steaming (or heat in a saucepan on the stovetop). Set aside.

2. Place rice in sieve and rinse. Transfer to a bowl and add water to cover. Let soak for 15 minutes. Drain.

3. In a medium saucepan, heat oil over medium heat. Add garlic and green onions; cook, stirring, for 2 minutes or until onion is softened.

4. Add rice, salt, saffron mixture and water; bring to a boil. Reduce heat to low, cover and simmer for 35 minutes or until rice is tender and liquid is absorbed. Let stand, covered, for 5 minutes. Fluff rice with a fork and serve sprinkled with almonds.

Nutritional Analysis per Serving

Calories..........231	Sodium.......344 mg	Fiber.............2 g
Fat...............9 g	Carbohydrate.....35 g	Protein...........5 g

Fragrant Coconut Rice

Makes 4 servings

This deliciously rich, sweet rice is creamy and fragrant, perfect for those with a sore mouth or reduced taste.

Tip

This dish is high in saturated fat, but the source is coconut, which appears to have many health benefits. Research into coconut oil is in the preliminary stages, but we do know that it contains a number of fatty acids that have anti-inflammatory properties.

Make Ahead

Transfer cooked rice to individual shallow airtight containers and refrigerate for up to 2 days or freeze for up to 2 months. If frozen, thaw in the microwave or refrigerator. Reheat individual portions in the microwave on Medium-High (70%) for 2 to 3 minutes, or in a saucepan over medium heat, stirring often and adding a little water as necessary to moisten, for 3 to 4 minutes or until very hot.

1½ cups	coconut milk	375 mL
1 cup	water	250 mL
1	stick cinnamon, about 2 inches (5 cm) long (or ¼ tsp/1 mL ground cinnamon)	1
1 cup	long-grain brown rice, rinsed and drained	250 mL

1. In a saucepan, bring coconut milk, water and cinnamon stick to a rapid boil over medium-high heat. Stir in rice and return to a boil. Cover, reduce heat to low and simmer for about 50 minutes or until rice is tender and liquid is absorbed. Let stand, covered, for 5 minutes.

Nutritional Analysis per Serving

Calories..........223	Sodium........ 14 mg	Fiber .... 1 g
Fat.............. 19 g	Carbohydrate..... 14 g	Protein .... 3 g

Makes 4 servings

Although it needs to bake for 30 minutes, this risotto method eliminates the tedious task of stirring until the liquid is absorbed.

Tips

If you don't have a saucepan with an ovenproof handle, transfer the mixture to a deep 6-cup (1.5 L) baking dish after completing step 1.

To partially thaw the spinach for this recipe, place the package in a microwave and heat on High for 3 minutes. It can easily be separated using a fork, but will still have some ice crystals. Do not drain.

Make Ahead

Transfer cooked rice to individual shallow airtight containers and refrigerate for up to 2 days or freeze for up to 2 months. If frozen, thaw in the microwave or refrigerator. Reheat individual portions in the microwave on Medium-High (70%) for 3 to 4 minutes, or in a saucepan over medium heat, stirring often and adding a little water as necessary to moisten, for 4 to 5 minutes or until very hot.

Spinach Risotto

- **Preheat oven to 400°F (200°C)**
- **Ovenproof saucepan (see tip, at left)**

2 tbsp	butter or olive oil	30 mL
1 cup	diced onion	250 mL
1 tbsp	minced garlic	15 mL
1 cup	Arborio rice	250 mL
1	package (10 oz/300 g) frozen spinach, partially thawed (see tip, at left)	1
3 cups	reduced-sodium ready-to-use vegetable broth	750 mL
3 tbsp	sun-dried tomato pesto	45 mL
	Grated Parmesan cheese	

1. In an ovenproof saucepan, melt butter over medium heat. Add onion and cook, stirring, for 3 minutes or until softened. Stir in garlic. Add rice and cook, stirring, until the grains of rice are coated with butter, about 1 minute. Add spinach and cook, breaking up with a spoon, until thoroughly integrated into the rice, about 2 minutes. Stir in broth and pesto. Bring to a boil.

2. Transfer saucepan to preheated oven and bake, stirring partway through, until rice has absorbed the liquid, about 30 minutes. Remove from oven and sprinkle Parmesan over top. Serve immediately.

Nutritional Analysis per Serving

Calories..........272	Sodium.......167 mg	Fiber.............5 g
Fat..............8 g	Carbohydrate.....45 g	Protein...........7 g

---

Makes 8 servings

Traditional risotto takes 30 minutes on the stovetop and needs constant attention. This simpler method finishes in the oven. The results are just as tasty.

Tip

Leftover risotto makes great rice cakes for another meal. Form cooled risotto into ½-inch (1 cm) rounds and flatten. Heat a skillet over medium-high heat and spray with nonstick cooking spray. Cook risotto cakes for 3 minutes per side or until golden.

Make Ahead

Transfer cooked rice to individual shallow airtight containers and refrigerate for up to 2 days or freeze for up to 2 months. If frozen, thaw in the microwave or refrigerator. Reheat individual portions in the microwave on Medium-High (70%) for 3 to 4 minutes, or in a saucepan over medium heat, stirring often and adding a little water as necessary to moisten, for 4 to 5 minutes or until very hot.

Oven-Baked Mushroom Risotto

- **Preheat oven to 350°F (180°C)**
- **12-cup (3 L) casserole dish with cover**
- **Baking sheet**

1 cup	assorted dried mushrooms	250 mL
2 cups	boiling water	500 mL
2 tbsp	olive oil	30 mL
8 oz	mushrooms, chopped	250 g
1	onion, chopped	1
1 cup	Arborio rice	250 mL
½ cup	dry white wine (optional)	125 mL
	Salt and freshly ground black pepper	
2 tbsp	freshly grated Parmesan cheese	30 mL
1 tbsp	butter or olive oil	15 mL

1. Soak dried mushrooms in boiling water for 30 minutes. Drain and reserve liquid. Chop mushrooms.

2. In a medium skillet, heat oil over medium heat. Add fresh mushrooms, onion and chopped soaked mushrooms; cook, stirring, for about 10 minutes or until lightly browned. Stir in rice. Transfer to casserole dish.

3. To the reserved mushroom liquid, add wine (if using) and enough water to make 3 cups (750 mL). Stir into mushroom mixture. Season to taste with salt and pepper. Cover casserole and place on baking sheet.

4. Bake in preheated oven for 20 minutes. Remove from oven and stir in cheese and butter. Cover and bake for 10 minutes or until rice is al dente (tender to the bite) and most of the liquid is absorbed.

This recipe courtesy of Eileen Campbell.

Nutritional Analysis per Serving

Calories..........204	Sodium........ 45 mg	Fiber .... 3 g
Fat.............. 6 g	Carbohydrate..... 36 g	Protein .... 4 g

Makes 6 servings

Polenta is a magnificent way to add whole grains to your diet. When properly cooked, it is a soothing comfort food that functions like a bowl of steaming mashed potatoes. Many people aren't keen to make polenta because they think it takes hours of stirring over a hot stove. In fact, you can produce excellent results in the oven with virtually no stirring at all.

Tip

This recipe can also be fully prepared on the stovetop. After step 1, reduce heat to low (placing a heat diffuser under the pot if your stove doesn't have a true simmer). Continue cooking, stirring frequently, while the mixture bubbles and thickens, for about 30 minutes for polenta or 1 hour for grits, until the grains are tender and creamy. Serve immediately.

Basic Polenta and Grits

- Preheat oven to 350°F (180°C)
- 8-cup (2 L) ovenproof saucepan or baking dish, lightly greased

4½ cups	water	1.125 L
¼ tsp	salt	1 mL
1 cup	coarse stone-ground cornmeal or coarse stone-ground grits	250 mL

1. In a saucepan, bring water and salt to a boil over medium heat. Gradually stir in cornmeal in a steady stream. Cook, stirring constantly, for about 5 minutes or until smooth and blended and mixture bubbles like lava.

2. Transfer pot to preheated oven, or if you don't have an ovenproof saucepan, transfer mixture to lightly greased baking dish. Bake, covered, for about 40 minutes for cornmeal and 1 hour for grits, until the grains are tender and creamy.

This recipe should be adjusted based on your symptoms. Follow this symptom guide:

For low blood pressure:
- Use ready-to-use vegetable or chicken broth (not reduced-sodium) in place of half of the water.

To encourage weight gain:
- Substitute 1 cup (250 mL) heavy or whipping (35%) cream for an equal amount of the water; and/or
- Stir ¼ cup (60 mL) to ⅓ cup (75 mL) shredded mozzarella or provolone cheese or 2 tbsp (30 mL) mascarpone cheese into each serving.

For reduced taste sensitivity:
- Stir ¼ cup (60 mL) basil pesto or ½ cup (125 mL) chopped fresh basil into the polenta after cooking.

Nutritional Analysis per Serving

Calories...........84	Sodium........98 mg	Fiber.............2 g
Fat..............0 g	Carbohydrate.....18 g	Protein..........2 g

Makes 4 servings

This soft casserole is a variation on Italian polenta. Look for whole-grain cornmeal to get all the benefits you can from this dish. Cornmeal comes in white, yellow and blue varieties; all are nutritious as long as the cornmeal is stone-ground (whole-grain).

Make Ahead

Transfer the cooked casserole to individual airtight containers and refrigerate for up to 2 days. Enjoy cold or reheat individual portions in the microwave on Medium-High (70%) for 4 to 5 minutes or until very hot.

Cornmeal Casserole

- **Preheat oven to 350°F (180°C)**
- **4-cup (1 L) baking dish, lightly greased**

1 tbsp	butter or margarine	15 mL
1	small onion, chopped	1
1	stalk celery, chopped	1
½ cup	yellow cornmeal	125 mL
½ tsp	salt	2 mL
½ tsp	granulated sugar	2 mL
Pinch	freshly ground black pepper	Pinch
2 cups	milk, heated until steaming	500 mL
1	egg, well beaten	1

1. In a skillet, melt butter over medium heat. Add onion and celery and cook, stirring, for about 5 minutes or until golden. Stir in cornmeal and mix until coated. Stir in salt, sugar and pepper.

2. Gradually pour in hot milk, stirring constantly. Reduce heat to medium-low and cook, stirring often, for about 5 minutes or until thickened. Remove from heat and let cool.

3. Stir in beaten egg until well blended. Spoon mixture into prepared baking dish. Bake in preheated oven for 35 to 40 minutes or until top is browned and casserole is set.

This recipe courtesy of Lydia Husak.

This recipe should be adjusted based on your symptoms. Follow this symptom guide:

To encourage weight gain:
- Replace the milk with evaporated milk, half-and-half (10%) cream or table (18%) cream; and/or
- Stir 1 cup (250 mL) shredded mozzarella, Cheddar or provolone cheese into the cornmeal mixture after the egg.

Nutritional Analysis per Serving

Calories..........178	Sodium.......368 mg	Fiber.............2 g
Fat..............7 g	Carbohydrate.....22 g	Protein..........7 g

Makes 4 to 6 servings

This is another one of those dishes that is synonymous with comfort food. Use your food processor to quickly slice the potatoes.

Tip

For the best results, choose oblong, starchy baking potatoes, such as russet (Idaho) or all-purpose yellow-fleshed potatoes.

Make Ahead

To make ahead, layer potatoes in cream sauce in dish, cover and refrigerate for up to 1 day.

Cover leftover baked scalloped potatoes and refrigerate for up to 2 days or freeze in individual airtight containers for up to 2 months. If frozen, thaw in the microwave or refrigerator. Reheat individual portions in the microwave on Medium-High (70%) for 3 to 4 minutes or until very hot.

Classic Scalloped Potatoes

- **Preheat oven to 350°F (180°C)**
- **10-cup (2.5 L) shallow baking dish, greased**

6	potatoes (about 2 lbs/1 kg)	6
2 tbsp	butter or olive oil	30 mL
1	large onion, halved lengthwise, thinly sliced	1
2 tbsp	all-purpose flour	30 mL
1½ cups	milk	375 mL
2 tsp	Dijon mustard	10 mL
½ tsp	salt	2 mL
Pinch	freshly grated nutmeg	Pinch
1 cup	shredded aged Cheddar or Swiss cheese	250 mL

1. Peel and thinly slice potatoes; rinse under cold water. Drain; wrap in a clean, dry towel to dry.

2. In a saucepan, melt butter over medium heat. Cook onion, stirring often, for 3 minutes or until softened. Sprinkle with flour and stir until blended. Gradually pour in milk, stirring constantly; stir in mustard, salt and nutmeg. Bring to a boil, stirring, until sauce thickens.

3. Stir potatoes into sauce; bring to a boil over medium heat. Spoon into prepared baking dish; sprinkle with cheese. Bake for 45 to 50 minutes or until potatoes are tender and top is golden.

This recipe should be adjusted based on your symptoms. Follow this symptom guide:

To encourage weight gain:
- Replace the milk with evaporated milk, half-and-half (10%) cream or table (18%) cream; and/or
- Increase the cheese to 2 cups (500 mL); stir half into the sauce before adding the potatoes.

Nutritional Analysis per Serving

Calories...........281	Sodium....... 422 mg	Fiber .... 3 g
Fat .... 12 g	Carbohydrate..... 34 g	Protein .... 10 g

Makes 6 servings

This tasty potato recipe is similar to a dish served in Greek restaurants. It will be just the thing to balance out your taste buds if food is tasting metallic or overly sweet.

Make Ahead

Wrap and refrigerate potatoes for up to 3 days. Reheat individual portions in the microwave on Medium-High (70%) for 3 to 4 minutes, or wrapped in foil in a 350°F (180°C) toaster oven or conventional oven for 15 to 20 minutes or until steaming.

Survivor Wisdom

Give yourself permission to have bad days, even 6 months after treatment when everyone thinks you should be okay.

Oven-Roasted Lemon Potatoes

- Preheat oven to 400°F (200°C)
- Large, shallow roasting pan

1½ lbs	potatoes, peeled and cut in chunks	750 g
3 tbsp	olive oil	45 mL
	Juice of 1 lemon	
½ tsp	dried oregano	2 mL
¼ tsp	freshly ground black pepper	1 mL
⅛ tsp	salt	0.5 mL
1½ cups	reduced-sodium ready-to-use chicken or vegetable broth (approx.)	375 mL

1. Place potatoes in a single layer in roasting pan. Add olive oil, lemon juice, oregano, pepper and salt; toss to coat. Pour in just enough broth to half-cover potatoes.

2. Bake in preheated oven for about 1 hour or until potatoes are tender, golden brown and crispy on the outside.

This recipe courtesy of dietitian Patti Thomson.

This recipe should be adjusted based on your symptoms. Follow this symptom guide:

If you have high blood pressure or fluid retention, or foods taste too salty:
- Use no-salt-added ready-to-use chicken broth or unsalted homemade Chicken Stock (page 167) or Basic Vegetable Stock (page 166).

Nutritional Analysis per Serving

Calories...........131	Sodium.......230 mg	Fiber.............1 g
Fat...............6 g	Carbohydrate.....18 g	Protein...........2 g

Makes 6 servings

When you make potatoes or sweet potatoes, make extra so that you can have this the next day. The sweet potato gives it a nice orange color. The combination of potato and cheese may appeal to those with low appetites.

Tip

Use plain mashed potato and sweet potato, without milk or butter added.

Make Ahead

Wrap and refrigerate potato cakes for up to 3 days. Reheat individual cakes in the microwave on Medium-High (70%) for 3 to 4 minutes, or wrapped in foil in a 350°F (180°C) toaster oven or conventional oven for 15 to 20 minutes or until steaming.

Potato Cakes with a Twist

1	egg, beaten	1
1 cup	mashed cooked potatoes	250 mL
1 cup	mashed cooked sweet potato	250 mL
1/2 cup	crumbled feta cheese or any mild shredded cheese	125 mL
	Nonstick cooking spray	

1. In a medium bowl, combine egg, mashed potatoes and mashed sweet potatoes until smooth. Stir in cheese.

2. Heat a skillet over medium heat and spray with cooking spray. Spoon 1/2 cup (125 mL) potato mixture into the pan and cook until bottom is golden. Flip and cook until bottom is golden and cake is heated through. Remove to a plate and repeat until all potato mixture is used, spraying pan and adjusting heat as needed between batches.

This recipe courtesy of dietitian Charissa McKay.

Nutritional Analysis per Serving

Calories..........119	Sodium.......166 mg	Fiber.............2 g
Fat..............4 g	Carbohydrate.....17 g	Protein...........4 g

Makes 6 servings

These traditional Irish mashed potatoes are made with butter and green onions and are another example of comfort food that can appeal to tired appetites.

Tip

Do not use a food processor in step 2 or the potatoes will turn into glue.

Make Ahead

Transfer potatoes to individual airtight containers and refrigerate for up to 2 days or freeze for up to 2 months. If frozen, thaw in the microwave or refrigerator. Reheat individual portions in the microwave on Medium-High (70%) for 3 to 4 minutes or until very hot.

Variation

Instead of green onions, use 1/3 cup (75 mL) snipped fresh chives or parsley.

Champ

6	russet or yellow-fleshed potatoes, peeled and quartered (about 2 lbs/1 kg)	6
3/4 cup	milk (approx.)	175 mL
3/4 cup	chopped green onions	175 mL
2 tbsp	butter or olive oil	30 mL
	Salt and freshly ground black pepper	
	Chopped green onion tops	

1. Place potatoes in a large saucepan and add salted cold water to cover. Bring to a boil over high heat. Reduce heat and boil gently for about 20 minutes or until fork-tender. Drain well and return to saucepan. Place over low heat and dry, shaking pan, for 1 to 2 minutes.

2. Press potatoes through a food mill or ricer or mash with potato masher or use an electric mixer at low speed until very smooth.

3. Meanwhile, in a small saucepan, combine milk, green onions and butter. Heat over medium-low heat for 5 minutes or until piping hot. Using an electric mixer or masher, beat milk mixture into potatoes, adding more milk if necessary, until potatoes are creamy. Season with salt and pepper to taste.

4. Place pan over medium-low heat, if necessary, to reheat until piping hot. Spoon into serving bowl and sprinkle with green onion tops.

This recipe should be adjusted based on your symptoms. Follow this symptom guide:

For lactose intolerance:
- Replace the milk with a lactose-free beverage, such as lactose-reduced milk or non-dairy milk (e.g., soy milk or rice milk).

To encourage weight gain:
- Replace the milk with evaporated milk, half-and-half (10%) cream or table (18%) cream; and/or
- Stir 1/4 cup (60 mL) shredded cheese into each serving; and/or
- Stir 2 tbsp (30 mL) sour cream into each serving.

Nutritional Analysis per Serving

Calories..........177	Sodium........ 59 mg	Fiber .... 2 g
Fat.............. 5 g	Carbohydrate..... 29 g	Protein .... 4 g

Makes 6 servings

The combination of sweet potatoes and apples accented with maple syrup provides that extra enticement when plain sweet potatoes don't seem appealing enough.

Tip

To prepare this recipe in the microwave, combine ingredients in an 8-cup (2 L) casserole dish. Microwave, covered, on High for 20 to 25 minutes, stirring once, until sweet potatoes are tender. Purée as directed in step 3.

Make Ahead

Transfer potatoes to individual airtight containers and refrigerate for up to 2 days. Reheat individual portions in the microwave on Medium-High (70%) for 3 to 4 minutes or until very hot.

Variation

Instead of sweet potatoes, use 2 lbs (1 kg) butternut squash, peeled and seeded.

Mashed Roasted Sweet Potatoes with Apples

- **Preheat oven to 375°F (190°C)**
- **13- by 9-inch (33 by 23 cm) baking dish, greased**
- **Food processor**

3	sweet potatoes (about 2 lbs/1 kg), peeled and cut into 1-inch (2.5 cm) chunks	3
2	apples, peeled and chopped	2
1	onion, chopped	1
	Salt and freshly ground black pepper	
2 tbsp	butter, melted, or olive oil	30 mL
¼ cup	pure maple syrup	60 mL

1. Place sweet potatoes, apples and onion in prepared baking dish. Season with salt and pepper. Drizzle with melted butter and maple syrup.

2. Bake in preheated oven, stirring occasionally, for 45 to 50 minutes or until sweet potatoes are very tender.

3. In a food processor, purée vegetable mixture in batches until smooth. Transfer to a heatproof serving dish.

This recipe should be adjusted based on your symptoms. Follow this symptom guide:

If food tastes too sweet:
- Use tart apples, such as Crispin (Mutsu), Granny Smith or McIntosh; and/or
- Reduce or eliminate the maple syrup; and/or
- Add cider vinegar or lemon juice to taste to each serving.

Nutritional Analysis per Serving

Calories.......... 276	Sodium....... 105 mg	Fiber .... 7 g
Fat .... 5 g	Carbohydrate..... 57 g	Protein .... 4 g

Makes 6 servings

This make-ahead mashed potato casserole is a welcome dish to have on hand when you don't have the energy to cook. For sore mouths that need lump-free mashed potatoes, use a food mill or ricer instead of a potato masher.

Tip

The type of potatoes used determines how fluffy your mashed potatoes will be. The starchy russet, or baking, variety produces fluffy mashed potatoes. Yellow-fleshed potatoes, such as Yukon gold, have a slightly buttery taste and make delicious mashed potatoes with a creamier texture. Regular white potatoes also make a creamy purée, although not as flavorful. New potatoes are not suitable for mashing, as they don't have the starch content of storage potatoes.

Creamy Mashed Potato Casserole

- **Preheat oven to 350°F (180°C)**
- **8-cup (2 L) casserole dish, greased**

6	large russet or yellow-fleshed potatoes (about 3 lbs/1.5 kg) (see tip, at left)	6
4 oz	light cream cheese, softened, cubed	125 g
¾ cup	hot milk (approx.)	175 mL
	Salt and freshly grated nutmeg	
½ cup	shredded Cheddar cheese	125 mL
¼ cup	fine dry bread crumbs	60 mL
½ tsp	paprika	2 mL

1. Peel potatoes and cut into 3-inch (7.5 cm) chunks. Place in a large saucepan and add salted cold water to cover. Bring to a boil over high heat. Reduce heat and boil gently for 20 to 25 minutes or until fork-tender. Drain well and return to saucepan. Place over low heat and dry, shaking pan, for 1 to 2 minutes.

2. Press potatoes through a food mill or ricer or mash with potato masher or use an electric mixer at low speed until very smooth. (Do not use a food processor or the potatoes will turn into glue.) Beat in cream cheese and milk until smooth; season with salt and nutmeg to taste. Spread evenly in prepared casserole dish.

3. In a small bowl, combine Cheddar cheese, bread crumbs and paprika. Sprinkle evenly over potatoes.

4. Bake, uncovered, in preheated oven for 40 to 50 minutes or until top is golden and a knife inserted in center is hot to the touch.

Make Ahead

Prepare the casserole through step 2, cover and refrigerate for up to 2 days. Sprinkle with crumb topping before baking. Increase the baking time by 10 minutes.

Transfer the baked casserole to individual airtight containers and refrigerate for up to 2 days or freeze for up to 2 months. If frozen, thaw in the microwave or refrigerator. Reheat individual portions in the microwave on Medium-High (70%) for 3 to 4 minutes, or in a baking dish covered in foil in a 350°F (180°C) toaster oven or conventional oven for 20 to 30 minutes or until very hot.

Survivor Wisdom

When you are in an environment with other people, they will be watchful. Know that their advice is well intended.

This recipe should be adjusted based on your symptoms. Follow this symptom guide:

For lactose intolerance:
- Replace the milk with a lactose-free beverage, such as lactose-reduced milk or non-dairy milk (e.g., soy milk or rice milk).

To encourage weight gain:
- Replace the milk with evaporated milk, half-and-half (10%) cream or table (18%) cream; and/or
- Use full-fat cream cheese rather than light.

Nutritional Analysis per Serving

Calories..........299	Sodium....... 218 mg	Fiber .... 4 g
Fat .... 7 g	Carbohydrate ..... 48 g	Protein .... 12 g

Makes 4 servings

When you are craving pasta, but not the tomato sauce, consider this stovetop recipe for thin pasta with fresh vegetables.

Tips

To save time, cook the pasta while you are preparing the other ingredients.

If you love spinach, add extra — the recipe will still turn out great.

Survivor Wisdom

I found, after surgery, that meat was the last thing I wanted.

Spinach Spaghettini

8 oz	whole wheat spaghettini	250 g
2 tbsp	olive oil	30 mL
½ cup	sliced mushrooms	125 mL
2	cloves garlic, chopped	2
Pinch	salt	pinch
Pinch	hot pepper flakes (optional)	Pinch
1 cup	chopped spinach	250 mL
2 tbsp	freshly grated Parmesan cheese	30 mL

1. In a large pot of boiling salted water, cook spaghettini according to package directions until al dente. Drain well.

2. Meanwhile, in a medium saucepan, heat oil over medium-low heat. Add mushrooms, garlic, salt and pepper flakes; cook, stirring, for about 5 minutes or until mushrooms are tender. Add spinach and cook, stirring, for about 3 minutes or until tender and wilted. Add spaghettini and toss until heated. Serve sprinkled with Parmesan.

This recipe courtesy of dietitian Carla Reid.

Nutritional Analysis per Serving

Calories..........302	Sodium....... 127 mg	Fiber .... 8 g
Fat.............. 9 g	Carbohydrate..... 48 g	Protein .... 11 g

Sustaining Snacks

Low energy levels are one of the most common side effects of cancer and its treatment. One of the recommendations to combat this problem is to go no more than four hours without eating. Enter the sustaining snack, that mini-meal between meals that keeps your blood sugars from bottoming out and gives you another opportunity to consume beneficial cancer-fighting nutrients, protein and calories.

Most of the sustaining snacks in this chapter are portable. As a nutrition professional, I am saddened to see that many hospitals have given in to the pressures of readily available fast food and junk food. Don't rely on your facility to have healthy snacks available. Instead, if you can, bring something from home.

This is a great chapter to share with a friend, neighbor or family member who has said, "Let me know if there is anything I can do to help." Ask them to make one of these recipes for you.

Makes 16 squares

These delicious squares are great as a breakfast bar or a mid-morning snack.

Tip

Brown rice syrup is available in the natural food section of your supermarket or at health food stores. If you cannot find it, use light (fancy) molasses instead.

Make Ahead

Wrap individual squares in plastic wrap and store in an airtight container or sealable plastic bag at room temperature for up to 5 days.

Variation

Replace the apricots with another dried fruit. Raisins, cranberries, cherries, chopped pitted dates and figs all work well.

Almond Butter Cereal Squares

- **9-inch (23 cm) square metal baking pan, lightly greased**

½ cup	crunchy almond butter or natural peanut butter	125 mL
½ cup	brown rice syrup	125 mL
½ cup	liquid honey	125 mL
1 tsp	vanilla extract	5 mL
1 cup	chopped dried apricots	250 mL
½ cup	sliced almonds	125 mL
¼ cup	sesame seeds	60 mL
¼ cup	ground flax seeds	60 mL
¼ cup	sunflower seeds	60 mL
2½ cups	high-fiber cereal, such as bran flakes	625 mL
1¼ cups	large-flake (old-fashioned) rolled oats	300 mL

1. In a large saucepan, over low heat, cook almond butter, rice syrup, honey and vanilla until blended. Add apricots, almonds, sesame seeds, flaxseed and sunflower seeds; mix well. Add cereal and oats; mix well.

2. Pour mixture into prepared pan. Press down with clean, damp hands to compact evenly. Let stand for 30 minutes, until firm, then cut into squares.

This recipe courtesy of Eileen Campbell.

Nutritional Analysis per Serving

Calories..........234	Sodium........ 89 mg	Fiber .... 4 g
Fat............. 10 g	Carbohydrate..... 35 g	Protein .... 6 g

Makes 18 servings

A twist on traditional peanut butter sandwiches, these healthy wraps are portable, easy to make and delicious as a breakfast, lunch or portable snack.

Tips

If possible, purchase whole-grain tortillas. These are even better than whole wheat, since the whole grain contains the germ, which is a source of beneficial phytonutrients.

To toast pecans, heat a skillet over medium-high heat. Add pecans and toast, shaking occasionally, for about 4 minutes or until lightly browned and fragrant.

If you are taking this along to appointments, cut each roll in half, rather than bite-size pieces, and wrap in plastic wrap.

Make Ahead

These twisters can be wrapped in plastic wrap and refrigerated for up to 2 days.

Chunky Peanut Butter Twisters

½ cup	peanut butter	125 mL
¼ cup	unsweetened shredded coconut	60 mL
¼ cup	pure maple syrup	60 mL
2 tbsp	finely chopped dried figs	30 mL
2 tbsp	finely chopped dried apricots	30 mL
2 tbsp	finely chopped dried cranberries	30 mL
Pinch	ground cinnamon	Pinch
3	10-inch (25 cm) whole wheat tortillas	3
3 tbsp	finely chopped toasted pecans (see tip, at left)	45 mL

1. In a small bowl, combine peanut butter, coconut, maple syrup, figs, apricots, cranberries and cinnamon.
2. Spread ⅓ cup (75 mL) peanut butter mixture on each tortilla. Sprinkle each with 1 tbsp (15 mL) pecans. Roll up tortillas and cut each into 6 pieces.

This recipe courtesy of Lydia Butler.

This recipe should be adjusted based on your symptoms. Follow this symptom guide:

To assist with constipation:
- Replace the apricots with pitted prunes; and/or
- Stir 3 tbsp (45 mL) natural bran into the peanut butter mixture; and/or
- Follow this snack with a hot drink, then a cold beverage.

Nutritional Analysis per Serving

Calories............95	Sodium........ 85 mg	Fiber .... 2 g
Fat .... 5 g	Carbohydrate..... 13 g	Protein .... 3 g

Makes 12 large muffins

Muffins are a great snack to take to an appointment, to keep you on your eating schedule. This recipe uses whole wheat flour and less oil than other recipes.

Tip

To boost the risk reduction properties of these muffins, use omega-3 eggs and add 1 tsp (5 mL) ground cinnamon with the flour.

Make Ahead

Place cooled muffins in an airtight container and store at room temperature for up to 2 days, or wrap individually in plastic wrap, then place in an airtight container or sealable plastic bag and freeze for up to 1 month.

Banana Applesauce Muffins

- **Preheat oven to 400°F (200°C)**
- **12-cup muffin pan, lightly greased or lined with paper liners**

2 cups	whole wheat flour	500 mL
1 tbsp	baking powder	15 mL
1 tsp	baking soda	5 mL
1/2 tsp	salt	2 mL
3	ripe bananas, mashed (about 1 1/3 cups/325 mL)	3
1	large egg, lightly beaten	1
1 cup	unsweetened applesauce	250 mL
1/2 cup	granulated sugar	125 mL
1/4 cup	vegetable oil	60 mL

1. In a large bowl, combine flour, baking powder, baking soda and salt.
2. In a medium bowl, combine bananas, egg, applesauce, sugar and oil. Stir into flour mixture until just combined.
3. Divide batter evenly among prepared muffin cups.
4. Bake in preheated oven for 15 to 20 minutes or until tops are firm to the touch and a tester inserted in the center of a muffin comes out clean. Let cool in pan on a wire rack for 10 minutes, then transfer to rack to cool completely.

This recipe courtesy of Glenyss Turner.

This recipe should be adjusted based on your symptoms. Follow this symptom guide:

To assist with constipation:
- Replace the applesauce with two 4 1/2-oz (128 mL) jars of baby food prunes and reduce the sugar to 1/3 cup (75 mL); and/or
- Add 1/4 cup (60 mL) ground flax seeds with the flour.

Nutritional Analysis per Serving

Calories..........183	Sodium....... 283 mg	Fiber .... 3 g
Fat............... 5 g	Carbohydrate..... 32 g	Protein .... 4 g

Makes 24 muffins

These tasty muffins are great to have on hand when you need a snack and don't have the energy to put one together; they're also the perfect snack to take along to appointments. This big-batch recipe allows you to have an ample supply.

Tips

Ripe bananas can be thrown in the freezer, peel and all. To use, just thaw, peel and mash. You can also mash bananas and freeze in airtight containers in amounts appropriate for your recipes.

To boost the risk reduction potential of these muffins, use omega-3 eggs.

Make Ahead

Place cooled muffins in an airtight container and store at room temperature for up to 2 days, or wrap individually in plastic wrap, then place in an airtight container or sealable plastic bag and freeze for up to 1 month.

Big-Batch Banana Blueberry Muffins

- Preheat oven to 350°F (180°C)
- Two 12-cup muffin pans, lightly greased or lined with paper liners

3 cups	whole wheat flour	750 mL
3 cups	ground flax seeds	750 mL
2 cups	lightly packed brown sugar	500 mL
1 tbsp	baking powder	15 mL
1 tbsp	baking soda	15 mL
Pinch	salt	Pinch
3	large eggs	3
3	ripe bananas, mashed (about 1⅓ cups/ 325 mL)	3
1	jar (4½ oz/128 mL) baby food prunes (or ½ cup/125 mL unsweetened applesauce)	1
⅔ cup	vegetable oil	150 mL
2 tsp	vanilla extract	10 mL
2 cups	fresh or frozen blueberries	500 mL

1. In a very large bowl, combine flour, flaxseed, brown sugar, baking powder, baking soda and salt.

2. In a large bowl, combine eggs, bananas, prunes, oil and vanilla. Stir into flour mixture until just combined. Fold in blueberries.

3. Divide batter evenly among prepared muffin cups.

4. Bake in preheated oven for 20 minutes, rotating pans halfway through, or until tops are firm to the touch and a tester inserted in the center of a muffin comes out clean. Let cool in pan on a wire rack for 10 minutes, then transfer to rack to cool completely.

This recipe courtesy of Jacqueline O'Keefe.

Nutritional Analysis per Serving

Calories..........226	Sodium........172 mg	Fiber.............5 g
Fat..............10 g	Carbohydrate.....31 g	Protein..........5 g

Makes 12 muffins

If nausea has you down, the ginger in these muffins may be just the ticket. As a bonus, cloves are ranked the highest in antioxidant content of all herbs and spices.

Tip

To boost the risk reduction properties of these muffins, use omega-3 eggs.

Make Ahead

Place cooled muffins in an airtight container and store at room temperature for up to 2 days, or wrap individually in plastic wrap, then place in an airtight container or sealable plastic bag and freeze for up to 1 month.

Variations

You can make 24 mini muffins and decrease the baking time to about 16 minutes.

For a sweeter and more intense ginger flavor, fold in ¼ cup (60 mL) chopped candied ginger at the end of step 3.

Gingerbread Muffins

- **Preheat oven to 325°F (160°C)**
- **12-cup muffin pan, lightly greased or lined with paper liners**

1½ cups	whole wheat flour	375 mL
1 cup	all-purpose flour	250 mL
1½ tsp	ground ginger	7 mL
1 tsp	ground cinnamon	5 mL
1 tsp	ground cloves	5 mL
½ cup	granulated sugar	125 mL
½ cup	canola oil	125 mL
1 cup	light (fancy) molasses	250 mL
1 cup	boiling water	250 mL
2 tsp	baking soda	10 mL
2	large eggs	2

1. In a large bowl, combine whole wheat flour, all-purpose flour, ginger, cinnamon and cloves. Set aside.
2. In a medium bowl, whisk together sugar and oil. Whisk in molasses and eggs until blended. In a glass measuring cup, combine water and baking soda. Stir to dissolve. Pour into egg mixture and whisk until blended. Stir into flour mixture just until combined.
3. Divide batter evenly among prepared muffin cups.
4. Bake in preheated oven for about 25 minutes or until a toothpick inserted in the center comes out clean. Let cool in pan on a wire rack for 15 minutes, then transfer to rack to cool completely.

Nutritional Analysis per Serving

Calories..........285	Sodium....... 270 mg	Fiber .... 2 g
Fat.............. 10 g	Carbohydrate..... 46 g	Protein .... 4 g

Makes 12 muffins

Eat one of these muffins whenever you require some bulk in your diet — or just because they're delicious!

Tips

To boost the risk reduction properties of these muffins, use omega-3 eggs.

Always measure the oil before measuring sticky sweeteners such as molasses or honey. For recipes that don't call for oil, spray the measure with nonstick vegetable spray or lightly coat with oil. Every last drop of sweetener will easily pour out.

Make Ahead

Place cooled muffins in an airtight container and store at room temperature for up to 2 days, or wrap individually in plastic wrap, then place in an airtight container or sealable plastic bag and freeze for up to 1 month.

Bran Muffins

- Preheat oven to 400°F (200°C)
- 12-cup muffin pan, well greased or lined with paper liners

1¼ cups	whole wheat flour	300 mL
1 cup	natural bran	250 mL
1 tsp	baking soda	5 mL
½ tsp	baking powder	2 mL
¼ tsp	salt	1 mL
2	large eggs	2
1 cup	buttermilk	250 mL
⅓ cup	packed brown sugar	75 mL
¼ cup	vegetable oil	60 mL
¼ cup	light (fancy) molasses	60 mL
½ cup	raisins or chopped dried apricots	125 mL

1. In a bowl, combine flour, bran, baking soda, baking powder and salt.
2. In another bowl, beat eggs. Add buttermilk, brown sugar, oil and molasses. Stir into flour mixture just until combined. Fold in raisins.
3. Divide batter evenly among prepared muffin cups.
4. Bake in preheated oven for 20 to 24 minutes or until tops spring back when lightly touched. Let cool in pan for 10 minutes, then transfer muffins to a wire rack to cool.

This recipe should be adjusted based on your symptoms. Follow this symptom guide:

To assist with constipation:
- Substitute a 4½-oz (128 mL) jar of baby food prunes for ½ cup (125 mL) of the buttermilk; and/or
- Replace the raisins with chopped dates or dried figs.

Nutritional Analysis per Serving

Calories...........190	Sodium.......203 mg	Fiber.............3 g
Fat...............7 g	Carbohydrate.....32 g	Protein..........5 g

Makes 12 muffins

These healthy muffins are a good choice for breakfast, a mid-morning snack or to take along to an appointment. With the lowest calories of all the muffin and bread recipes, they're perfect for those whose goal is weight loss.

Tip

To boost the risk reduction properties of these muffins, use omega-3 eggs.

Make Ahead

Place cooled muffins in an airtight container and store at room temperature for up to 2 days, or wrap individually in plastic wrap, then place in an airtight container or sealable plastic bag and freeze for up to 1 month.

Survivor Wisdom

I could only eat junk food. Healthy food did not appeal to me at all.

Triple B Health Muffins

- Preheat oven to 400°F (200°C)
- 12-cup muffin pan, lightly greased or lined with paper liners

1 cup	whole wheat flour	250 mL
1 cup	natural wheat bran or oat bran	250 mL
1 cup	fresh or frozen blueberries	250 mL
1 tsp	baking soda	5 mL
1 tsp	baking powder	5 mL
2	ripe bananas, mashed (about 1 cup/250 mL)	2
1	large egg, lightly beaten	1
½ cup	granulated sugar	125 mL
½ cup	milk	125 mL
¼ cup	vegetable oil	60 mL
1 tsp	vanilla extract	5 mL

1. In a large bowl, combine flour, wheat bran, blueberries, baking soda and baking powder.
2. In a medium bowl, combine bananas, egg, sugar, milk, oil and vanilla. Stir into flour mixture until just combined.
3. Divide batter evenly among prepared muffin cups.
4. Bake in preheated oven for 20 to 25 minutes or until tops are firm to the touch and a tester inserted in the center of a muffin comes out clean. Let cool in pan for 10 minutes, then remove to a wire rack to cool completely.

This recipe courtesy of Barbara Kajifasz.

Nutritional Analysis per Serving

Calories..........152	Sodium.......141 mg	Fiber.............4 g
Fat...............6 g	Carbohydrate.....26 g	Protein...........3 g

Makes 8 slices

This moist, flavorful bread makes a delicious snack. You can also enjoy it as dessert or for breakfast on the run.

Tips

A variety of baking pans work well for this bread: a small loaf pan (about 8 by 4 inches/20 by 10 cm) makes a traditionally shaped bread; a round 6-cup (1.5 L) soufflé dish or a square 7-inch (18 cm) baking dish produces slices of different shapes.

Preparing this bread in a loaf pan inside a slow cooker allows for a soft bread without a crust on top, which is ideal if you have a sore mouth. If your taste buds are run down and you rely on texture to enjoy your meal, prepare this bread the traditional way, in the oven (see variation, below).

Variation

Instead of baking in the slow cooker, use a metal loaf pan and bake bread in a 350°F (180°C) oven for about 55 minutes or until a tester inserted in the center comes out clean. Let cool in pan on a wire rack for 15 minutes, then turn out and serve warm or let cool.

Banana Walnut Oat Bread

- Large (minimum 5 quart) oval slow cooker
- 8- by 4-inch (20 by 10 cm) loaf pan or 6-cup (1.5 L) soufflé or baking dish, greased (see tip, at left)

¾ cup	all-purpose flour	175 mL
¾ cup	large-flake (old-fashioned) rolled oats	175 mL
2 tbsp	ground flax seeds	30 mL
2 tsp	baking powder	10 mL
½ tsp	salt	2 mL
¼ tsp	baking soda	1 mL
⅓ cup	butter, softened	75 mL
⅔ cup	packed brown sugar	150 mL
2	large eggs	2
3	ripe bananas, mashed (about 1¼ cups/ 300 mL)	3
½ cup	finely chopped walnuts	125 mL
	Boiling water	

1. In a bowl, combine flour, oats, flax seeds, baking powder, salt and baking soda.

2. In a separate bowl, using an electric mixer, beat butter and sugar until light and creamy. Add eggs, one at a time, beating until incorporated. Beat in bananas.

3. Stir flour mixture into banana mixture just until combined. Fold in walnuts.

4. Spoon batter into prepared pan. Cover tightly with foil and secure with a string. Place pan in slow cooker stoneware and pour in enough boiling water to come 1 inch (2.5 cm) up the sides. Cover and cook on High for 3 hours, until a tester inserted in the center comes out clean. Unmold and serve warm or let cool.

Nutritional Analysis per Serving

Calories..........249	Sodium....... 439 mg	Fiber .... 3 g
Fat .... 7 g	Carbohydrate ..... 42 g	Protein .... 7 g

Makes 8 slices

Preparing this bread in a loaf pan inside a slow cooker allows for a soft bread without a crust on top, which is ideal if you have a sore mouth. If your taste buds are run down and you rely on texture to enjoy your meal, prepare this bread the traditional way, in the oven (see variation, opposite).

Tip

A variety of baking pans work well for this bread: a small loaf pan (about 8 by 4 inches/20 by 10 cm) makes a traditionally shaped bread; a round 6-cup (1.5 L) soufflé dish or a square 7-inch (18 cm) baking dish produces slices of different shapes.

Apple Cranberry Bread

- Large (minimum 5 quart) oval slow cooker
- 8- by 4-inch (20 by 10 cm) loaf pan or 6-cup (1.5 L) soufflé or baking dish, greased (see tip, at left)

1 cup	all-purpose flour	250 mL
1 cup	whole wheat flour	250 mL
1/4 cup	ground flax seeds	60 mL
2 tsp	baking powder	10 mL
1/2 tsp	salt	2 mL
1/2 tsp	ground cinnamon	2 mL
3/4 cup	packed brown sugar	175 mL
1/4 cup	olive oil	60 mL
1	large egg	1
2 tbsp	finely grated orange zest (2 oranges)	30 mL
3/4 cup	freshly squeezed orange juice (1 large navel orange)	175 mL
1 tsp	vanilla extract	5 mL
1 cup	finely chopped peeled apple	250 mL
1 cup	fresh or frozen cranberries	250 mL
	Boiling water	

1. In a large bowl, combine all-purpose flour, whole wheat flour, flax seeds, baking powder, salt and cinnamon.
2. In a medium bowl, whisk together sugar, oil, egg, orange zest, orange juice and vanilla until thoroughly blended. Stir into flour mixture just until blended. Fold in apple and cranberries.

Sprinkled over your morning cereal or added to baked goods or smoothies, nutrient-dense flax seeds are an excellent supplement to your diet. In addition to being a source of iron, magnesium and potassium, flax seeds are high in fiber, so they help you to stay regular and keep your cholesterol levels under control. Moreover, flax seeds are one of the best plant sources of heart-healthy omega-3 fats. They also contain lignans, a plant fiber that protects against cancer. In fact, the USDA lists 27 anticancer agents in flax. When using flax seeds, you can grind them yourself. If you buy the ground (milled) variety, choose prepackaged, not bulk, to ensure freshness.

Variation

Instead of baking in the slow cooker, use a metal loaf pan and bake bread in a 350°F (180°C) oven for 65 to 75 minutes or until a tester inserted in the center comes out clean. Let cool in pan on a wire rack for 15 minutes, then turn out and serve warm or let cool.

3. Spoon batter into prepared pan. Cover tightly with foil and secure with a string. Place in slow cooker stoneware and pour in enough boiling water to come 1 inch (2.5 mL) up the sides of the dish. Cover and cook on High for 4 hours, until a tester inserted in the center comes out clean. Unmold and serve warm or let cool.

Nutritional Analysis per Serving

Calories..........310	Sodium....... 444 mg	Fiber .... 4 g
Fat.............. 10 g	Carbohydrate..... 53 g	Protein .... 6 g

Recommended for:
• Constipation
• Low appetite
Bonus features:
• High fiber
• High protein
• Portability
• Risk reduction

Makes 12 slices

This yummy bread is great for breakfast, as a snack or for dessert and combines both soluble and insoluble fibers, for a bread that will feed a healthy digestive tract as well as it feeds you.

Tips

The omega-3 fatty acids DHA and EPA are important anti-inflammatories. When hens are fed flax seeds, they convert the ALA type of omega-3 to DHA and EPA, the types most beneficial to us. A dozen omega-3 eggs may cost more, but you get about 400 mg of omega-3 per egg, about eight times more than is present in eggs produced by hens not fed flax.

To increase the omega-3 content, fiber and phytonutrients, fold ½ cup (125 mL) chopped walnuts into the batter at the end of step 2.

Oat Bran Banana Bread

- **Preheat oven to 325°F (160°C)**
- **9- by 5-inch (23 by 12.5 cm) metal loaf pan, lightly greased**

1½ cups	whole wheat flour	375 mL
½ cup	oat bran	125 mL
⅓ cup	ground flax seeds	75 mL
1 tsp	baking powder	5 mL
1 tsp	baking soda	5 mL
2	large egg whites (or 1 whole egg)	2
1	whole egg	1
½ cup	granulated sugar	125 mL
¼ cup	canola oil	60 mL
1 tsp	vanilla extract	5 mL
¾ cup	low-fat plain yogurt	175 mL
3	ripe bananas, mashed (about 1⅓ cups/ 325 mL)	3
2 tbsp	whole flax seeds (optional)	30 mL

1. In a medium bowl, combine flour, oat bran, ground flax seeds, baking powder and baking soda.
2. In a large bowl, using an electric mixer, beat egg whites, whole egg, sugar, oil and vanilla for 3 to 4 minutes or until creamy. Stir in yogurt until well combined. Stir in bananas. Gradually fold in flour mixture.
3. Spoon batter into prepared loaf pan and smooth top. Sprinkle with whole flax seeds (if using).
4. Bake in preheated oven for 50 to 60 minutes or until top is firm to the touch and a tester inserted in the center comes out clean. Let cool in pan on a wire rack for 10 minutes, then transfer to rack to cool completely.

This recipe courtesy of dietitian Melanie Faust.

Nutritional Analysis per Serving

Calories...........193	Sodium....... 157 mg	Fiber .... 4 g
Fat............... 7 g	Carbohydrate..... 31 g	Protein .... 6 g

Makes 1½ cups (375 mL)

When you need to gain some weight and sweetness is appealing to you, add this honey butter to any food you like.

Tips

If you don't have a food processor with a mini bowl attachment, or a mini chopper, combine the ingredients in a bowl and use an electric mixer to beat until creamy.

Make sure your butter is unsalted or you will have salty-tasting honey butter.

Make Ahead

Transfer honey butter to an airtight container and refrigerate for up to 1 week or freeze for up to 2 months. If frozen, thaw in the refrigerator. Let soften slightly at room temperature before spreading.

Variation

Try using a different-flavored honey, such as lavender or clove.

Honey Butter

- **Food processor with mini bowl attachment or mini chopper (see tip, at left)**

1 cup	unsalted butter, softened	250 mL
½ cup	liquid honey	125 mL
1 tsp	ground cinnamon	5 mL
½ tsp	ground nutmeg	2 mL

1. In mini bowl of food processor, combine butter, honey, cinnamon and nutmeg; process until smooth, stopping and scraping down sides of the bowl as necessary, about 2 minutes. Spoon into a ramekin or small bowl and chill until firm, about 30 minutes.

Nutritional Analysis per 2 tbsp (30 mL)

Calories..........182	Sodium..........2 mg	Fiber.............0 g
Fat..............15 g	Carbohydrate.....12 g	Protein...........0 g

Makes about 1½ cups (375 mL)

Egg and Olive Spread

4	hard-cooked eggs, peeled and chopped	4
2 tbsp	mayonnaise	30 mL
6	pimento-stuffed green olives, finely chopped	6
	Salt and freshly ground black pepper	
	Pumpernickel rounds or dark rye bread	

1. In a bowl, combine eggs, mayonnaise and olives. Mix well. Season with salt and pepper to taste.
2. Mound into a small serving bowl. Accompany with pumpernickel rounds or dark rye bread.

Finding protein to snack on between meals can be a challenge, but it's important to include protein whenever you eat, to help maintain good blood sugar control and sustain energy.

Tip

For a visually appealing presentation, sprinkle with paprika.

Make Ahead

Cover and refrigerate spread for up to 2 days.

This recipe should be adjusted based on your symptoms. Follow this symptom guide:

If food tastes too salty:
- Replace the olives with 1 tbsp (15 mL) finely chopped fresh chives or 2 small roasted red peppers, finely chopped.

To encourage weight gain:
- Spread the filling between two slices of thickly buttered whole-grain bread.

For sore mouth or throat:
- Serve on soft bread or eat the spread on its own.

Nutritional Analysis per 2 tbsp (30 mL)

Calories............38	Sodium....... 100 mg	Fiber .... 0 g
Fat.............. 3 g	Carbohydrate...... 1 g	Protein .... 2 g

Makes 3 to 4 servings

This bean purée is a great solution for days when you need protein but meat does not appeal. Spread it on bread, use it as a dip for vegetables or serve it in a bowl with a spoon. It's very soft and moist, so even a sore mouth should be able to handle it. Double or triple the recipe to meet your needs.

Tip

To make this into a complete protein, eat it along with a whole-grain choice or a vegetable; that way, all of the essential amino acids will be represented.

Make Ahead

Transfer bean purée to an airtight container and refrigerate for up to 3 days. Reheat in the microwave on Medium-High (70%) for 2 to 3 minutes or until warmed.

Variation

Substitute chickpeas, red kidney beans, black beans or pinto beans for the white beans.

Easy White Bean Purée

- **Food processor**

2 cups	drained rinsed cooked or canned white beans	500 mL
½ cup	fresh Italian flat-leaf parsley leaves	125 mL
2	green onions, white part only, coarsely chopped	2
2 tbsp	extra virgin olive oil	30 mL
	Salt and freshly ground black pepper	

1. Place beans in a saucepan and add water to cover. Bring to a boil over medium heat. Reduce heat and simmer for about 5 minutes or until beans are nicely hot. Drain.

2. Meanwhile, in food processor, pulse parsley, green onions and olive oil until chopped, about 5 times, stopping and scraping down sides of the bowl once or twice. Add warm beans and pulse until beans are the consistency you prefer. Season with salt and pepper to taste. Serve hot.

This recipe should be adjusted based on your symptoms. Follow this symptom guide:

If food tastes too sweet or metallic:
- Add 1 to 2 tbsp (15 to 30 mL) lemon juice to taste with the salt and pepper.

Nutritional Analysis per ¼ cup (60 mL)

Calories...........175	Sodium....... 405 mg	Fiber .... 7 g
Fat............... 7 g	Carbohydrate..... 21 g	Protein .... 8 g

Makes 2¾ cups (675 mL)

This version of the Middle Eastern dip uses probiotic yogurt to replace much of the traditional olive oil. It's an excellent choice when you need a protein that is soft and moist, and when meat doesn't appeal.

Tips

If using dried chickpeas, soak and cook 1 cup (250 mL).

Tahini, a sesame seed paste, is widely available in health food stores. If you cannot find tahini, substitute toasted sesame seeds and process with the chickpeas.

Portion hummus into individual airtight containers and refrigerate. Pack a container in a small cooler with crackers, soft bread or raw vegetables for a portable, high-protein snack.

Make Ahead

Transfer hummus to an airtight container and refrigerate for up to 3 days.

Hummus with Tahini

- **Food processor or blender**

2 cups	drained rinsed canned or cooked chickpeas	500 mL
2	green onions	2
2 to 4	large cloves garlic	2 to 4
¼ cup	freshly squeezed lemon juice	60 mL
¼ cup	tahini (see tip, at left)	60 mL
½ tsp	ground cumin	2 mL
½ tsp	salt	2 mL
	Freshly ground black pepper	
½ cup	lower-fat plain probiotic yogurt	125 mL
	Chopped onion, tomato and fresh parsley	

1. In a food processor or blender, combine chickpeas, green onions, garlic, lemon juice, tahini, cumin, salt and pepper to taste and process until smooth.

2. Transfer to a bowl and stir in yogurt. Garnish with onion, tomato and parsley. Serve at room temperature or cover and refrigerate for about 1 hour, until chilled.

This recipe courtesy of Brenda Steinmetz.

This recipe should be adjusted based on your symptoms. Follow this symptom guide:

For sore mouth or throat:
- Omit the garlic or use roasted garlic; and/or
- Reduce or omit the lemon juice.

Nutritional Analysis per 2 tbsp (30 mL)

Calories............40	Sodium........109 mg	Fiber.............1 g
Fat...............2 g	Carbohydrate......5 g	Protein..........2 g

Makes about 2 cups (500 mL)

This delicious, easy pâté will give you an extra boost of iron, helping you to correct low iron levels.

Tips

You can eat this by itself, on crackers or bread, or instead of butter or mayonnaise on a sandwich.

Portion pâté into individual airtight containers and refrigerate. Pack a container in a small cooler with crackers, soft bread or raw vegetables for a portable, high-protein snack.

Survivor Wisdom

Understand that your pathway is unique.

Instant Pâté

- **Food processor**

1 lb	chicken livers, trimmed	500 g
¾ cup	butter, softened	175 mL
¼ cup	coarsely chopped sweet onion, such as Vidalia	60 mL
2	cloves garlic	2
2 tbsp	fresh thyme leaves (or 1 tsp/5 mL dried)	30 mL
2 tbsp	cognac, brandy or white wine vinegar	30 mL
1 tsp	salt	5 mL
1 tsp	cracked black peppercorns	5 mL
	Baguette or crackers	

1. In a pot of boiling water, cook chicken livers until just a hint of pink remains in the center, about 3 minutes. Drain.
2. Transfer to food processor. Add butter, onion and garlic; purée until smooth. Add thyme, cognac, salt and peppercorns and process until blended.
3. Transfer to a serving dish. Cover and refrigerate for at least 3 hours or for up to 2 days. Serve on sliced baguette or your favorite crackers.

This recipe should be adjusted based on your symptoms. Follow this symptom guide:

For sore mouth or throat:
- Omit the cognac, brandy or vinegar; and/or
- Omit or reduce the black pepper; and/or
- Cook the onion in a small amount of butter or canola oil until softened before adding it to food processor.

Nutritional Analysis per 2 tbsp (30 mL)

Calories..........137	Sodium.......168 mg	Fiber.............0 g
Fat..............12 g	Carbohydrate......1 g	Protein..........5 g

Makes about 3½ cups (875 mL)

Preventing and treating constipation with dietary changes may reduce your need for laxatives. This spread can be used on toast or mixed into hot cereal or plain yogurt.

Make Ahead

Transfer to an airtight container and refrigerate for up to 2 weeks or freeze for up to 3 months. If frozen, thaw in the microwave or refrigerator.

Fiberful Fruit Spread

- **Blender or food processor**

2 cups	pitted prunes	500 mL
1 cup	dates or chopped dried figs	250 mL
1½ cups	chopped rhubarb (fresh or frozen)	375 mL
⅔ cup	unsweetened orange juice or apple juice	150 mL
½ cup	water	125 mL
1 cup	natural wheat bran	250 mL

1. In a saucepan, combine prunes, dates, rhubarb, orange juice and water. Bring to a boil over medium-high heat, stirring often. Reduce heat to medium-low, cover and boil gently for about 15 minutes or until rhubarb is very soft. Transfer to a bowl and stir in bran. Cover and refrigerate for at least 4 hours or overnight.

2. Transfer to blender and purée until smooth.

Nutritional Analysis per 2 tbsp (30 mL)

Calories............54	Sodium..........2 mg	Fiber ....2 g
Fat...............0 g	Carbohydrate.....14 g	Protein ....1 g

---

Nurturing Desserts

Pumpkin, bananas, apples, berries, lemon, ginger, cinnamon, vanilla, rolled oats, cornmeal, rice, split peas and nuts — all are healthy, and all are included in this chapter, along with some sugar. Don't be surprised if your tastes have changed since before you had cancer. This common effect may include either an aversion to sweet things or a heightened appreciation for them. For some, sugar really does make the medicine go down; if you are one of those people, this chapter is just what the doctor ordered. While sugar can hardly be called a cancer-fighting ingredient, if it encourages you to eat, then it's helping your body get the nutrients it needs. Desserts can play a key role in adding much-needed protein and calories to your day.

Makes 24 servings

This moist, spice-filled cake is as rich in fiber as it is in flavor. It's also an excellent source of phytonutrients from the pumpkin, raisins, spices and whole grains.

Tip

If a 14-oz (398 mL) can of pumpkin isn't available, buy a larger can and measure out 1¾ cups (425 mL). Transfer extra pumpkin to an airtight container and refrigerate for up to 5 days or freeze for up to 3 months (the texture will be softer after thawing, but fine for baked goods such as this recipe or other muffins or quick breads).

Make Ahead

Place the cooled cake in an airtight container and store at room temperature for up to 2 days, or wrap quarters or individual pieces in plastic wrap, then place in an airtight container or sealable plastic bag and freeze for up to 1 month. Wrap slices individually before placing them in the container, if desired, to make them easier to grab on the go.

Harvest Raisin Cake

- **Preheat oven to 350°F (180°C)**
- **13- by 9-inch (33 by 23 cm) metal baking pan, lightly greased**

1½ cups	granulated sugar	375 mL
1 cup	whole wheat flour	250 mL
1 cup	all-purpose flour	250 mL
2 tsp	baking powder	10 mL
1½ tsp	ground cinnamon	7 mL
1 tsp	baking soda	5 mL
½ tsp	salt	2 mL
¼ tsp	ground cloves	1 mL
¼ tsp	ground nutmeg	1 mL
¼ tsp	ground ginger	1 mL
4	large eggs	4
1	can (14 oz/398 mL) pumpkin purée (not pie filling)	1
½ cup	vegetable oil	125 mL
1 cup	high-fiber bran cereal, such as All-Bran	250 mL
1 cup	raisins	250 mL

1. In a large bowl, combine sugar, whole wheat flour, all-purpose flour, baking powder, cinnamon, baking soda, salt, cloves, nutmeg and ginger.

2. In another large bowl, whisk together eggs, pumpkin, oil and cereal. Stir in flour mixture just until combined. Fold in raisins.

3. Spread evenly in prepared baking pan. Bake in preheated oven for about 40 minutes or until tester inserted in center comes out clean. Let cool completely in pan on a wire rack.

This recipe courtesy of Maryanne Cattrysse.

Nutritional Analysis per Serving

Calories..........119	Sodium...... 225 mg	Fiber .... 3 g
Fat.............. 1 g	Carbohydrate..... 27 g	Protein .... 3 g

Makes 9 servings

If your appetite is waning or nausea is threatening to derail your day, the smell of ginger, cinnamon and cloves may be just what you need to entice you to eat.

Tips

For an extra ginger hit, add 2 to 4 tbsp (30 to 60 mL) finely chopped crystallized ginger to the flour mixture.

Cloves have the most antioxidants of any spice, so look for ways to incorporate them into your recipes.

Make Ahead

Place the cooled cake in an airtight container and store at room temperature for up to 2 days, or wrap quarters or individual pieces in plastic wrap, then place in an airtight container or sealable plastic bag and freeze for up to 1 month. Wrap slices individually before placing them in the container, if desired, to make them easier to grab on the go.

Gingerbread Cake

- **Preheat oven to 350°F (180°C)**
- **8-inch (20 cm) square metal baking pan, greased**

¾ cup	all-purpose flour	175 mL
¾ cup	whole wheat flour	175 mL
1½ tsp	ground ginger	7 mL
1 tsp	baking soda	5 mL
¾ tsp	ground cinnamon	3 mL
¼ tsp	ground cloves	1 mL
¼ tsp	salt	1 mL
⅔ cup	packed brown sugar	150 mL
⅓ cup	butter or non-hydrogenated margarine, softened	75 mL
½ cup	light (fancy) molasses	125 mL
1	large egg	1
⅔ cup	hot water	150 mL

1. In a bowl, stir together all-purpose flour, whole wheat flour, ginger, baking soda, cinnamon, cloves and salt.

2. In another bowl, using an electric mixer, beat brown sugar and butter until fluffy. Beat in molasses and egg. Add flour mixture; beat on low speed until well blended. Beat in hot water.

3. Spread batter in prepared baking pan. Bake in preheated oven for 35 to 40 minutes or until tester inserted in center comes out clean. Let cool in pan on a wire rack. Cut into squares. Serve warm or let cool completely.

This recipe should be adjusted based on your symptoms. Follow this symptom guide:

To encourage weight gain:
- Serve the cake with a scoop of vanilla ice cream.

Nutritional Analysis per Serving

Calories..........270	Sodium....... 364 mg	Fiber .... 2 g
Fat.............. 9 g	Carbohydrate..... 45 g	Protein .... 3 g

Makes 12 servings

This cake contains both soluble and insoluble fibre. The banana flavour is subtle, and the texture is soft as a result of presoaking the oats and bran. The optional glaze poured over top makes the cake extra-moist and adds a sweetness that some palates need, as well as extra calories.

Tip

This recipe is a great way to use overripe bananas. If you can't use bananas that are becoming ripe, pop them into a sealable plastic bag and freeze them. They will turn black, but once they are thawed and the skins are removed, they will be perfect for this recipe.

Buttermilk Oat Banana Cake

- **Preheat oven to 350°F (180°C)**
- **8-inch (20 cm) square metal baking pan, lightly greased and floured**

1 cup	buttermilk	250 mL
²⁄₃ cup	quick-cooking rolled oats	150 mL
¹⁄₃ cup	oat bran or natural wheat bran	75 mL
¾ cup	all-purpose flour	175 mL
¾ cup	whole wheat flour	175 mL
1 tsp	baking soda	5 mL
1 tsp	baking powder	5 mL
¼ cup	butter or non-hydrogenated margarine	60 mL
1 cup	granulated sugar	250 mL
1	large egg	1
1 tsp	vanilla	5 mL
2	ripe bananas, mashed	2

Glaze (Optional)

½ cup	granulated sugar	125 mL
½ cup	buttermilk	125 mL
¼ cup	butter or non-hydrogenated margarine	60 mL
½ tsp	baking soda	2 mL

1. In a small bowl, pour buttermilk over oats and oat bran. Let stand for 10 minutes.

2. In another small bowl, combine all-purpose flour, whole wheat flour, baking soda and baking powder. In a medium bowl, using an electric mixer, cream butter and sugar until fluffy. Beat in egg and vanilla. Beat in bananas and buttermilk mixture until blended. Stir in dry ingredients until combined.

3. Pour batter into prepared pan. Bake in preheated oven for 45 minutes or until tester inserted in center comes out clean. Let stand for 5 minutes.

4. *Glaze (if using):* In a small saucepan, combine sugar, buttermilk, butter and baking soda; bring just to a boil over medium heat, stirring often. (Watch closely; mixture will foam.)

Make Ahead

Place the cooled glazed cake in an airtight container and store at room temperature for up to 2 days. To freeze, omit the glaze or add just before serving. Wrap quarters or individual pieces of unglazed cake in plastic wrap, then place in an airtight container or sealable plastic bag and freeze for up to 1 month. Wrap slices individually before placing them in the container, if desired, to make them easier to grab on the go.

Survivor Wisdom

Pain also affects the appetite. I was on painkillers for quite a long time — that didn't help my appetite.

5. Poke holes with a metal skewer or a wooden toothpick all over cake surface; pour glaze over cake while still warm. Let cake cool completely in pan on a wire rack before cutting.

This recipe courtesy of Helen Sutton.

This recipe should be adjusted based on your symptoms. Follow this symptom guide:

To assist with constipation:
- Use the wheat bran instead of oat bran; and/or
- Replace one of the bananas with a 4½-oz (128 mL) jar of baby food prunes; and/or
- Follow this cake with a hot drink, then a cold beverage.

For diarrhea:
- Use the oat bran instead of wheat bran and omit the glaze; and/or
- Serve cake topped with probiotic yogurt.

Nutrients per serving

Calories..........198	Sodium.......258 mg	Fiber.............3 g
Fat..............6 g	Carbohydrate.....34 g	Protein...........5 g

Makes 12 slices

This cake doesn't contain flour, but you would never know it. The eggs and hazelnuts combine to provide more protein than most cakes.

Tips

Vanilla sugar is available in small paper envelopes in the baking section of well-stocked supermarkets and at some specialty baking stores. If you don't have it, add 2 tsp (10 mL) more granulated sugar and stir in 1½ tsp (7 mL) vanilla extract with the hazelnuts.

If ground hazelnuts aren't available, buy whole hazelnuts and pulse them in a food processor until finely ground.

Make Ahead

Place the cooled cake in an airtight container and refrigerate for up to 3 days, or wrap individual pieces in plastic wrap, then place in an airtight container or sealable plastic bag and freeze for up to 1 month. Wrap slices individually before placing them in the container, if desired, to make them easier to grab on the go.

Hazelnut Loaf Cake

- **Preheat oven to 350°F (180°C)**
- **9- by 5-inch (23 by 12.5 cm) metal loaf pan, greased and lined with parchment paper**

6	large eggs	6
¾ cup	granulated sugar	175 mL
1	package (0.32 oz/9 g) vanilla sugar (see tip, at left)	1
3½ cups	ground hazelnuts (about 14 oz/400 g)	875 mL
2½ tbsp	dry bread crumbs	37 mL
2 tsp	baking powder	10 mL

1. In a large bowl, beat eggs, granulated sugar and vanilla sugar until frothy and pale. Add hazelnuts, bread crumbs and baking powder and fold until well combined. Pour into prepared loaf pan, smoothing top.

2. Bake in preheated oven for 55 minutes or until a tester inserted in the center comes out clean. Let cool in pan on a wire rack for 15 minutes, then turn out onto rack to cool completely.

This recipe courtesy of Traude Ohle.

This recipe should be adjusted based on your symptoms. Follow this symptom guide:

To encourage weight gain:
- Serve topped with chocolate hazelnut spread; or
- Serve topped with lightly sweetened whipped cream.

Nutritional Analysis per Slice

Calories..........214	Sodium........ 96 mg	Fiber .... 2 g
Fat.............. 15 g	Carbohydrate..... 15 g	Protein .... 7 g

Makes 16 squares

When your iron levels are low but red meat doesn't appeal, make a batch of these chewy squares and enjoy them knowing you are providing your body with several good sources of non-heme iron. Each square has 4.3 mg.

Tips

In terms of iron content, pumpkin seed butter is the best choice for this recipe.

When buying the rice and corn flakes cereals, check the labels to make sure you are getting the brand with the highest iron fortification. If you are making this as an iron source, don't buy brown rice or whole-grain versions. Also, don't drink coffee or tea with these squares, as compounds in these drinks can reduce the amount of iron absorbed from non-heme sources.

If your upper body is weak from surgery or for another reason, get someone else to stir this for you, as the stickiness makes it challenging to stir.

Chewy Molasses Squares

- 9-inch (23 cm) square metal baking pan, lined with foil with 2-inch (5 cm) overhang, foil greased

½ cup	blackstrap molasses	125 mL
¼ cup	packed brown sugar	60 mL
Pinch	salt	Pinch
1 cup	pumpkin seed butter, almond butter or natural peanut butter	250 mL
1 tsp	vanilla extract	5 mL
2 cups	crisp rice cereal	500 mL
1 cup	corn flakes cereal, slightly crushed	250 mL
¾ cup	raisins	175 mL

1. In a large saucepan, combine molasses, sugar and salt. Bring to a full boil over medium-high heat, stirring often. Stir in pumpkin seed butter and vanilla. Remove from heat.

2. Stir in rice cereal, corn flakes and raisins until evenly coated. Using a greased spatula, press into prepared pan. Let cool completely in pan on a wire rack. Using foil as handles, lift square out of pan and transfer to a cutting board, then cut into squares.

3. Place squares in an airtight container and store in the refrigerator for up to 5 days. Wrap them individually before placing them in the container, if desired, to make them easier to grab on the go.

This recipe courtesy of Bev LaMantia.

Nutritional Analysis per Square

Calories 216	Sodium . . . . 83 mg	Fiber . . . . 1 g
Fat . . . . 9 g	Carbohydrate . . . . . 30 g	Protein . . . . 8 g

Makes 30 cookies

These crisp, spicy cookies, perfect for those who like the flavor of gingerbread, may be especially welcomed by those with nausea.

Make Ahead

Place cooled cookies in a cookie tin (to keep them crispy) or an airtight container (to keep them soft) and store at room temperature for up to 5 days, or layer with parchment paper in an airtight container and freeze for up to 2 months.

Ginger Cookies

- Preheat oven to 350°F (180°C)
- Baking sheets, lightly greased or lined with parchment paper

1¾ cups	all-purpose flour	425 mL
1½ tsp	baking powder	7 mL
1 tsp	ground ginger	5 mL
1 tsp	ground cinnamon	5 mL
½ tsp	baking soda	2 mL
½ tsp	salt	2 mL
¼ tsp	ground cloves	1 mL
1	large egg	1
½ cup	granulated sugar	125 mL
½ cup	vegetable oil	125 mL
½ cup	light (fancy) molasses	125 mL

1. In a small bowl, combine flour, baking powder, ginger, cinnamon, baking soda, salt and cloves.
2. In a medium bowl, whisk egg, sugar, oil and molasses until blended. Fold in flour mixture until a moist dough forms.
3. Shape dough into balls, using about 1 tbsp (15 mL) dough per cookie, and place 2 inches (5 cm) apart on prepared baking sheets.
4. Bake, one sheet at a time, in preheated oven for 10 to 12 minutes or until lightly browned and crisp. Let cool on baking sheets on a wire rack for 5 minutes, then remove to rack to cool completely.

This recipe courtesy of dietitian Phyllis Levesque.

Nutritional Analysis per Cookie

Calories...........91	Sodium........ 79 mg	Fiber .... 0 g
Fat.............. 4 g	Carbohydrate..... 13 g	Protein .... 1 g

Makes 4 servings

This variation on a traditional crisp uses shredded wheat cereal biscuits instead of rolled oats. Packed with fruit and whole grains, each serving supplies 2 servings from the Vegetables and Fruit group, as well as plenty of fiber. It is equally delicious made with fresh or frozen berries.

Tips

Choose tart baking apples that hold their shape when baked, such as Crispin (Mutsu), Empire, Granny Smith, Ida Red or Northern Spy.

For an all-apple version, omit the berries and add an extra sliced apple.

Country Apple Berry Crisp

- **Preheat oven to 375°F (190°C)**
- **4-cup (1 L) baking dish with lid, greased**

3	large baking apples, thinly sliced	3
2 cups	mixed berries, sliced if large	500 mL
1 tbsp	cornstarch	15 mL
3	large shredded wheat cereal biscuits, crumbled	3
¼ cup	packed brown sugar	60 mL
¼ cup	butter or non-hydrogenated margarine	60 mL
1 tsp	ground cinnamon	5 mL

1. In a bowl, combine apples, berries and cornstarch.
2. In another bowl, combine crumbled biscuits, brown sugar, butter and cinnamon. Rub with fingers until crumbly. Set aside 1 cup (250 mL) of the crumble mixture.
3. Toss remaining crumble mixture with fruit. Place fruit mixture in prepared baking dish. Sprinkle remaining crumb mixture over top.
4. Cover and bake in preheated oven for 20 minutes. Remove cover and bake for 10 minutes or until apples are tender. Serve warm.

This recipe courtesy of dietitian Marilynn Small of Post Cereals.

This recipe should be adjusted based on your symptoms. Follow this symptom guide:

To encourage weight gain:
- Serve with vanilla ice cream.

Nutritional Analysis per Serving

Calories..........366	Sodium..........6 mg	Fiber.............6 g
Fat..............15 g	Carbohydrate.....60 g	Protein...........3 g

Recommended for:
- Constipation
- Taste alterations

Bonus features:
- High fiber
- Risk reduction

Makes 6 servings

Using several fruits instead of just one makes a crisp more colorful and adds flavor. Depending on the natural sweetness of each fruit, more or less sugar may be required. Large-flake rolled oats give this crisp a deliciously old-fashioned, crunchy topping. The sweetness of this dessert may appeal to those with metallic or bitter taste changes.

Tips

Choose tart baking apples that hold their shape when baked, such as Crispin (Mutsu), Empire, Granny Smith, Ida Red or Northern Spy. For a softer texture, use a soft apple, such as McIntosh.

If desired, replace the cranberries with 2 tbsp (30 mL) dried cranberries that have been soaked in 1 tbsp (15 mL) orange juice for 10 to 15 minutes.

This crisp offers lots of nutrients, and the bran and rolled oats make it a good source of fiber.

Winter Fruit Crisp

- **Preheat oven to 400°F (200°C)**
- **6-cup (1.5 L) shallow glass baking dish**

3	large baking apples, peeled and sliced	3
2	large pears, peeled and sliced	2
½ cup	fresh or frozen cranberries	125 mL
2 tbsp	granulated sugar or packed brown sugar (or to taste)	30 mL
1 cup	large-flake (old-fashioned) rolled oats	250 mL
¼ cup	packed brown sugar	60 mL
¼ cup	natural wheat bran	60 mL
½ tsp	ground cinnamon	2 mL
⅓ cup	butter or non-hydrogenated margarine	75 mL

1. Place apples, pears and cranberries in a baking dish. Sprinkle with granulated sugar to taste.

2. In a medium bowl, combine oats, brown sugar, bran and cinnamon. With pastry blender or two knives, cut in butter until crumbly. Sprinkle over fruit mixture.

3. Bake in preheated oven for about 40 minutes or until mixture is bubbling and fruit is barely tender.

This recipe courtesy of dietitian Laurie A. Wadsworth.

Nutritional Analysis per Serving

| Calories..........284 | Sodium..........3 mg | Fiber.............6 g |
| Fat..............13 g | Carbohydrate.....42 g | Protein..........3 g |

Makes 4 to 6 servings

Most baked custards have two or more eggs. This custard uses 2% evaporated milk and one egg to create a slightly softer version.

Tip

Transfer extra pumpkin to an airtight container and refrigerate for up to 5 days or freeze for up to 3 months (the texture will be softer after thawing, but fine for baked goods such as muffins or quick breads).

Make Ahead

Cover cooled custards and refrigerate for up to 3 days, or wrap tightly in plastic wrap, then in foil (or place in an airtight container), and freeze for up to 1 month. Thaw in the microwave or refrigerator.

Pumpkin Custard

- **Preheat oven to 325°F (160°C)**
- **Blender or food processor**
- **4 large or 6 small custard cups**

1 cup	2% evaporated milk	250 mL
1 cup	pumpkin purée (not pie filling)	250 mL
2 tbsp	granulated sugar	30 mL
1	large egg	1
¼ tsp	ground nutmeg	1 mL
¼ tsp	ground ginger	1 mL

1. In blender, combine milk, pumpkin, sugar, egg and spices; process until well blended. Pour into 4 large or 6 small custard cups and place on a baking sheet.

2. Bake in preheated oven for about 30 minutes or until knife inserted in center comes out clean. Serve warm or cover and refrigerate for about 4 hours or until chilled to serve cold.

This recipe courtesy of Cynthia Chace.

This recipe should be adjusted based on your symptoms. Follow this symptom guide:

To encourage weight gain:
- Replace the 2% evaporated milk with whole evaporated milk or half-and-half (10%) cream; and/or
- Serve topped with lightly sweetened whipped cream or ice cream.

Nutritional Analysis per Serving

Calories............70	Sodium........ 60 mg	Fiber .... 2 g
Fat............... 2 g	Carbohydrate..... 10 g	Protein .... 4 g

Makes 4 servings

Creamy puddings are nutritious and economical desserts that are incredibly easy to make and may appeal to those with poor appetites.

Tips

Pour pudding directly into individual airtight containers with tight-fitting lids, let cool, then cover and refrigerate to pack in a cooler to take along to appointments. Don't forget to pack a spoon.

To boost the protein in this pudding, whisk ½ cup (125 mL) unflavored or vanilla-flavored protein powder into the milk before adding the egg yolks.

Make Ahead

Refrigerate pudding, covered, for up to 3 days.

Easy Vanilla Pudding

2 cups	milk	500 mL
2	large egg yolks	2
⅓ cup	granulated sugar	75 mL
3 tbsp	cornstarch	45 mL
2 tsp	vanilla extract	10 mL

Stovetop Method

1. In a small saucepan, whisk together milk and egg yolks. Stir in sugar and cornstarch until smooth. Place over medium heat and cook, stirring constantly, for 5 minutes or until pudding comes to a full boil and thickens. Remove from heat. Stir in vanilla.

2. Pour pudding into individual serving dishes. Serve warm or cold. If serving cold, let cool slightly, and place plastic wrap directly on the surface to prevent the formation of a skin.

Microwave Method

1. Using an 8-cup (2 L) glass bowl or casserole dish, whisk together milk and egg yolks. Stir in sugar and cornstarch until smooth. Microwave, uncovered, on High for 2 minutes. Whisk well. Continue to microwave on High for 2 to 4 minutes, whisking every minute, until pudding comes to a full boil and thickens. Stir in vanilla.

2. Pour pudding into individual serving dishes. Serve warm or cold. If serving cold, let cool slightly, and place plastic wrap directly on the surface to prevent the formation of a skin.

This recipe should be adjusted based on your symptoms. Follow this symptom guide:

To encourage weight gain:
- Use whole milk or replace the milk with half-and-half (10%) cream or table (18%) cream; and/or
- Serve topped with lightly sweetened whipped cream.

Nutritional Analysis per Serving

Calories..........165	Sodium........ 86 mg	Fiber .... 0 g
Fat.............. 4 g	Carbohydrate..... 24 g	Protein .... 7 g

Makes 4 servings

This nourishing chocolate pudding takes little time to make on the stovetop or in the microwave and provides a good source of protein.

Tips

For an even deeper chocolate flavor and a bigger boost of flavonoids, use 70% cacao or dark chocolate chips.

If cooking pudding in the microwave, be sure to use a large bowl to prevent boilovers.

To boost the protein in this pudding, whisk ½ cup (125 mL) unflavored or vanilla-flavored protein powder into the milk with the cornstarch.

Pour pudding directly into individual airtight containers with tight-fitting lids, let cool, then cover and refrigerate to pack in a cooler to take along to appointments. Don't forget to pack a spoon.

Make Ahead

Refrigerate pudding, covered, for up to 3 days.

Homemade Chocolate Pudding

⅓ cup	granulated sugar	75 mL
¼ cup	cornstarch	60 mL
2¼ cups	milk	550 mL
⅓ cup	semisweet chocolate chips	75 mL
1 tsp	vanilla extract	5 mL

Stovetop Method

1. In a medium saucepan, whisk together sugar and cornstarch; add milk, whisking until smooth. Place over medium heat; cook, stirring, for 5 minutes or until mixture comes to a full boil; cook for 15 seconds. Remove from heat. Stir in chocolate chips and vanilla until smooth.

Microwave Method

1. In a deep 8-cup (2 L) glass bowl or casserole dish, whisk together sugar and cornstarch; add milk, whisking until smooth. Microwave, uncovered, on High for 2 minutes. Whisk well; microwave on High for 2 to 4 minutes more, whisking every minute, until pudding comes to a full boil and thickens. Stir in chocolate chips and vanilla.

For Both Methods

2. Pour pudding into individual serving dishes. Let cool slightly and serve warm. To serve cold, cover surface with plastic wrap to prevent skins from forming on surface and refrigerate for about 4 hours or until chilled.

This recipe should be adjusted based on your symptoms. Follow this symptom guide:

To encourage weight gain:
- Use whole milk or replace the milk with half-and-half (10%) cream or table (18%) cream; and/or
- Serve topped with lightly sweetened whipped cream.

Nutritional Analysis per Serving

Calories..........242	Sodium........ 57 mg	Fiber .... 0 g
Fat .... 8 g	Carbohydrate..... 38 g	Protein .... 6 g

Makes 6 servings

When your appetite is waning and only comfort food will do, this classic pudding with its cozy butterscotch flavor fits the bill.

Tips

To boost the protein in this pudding, whisk ½ cup (125 mL) unflavored or vanilla-flavored protein powder into the milk with the cornstarch.

Pour pudding directly into individual airtight containers with tight-fitting lids, let cool, then cover and refrigerate to pack in a cooler to take along to appointments. Don't forget to pack a spoon.

Make Ahead

Refrigerate pudding, covered, for up to 3 days.

Butterscotch Pudding

2½ cups	milk	625 mL
3	large egg yolks	3
⅔ cup	packed brown sugar (preferably dark brown)	150 mL
¼ cup	cornstarch	60 mL
2 tbsp	butter, cut into small pieces	30 mL
2 tsp	vanilla extract	10 mL

Stovetop Method

1. In a medium saucepan, whisk together milk and egg yolks. Stir in sugar and cornstarch until smooth. Cook over medium heat, stirring constantly, for about 7 minutes or until pudding comes to a full boil and thickens. Remove from heat. Stir in butter and vanilla until butter is melted.

Microwave Method

1. In an 8-cup (2 L) glass bowl or casserole dish, whisk together milk and egg yolks. Stir in sugar and cornstarch until smooth. Microwave, uncovered, on High for 3 minutes. Whisk well. Microwave on High for 2 to 4 minutes, whisking every minute, until pudding comes to a full boil and thickens. Stir in butter and vanilla until butter is melted.

For Both Methods

2. Pour pudding into individual serving dishes. Serve warm or cold. If serving cold, let cool slightly, and place plastic wrap directly on the surface to prevent the formation of a skin.

This recipe should be adjusted based on your symptoms. Follow this symptom guide:

To encourage weight gain:
- Use whole milk or replace the milk with half-and-half (10%) cream or table (18%) cream; and/or
- Serve topped with lightly sweetened whipped cream.

Nutritional Analysis per Serving

Calories...........235	Sodium........ 53 mg	Fiber .... 0 g
Fat............... 9 g	Carbohydrate..... 33 g	Protein .... 5 g

Makes 4 servings

This is a less sweet version of an old-fashioned family favorite.

Tips

Placing puddings in a water bath to bake helps them to stay moist and cook evenly.

Serve with fresh berries to add vitamins and antioxidants.

This pudding is best eaten warm the day it's made. Leftovers can be covered and refrigerated for up to 1 day.

Survivor Wisdom

When my mother-in-law had cancer, I thought, What would taste good? So I made custard and brought it over. She said, "Oh, I hate custard." I should have asked first.

Lemon Pudding

- **Preheat oven to 350°F (180°C)**
- **4-cup (1 L) baking dish, lightly greased**
- **Larger pan to fit baking dish**

⅓ cup	granulated sugar	75 mL
2 tbsp	all-purpose flour	30 mL
Pinch	salt	Pinch
	Grated zest and juice of 1 lemon	
2	large eggs, separated, yolks beaten	2
1 cup	milk	250 mL
	Boiling water	

1. In a bowl, combine sugar, flour and salt. Stir in lemon zest, lemon juice, egg yolks and milk.
2. In a separate, straight-sided bowl, using an electric mixer, beat egg whites until stiff but not dry; fold into lemon mixture.
3. Pour into prepared baking dish. Place in larger pan; pour in boiling water to about 1-inch (2.5 cm) depth. Bake in preheated oven for about 30 minutes or until topping is set and golden brown. Serve warm.

This recipe courtesy of Valerie Caldicott.

Nutritional Analysis per Serving

Calories..........124	Sodium.......171 mg	Fiber.............1 g
Fat...............3 g	Carbohydrate.....19 g	Protein...........6 g

Makes 6 servings

This tasty pudding, combining luscious apples with hearty oatmeal, is an adaptation of a traditional Irish recipe. If you need extra calories, add a dollop of freshly whipped cream.

Tips

Regular milk may curdle in the slow cooker, but evaporated milk stays nice and creamy. For a non-dairy choice, rice milk or almond milk work best in this recipe, as they have a milder flavor than soy milk.

Choose tart baking apples that hold their shape when baked, such as Empire, Granny Smith, Ida Red or Northern Spy.

This pudding is best eaten warm the day it's made. Leftovers can be covered and refrigerated for up to 2 days.

Rolled and steel-cut oats contain the bran layer of the grain, which provides minerals, antioxidants, plant lignans and fiber. Plant lignans appear to protect against breast cancer. Enjoying oatmeal in a dessert is one way to increase your intake of healthy whole grains.

Apple Oatmeal Pudding

- **Works best in a small (3½ quart) slow cooker**
- **Greased slow cooker stoneware**

2 tbsp	melted butter	30 mL
1 cup	large-flake (old-fashioned) rolled oats	250 mL
⅓ cup	packed brown sugar	75 mL
½ cup	all-purpose flour	125 mL
1 tsp	baking soda	5 mL
Pinch	salt	Pinch
2	large eggs, beaten	2
1 cup	2% evaporated milk or rice or almond milk	250 mL
6	apples, peeled, thinly sliced	6
1 tbsp	freshly squeezed lemon juice	15 mL
1 tbsp	packed brown sugar	15 mL
1 tsp	ground cinnamon	5 mL

1. In a bowl, mix together butter, oats and ⅓ cup (75 mL) sugar. Stir in flour, baking soda and salt. Gradually add eggs and milk, mixing until blended. Spoon into prepared slow cooker stoneware.

2. In a separate bowl, combine apples, lemon juice, 1 tbsp (15 mL) sugar and cinnamon. Spread evenly over oatmeal mixture. Cover and cook on High for 3½ to 4 hours, until apples are tender. Let cool slightly; serve warm.

This recipe should be adjusted based on your symptoms. Follow this symptom guide:

For sore mouth or throat:
- Use apples that soften and lose their shape when cooked, such as McIntosh or Cortland.

To encourage weight gain:
- Serve with vanilla ice cream; and/or
- Sprinkle with toasted chopped pecans.

Nutritional Analysis per Serving

Calories.......... 350	Sodium....... 462 mg	Fiber .... 5 g
Fat............... 8 g	Carbohydrate..... 64 g	Protein .... 8 g

Makes 6 to 8 servings

Not only is this old-fashioned dessert great comfort food, it is also very versatile. It is delicious served with fresh berries, a dollop of whipped cream or a scoop of vanilla ice cream.

Tip

Stone-ground cornmeal is a whole grain and is therefore more nutritious than refined varieties. Look for it in the natural foods section of well-stocked supermarkets or at bulk or health food stores. Store in a sealable plastic bag in the refrigerator or freezer for up to 1 year.

Make Ahead

Portion the pudding into airtight containers, let cool, cover and refrigerate for up to 3 days. Reheat in the microwave on Medium-High (70%) for 2 to 3 minutes or until steaming. Stir in additional milk or water to thin to desired consistency.

Cornmeal Pudding

- **Works best in a small (3½ quart) slow cooker**
- **Greased slow cooker stoneware**

4 cups	milk	1 L
½ cup	stone-ground yellow cornmeal	125 mL
2	large eggs	2
1 tbsp	extra virgin olive oil	15 mL
½ cup	light (fancy) molasses	125 mL
½ tsp	ground ginger	2 mL
½ tsp	ground cinnamon	2 mL
½ tsp	freshly grated nutmeg	2 mL
½ tsp	salt	2 mL
	Fresh berries (optional)	

1. In a saucepan, heat milk over medium-high heat, stirring often to prevent scorching, until boiling. Gradually whisk in cornmeal in a steady stream. Cook, stirring, until mixture begins to thicken and bubbles like lava, about 5 minutes. Remove from heat.

2. In a small bowl, whisk eggs until blended. Pour in about ½ cup (125 mL) of the hot cornmeal, whisking until combined. Gradually return to pot, mixing well. Stir in olive oil, molasses, ginger, cinnamon, nutmeg and salt. Transfer to prepared slow cooker stoneware.

3. Cover and cook on High for 3 hours, until set. Spoon into individual serving bowls and top with fresh berries, if using. Serve warm.

This recipe should be adjusted based on your symptoms. Follow this symptom guide:

To encourage weight gain:
- Use whole milk or replace 1 to 2 cups (250 to 500 mL) of the milk with half-and-half (10%) cream or table (18%) cream; and/or
- Serve topped with ice cream or sweetened whipped cream.

Nutritional Analysis per Serving

Calories..........188	Sodium....... 223 mg	Fiber .... 1 g
Fat .... 5 g	Carbohydrate..... 28 g	Protein .... 6 g

Makes 8 servings

This traditional Indian pudding has an unusual thickener: dried split peas. The benefits? Added protein, fiber and nutrients. Exotic and delicious, the pudding has a light banana flavor enhanced by sweet dates and the texture of crunchy toasted almonds.

Tips

The dates in this pudding add sweetness, fiber and a range of minerals, including potassium.

Almonds deliver more than just flavor and texture; they also provide significant health benefits. They are one of the best food sources of vitamin E, an antioxidant. They also contain magnesium, folate, iron and several important phytonutrients, as well as healthy monounsaturated fats.

Indian Banana Pudding

- **Works best in a small (3½ quart) slow cooker**
- **Greased slow cooker stoneware**
- **Blender or food processor**

½ cup	yellow split peas, rinsed and picked through	125 mL
1½ cups	water	375 mL
1 tbsp	minced gingerroot	15 mL
¼ cup	packed brown sugar	60 mL
1	can (14 oz/398 mL) coconut milk	1
½ tsp	almond extract	2 mL
1 tsp	ground cardamom or cinnamon	5 mL
2	ripe bananas, chopped	2
¼ cup	finely chopped pitted soft dates, preferably Medjool	60 mL
½ cup	toasted slivered almonds, divided	125 mL
	Whipped cream, optional	

1. In a saucepan, combine split peas and water. Cover and bring to a boil over high heat. Reduce heat and boil for 3 minutes. Turn off heat and let soak for 1 hour. Drain and rinse thoroughly under cold water.

2. In blender, combine soaked peas, ginger, sugar and ½ cup (125 mL) of the coconut milk; blend until smooth. Add remaining coconut milk, almond extract and cardamom; blend to combine. Pour into prepared slow cooker stoneware.

3. Place a tea towel folded in half (so you will have two layers) over top of stoneware to absorb moisture. Cover and cook on High for 3 hours, until peas are tender and mixture begins to thicken. Stir in bananas. Replace folded towel and cook on High for 30 minutes.

Tip

Pour pudding directly into individual airtight containers with tight-fitting lids, let cool, then cover and refrigerate to pack in a cooler to take along to appointments. Don't forget to pack a spoon.

Make Ahead

Refrigerate pudding, covered, for up to 3 days. Serve cold or reheat in the microwave on Medium-High (70%) for 2 to 3 minutes or until steaming. Stir in some milk or water to thin to desired consistency.

Survivor Wisdom

When I was sick, I asked my mom to make Jell-O for me. She made a double portion in a large metal pan and told me it was in the fridge. I wish she had portioned it out for me in little fruit cups, because once I saw that big metal pan, I couldn't eat any of it.

4. Remove stoneware from casing and, using a wooden spoon, beat mixture vigorously. Fold in dates and half the almonds. Transfer to a bowl or airtight container. Cover and refrigerate for about 1½ hours or until thoroughly chilled. Serve sprinkled with remaining almonds and a dollop of whipped cream (if using).

This recipe should be adjusted based on your symptoms. Follow this symptom guide:

For sore mouth or throat or dry mouth:
- Omit the toasted almonds and stir 2 to 3 tsp (10 to 15 mL) smooth almond butter into each serving.

Nutritional Analysis per Serving

Calories..........255	Sodium..........9 mg	Fiber.............5 g
Fat..............15 g	Carbohydrate.....28 g	Protein...........6 g

Makes 6 servings

When it comes to comfort food, many people put rice pudding at the top of the list. It's creamy, luscious and oh so satisfying.

Tips

If short-grain rice is unavailable, use long-grain rice (not converted). Long-grain rice is not as starchy, so reduce the amount of milk to 4 cups (1 L) total. Combine the rice with 3½ cups (875 mL) of the milk and continue with the recipe as directed.

Add 1 tbsp (15 mL) butter to the rice mixture to reduce the amount of foam.

Make Ahead

Portion the pudding into airtight containers, let cool, cover and refrigerate for up to 2 days. Serve cold or reheat in the microwave on Medium-High (70%) for 2 to 3 minutes or until steaming. Stir in additional milk or water to thin to desired consistency.

Creamy Rice Pudding

½ cup	short-grain rice, such as Arborio	125 mL
5 cups	whole milk, divided	1.25 L
⅓ cup	granulated sugar	75 mL
¼ tsp	salt	1 mL
1	large egg yolk	1
¼ cup	sultana raisins	60 mL
1 tsp	vanilla extract	5 mL
	Ground cinnamon (optional)	

1. In a large saucepan, combine rice, 4½ cups (1.125 L) milk, sugar and salt. Bring to a boil; reduce heat to medium-low and simmer, partially covered, stirring occasionally, for 45 to 50 minutes or until rice is tender and mixture has thickened.

2. Beat together remaining ½ cup (125 mL) milk and egg yolk; stir into rice mixture, stirring, for 1 minute or until creamy. Remove from heat. Stir in raisins and vanilla.

3. Serve either warm or at room temperature. (Pudding thickens slightly as it cools.) Sprinkle with cinnamon, if desired.

This recipe should be adjusted based on your symptoms. Follow this symptom guide:

To encourage weight gain:
- Replace 1 to 2 cups (250 to 500 mL) of the milk with half-and-half (10%) cream or table (18%) cream.

If food tastes metallic or bitter:
- Omit the vanilla and add two 2-inch (5 cm) strips of lemon zest to the rice mixture before cooking. Discard before serving.

Nutritional Analysis per Serving

Calories...........236	Sodium....... 187 mg	Fiber .... 1 g
Fat .... 7 g	Carbohydrate ..... 35 g	Protein .... 8 g

Makes 8 servings

Rice pudding is a comfort food favorite that never seems to go out of style. This version uses brown rice and is enhanced with spices, dried fruits and nuts.

Tips

For 1 cup (250 mL) cooked brown rice, cook ⅓ cup (75 mL) long-grain brown rice with ⅔ cup (150 mL) water. For other types of rice, follow package directions.

Freshly grated nutmeg has more aroma and flavor than ground. If you only have ground, it is fine to use it, but try grinding fresh sometime — you will really taste and smell the difference.

Make Ahead

Portion the pudding into airtight containers, let cool, cover and refrigerate for up to 2 days. Serve cold or reheat in the microwave on Medium-High (70%) for 2 to 3 minutes or until steaming. Stir in additional milk or water to thin to desired consistency.

Indian-Style Rice Pudding

- **Preheat oven to 350°F (180°C)**
- **8-cup (2 L) glass baking dish with cover**
- **Baking sheet**

1 cup	cooked brown rice (any type)	250 mL
1	can (14 oz/398 mL) light coconut milk	1
3 cups	milk	750 mL
½ cup	raisins	125 mL
¼ cup	finely chopped almonds	60 mL
¼ cup	unsweetened shredded coconut	60 mL
¼ cup	granulated sugar	60 mL
½ tsp	ground cardamom	2 mL
1	cinnamon stick, about 4 inches (10 cm) long	1
½ tsp	grated nutmeg (see tip, at left)	2 mL

1. Place rice in baking dish. Add coconut milk, milk, raisins, almonds, coconut, sugar, cardamom and cinnamon stick.

2. Cover dish and place on baking sheet. Bake in preheated oven for 1 hour or until sauce has thickened. Discard cinnamon stick. Serve warm or refrigerate for about 4 hours, until chilled. Sprinkle with nutmeg.

This recipe courtesy of Eileen Campbell.

This recipe should be adjusted based on your symptoms. Follow this symptom guide:

To encourage weight gain:
- Use regular (full-fat) coconut milk instead of light; and/or
- Use whole milk or replace 1 to 2 cups (250 to 500 mL) of the milk with half-and-half (10%) cream or table (18%) cream; and/or
- Stir 1 to 2 tbsp (15 to 30 mL) butter into the hot pudding after baking.

Nutritional Analysis per Serving

Calories..........208	Sodium........ 64 mg	Fiber .... 2 g
Fat .... 9 g	Carbohydrate ..... 28 g	Protein .... 5 g

Makes 8 servings

On a comfort scale, bread pudding, with its old-fashioned appeal, rates as one of the most-loved desserts. This simple version, featuring cinnamon bread in a custard base, takes no time to put together.

Make Ahead

Portion the pudding into airtight containers, let cool, cover and refrigerate for up to 2 days or freeze for up to 2 months. If frozen, thaw in the microwave or refrigerator. Serve cold or reheat in the microwave on Medium-High (70%) for 2 to 3 minutes or until steaming. Moisten with additional milk, if desired.

Cinnamon Raisin Bread Pudding

- Preheat oven to 375°F (190°C)
- Rimmed baking sheets
- 10-cup (2.5 L) shallow glass baking dish, generously buttered
- Large shallow roasting pan or deep broiler pan

12	slices cinnamon raisin swirl bread (1 lb/500 g loaf)	12
6	large eggs	6
2 cups	whole milk	500 mL
1 cup	half-and-half (10%) cream	250 mL
¾ cup	granulated sugar	175 mL
2 tsp	vanilla extract	10 mL
	Boiling water	

Topping

2 tbsp	granulated sugar	30 mL
½ tsp	ground cinnamon	2 mL

1. Place bread slices in a single layer on baking sheets and lightly toast in preheated oven for 10 to 12 minutes. Let cool. Leave oven on. Cut bread into cubes and place in prepared baking dish.

2. In a bowl, whisk together eggs, milk, cream, ¾ cup (175 mL) sugar and vanilla. Pour over bread. Let soak for 10 minutes, pressing down gently with a spatula.

3. *Topping:* In a small bowl, combine 2 tbsp (30 mL) sugar and cinnamon. Sprinkle over top.

4. Place baking dish in roasting or broiler pan; add enough boiling water to come halfway up sides of dish. Bake in preheated oven for 45 to 50 minutes or until top is puffed and custard is set in center. Remove from water bath; place on a wire rack to cool. Serve warm or at room temperature.

Nutritional Analysis per Serving

Calories..........291	Sodium.......243 mg	Fiber.............2 g
Fat..............10 g	Carbohydrate.....42 g	Protein..........11 g

---

Soothing Ice Pops and Refreshing Beverages

Hydration, hydration, hydration. This should be the mantra of the cancer patient. Maintaining hydration has many benefits: flushing out by-products of toxic chemotherapy, maintaining blood pressure, replacing lost fluids, keeping the bowels regular and keeping nausea at bay. In addition, fluids are usually better accepted than solid food when your appetite is off and, of course, are much more appealing to those with a sore mouth or throat. Some patients have such a bad taste lingering in their mouth that numbing it is their best approach. That's where ice pops come in handy. These ice pops and beverages provide great taste, as well as nourishment and hydration.

Fruit Frenzy Pops

Makes 16 small pops

If you are only able to consume liquids and frozen pops and are worried about where the bulk in your diet might come from, give these fiber-full frozen fruit pops a try.

Tips

If you can't use bananas that are becoming ripe, pop them into a sealable plastic bag and freeze them. They will turn black, but once they are thawed and the skins are removed, they make a perfect addition to smoothies.

Bananas are one of the few fruits that are recommended if you have diarrhea.

Survivor Wisdom

When your immune system is fried and you get a cold, having a frozen fruit pop on hand is helpful.

- **Food processor or blender**
- **Small ice pop molds**

1	very ripe banana	1
1½ cups	bran cereal or bran flakes cereal	375 mL
1 cup	hulled strawberries	250 mL
10 oz	silken tofu	300 g
2 cups	probiotic plain yogurt	500 mL
¾ cup	frozen orange juice concentrate (½ can)	175 mL

1. In food processor or blender, combine banana, bran cereal and strawberries and blend until smooth (if using a blender, you may have to add the orange juice concentrate to help purée). Add tofu, yogurt and orange juice concentrate and blend until well combined.

2. Pour into molds and freeze until firm, about 6 hours. Keep frozen for up to 2 weeks.

This recipe courtesy of Anne-Christine Giguère, Sabrina Tremblay and Cindy Martel.

Nutritional Analysis per Pop

Calories............56	Sodium........ 29 mg	Fiber .... 1 g
Fat............... 2 g	Carbohydrate...... 8 g	Protein .... 3 g

These refreshing pops are a nutritious alternative to sweeter frozen treats. Use different puréed fruits or frozen fruit juice concentrates to vary the flavors. Transfer from the freezer to the refrigerator a few minutes before serving.

Icy Yogurt Pops

- **Large ice pop molds or paper cups**

1 cup	probiotic plain yogurt	250 mL
¾ cup	frozen juice concentrate, thawed, or puréed fruit	175 mL
¾ cup	milk	175 mL

1. Combine yogurt, fruit juice concentrate and milk. Pour into ice pop molds (or small paper cups, freeze until partially frozen and insert a wooden stick into center of each). Freeze for about 6 hours or until firm. Keep frozen for up to 2 weeks.

This recipe courtesy of Barbara Hudec.

Nutritional Analysis per Pop

Calories............41	Sodium........ 24 mg	Fiber .... 0 g
Fat............... 2 g	Carbohydrate...... 5 g	Protein .... 2 g

This great treat is healthier than store-bought Popsicles. Adapt the recipe to suit your preferences in fruit and yogurt. Papaya contains the enzyme papase, which may help with thick, ropey saliva.

Healthy Frozen Pops

- **Large ice pop molds**

1 cup	probiotic vanilla-flavored yogurt	250 mL
1 cup	finely chopped fruit (strawberry, blueberry, raspberry, mango, papaya, etc.)	250 mL

1. Spoon half of the yogurt into the bottom of ice pop molds, dividing equally. Top with fruit, then spoon in remaining yogurt. Freeze for about 6 hours or until firm. Keep frozen for up to 2 weeks.

This recipe courtesy of Doris Oullet.

Nutritional Analysis per Pop

Calories............49	Sodium........ 27 mg	Fiber .... 1 g
Fat............... 1 g	Carbohydrate...... 9 g	Protein .... 2 g

Makes 4 large pops

You'll love this unusual recipe, whether it's frozen or served as a pudding (just refrigerate in bowls until chilled instead of freezing). You don't even have to like avocado!

Tips

Pure vanilla contains a nutraceutical called vanillin. Nutraceuticals are nutrients that provide a medical or health benefit.

About 70% of the calories in an avocado come from fat, but most of this is the beneficial monounsaturated fat. In addition, they contain more potassium than a banana, B vitamins and the fat-soluble vitamins E and K.

Cocoa contains a type of flavanol called proanthocyanidins, which are natural antioxidants. To get the highest amount of these beneficial components, choose natural dark cocoa, not "dutched" or alkalized cocoa powder.

Chocolate Surprise Pudding Pops

- **Blender**
- **Large ice pop molds**

1	large avocado, peeled and pitted	1
1	very ripe banana	1
½ cup	milk	125 mL
2 tbsp	unsweetened cocoa powder	30 mL
1 tbsp	liquid honey	15 mL
1 tsp	vanilla extract	5 mL

1. In blender, combine avocado, banana, milk, cocoa powder, honey and vanilla and blend until smooth.
2. Pour into ice pop molds and freeze for about 6 hours or until firm. Keep frozen for up to 2 weeks.

This recipe courtesy of Donna Suerich.

Nutritional Analysis per Pop

Calories..........148	Sodium........ 17 mg	Fiber .... 5 g
Fat............... 8 g	Carbohydrate..... 18 g	Protein .... 3 g

Makes 8 pops

Here's a unique and fun way to enjoy the beneficial effects of green tea.

Tip

Japanese green tea tends to test higher in beneficial EGCG than other green teas. In their book *Foods That Fight Cancer*, Richard Béliveau and Denis Gingras found that the tea that ranked highest in EGCG content was Sencha-Uchiyama.

Survivor Wisdom

I had to take terrible-tasting contrast dye before my ultrasounds, and having a frozen pop beforehand helped to numb my mouth so that I wouldn't taste the dye.

Green Tea Pops

- Small ice pop molds

1 tbsp	green tea leaves (or 2 tea bags)	15 mL
1 cup	boiling water	250 mL
2 tbsp	agave nectar or liquid honey	30 mL
¾ cup	orange juice	175 mL
2 tbsp	freshly squeezed lemon juice	30 mL

1. In a measuring cup or tea pot, combine green tea and boiling water; let steep for 5 to 8 minutes or until flavorful. Strain through a fine sieve (or discard tea bags), without squeezing leaves, into another measuring cup or container with a pouring spout.

2. Stir in agave nectar until nectar is dissolved. Let cool to room temperature. Stir in orange juice and lemon juice.

3. Pour into molds and freeze until firm, about 4 hours or overnight. Keep frozen for up to 2 weeks.

Nutritional Analysis per Pop

Calories............28	Sodium..........0 mg	Fiber..............0 g
Fat...............0 g	Carbohydrate......7 g	Protein...........0 g

This shake, with only three ingredients, goes together quickly, for a carbohydrate and protein combination you can enjoy any time of day. The skim milk powder adds thickness and boosts the calcium and protein content.

Sunny Orange Shake

- Blender

¾ cup	probiotic vanilla-flavored yogurt	175 mL
2 tbsp	instant skim milk powder	30 mL
½ cup	orange juice	125 mL

1. In blender, combine yogurt, skim-milk powder and orange juice; blend until smooth.

This recipe courtesy of Dairy Farmers of Canada.

Nutritional Analysis per Serving

Calories..........199	Sodium.......133 mg	Fiber.............0 g
Fat...............6 g	Carbohydrate.....26 g	Protein..........10 g

Combining banana, which contains prebiotic fiber, with a probiotic yogurt is an excellent way to improve the balance of healthy bacteria in your digestive tract.

Variation

Instead of the vanilla-flavored yogurt, use any flavor that complements the berries you chose.

Banana Berry Wake-Up Shake

- Blender

1	banana	1
1 cup	fresh or frozen berries (any combination)	250 mL
1 cup	milk or vanilla-flavored soy beverage	250 mL
¾ cup	probiotic vanilla-flavored yogurt	175 mL

1. In blender, combine fruit with a small amount of the milk and blend until smooth. Add remaining milk and yogurt; blend until smooth. If shake is too thick, add extra milk to achieve desired consistency. Serve immediately.

This recipe courtesy of Ann Merritt.

Nutritional Analysis per Serving

Calories..........207	Sodium.......112 mg	Fiber.............3 g
Fat...............5 g	Carbohydrate.....35 g	Protein..........8 g

Whoever said milkshakes aren't healthy hasn't tried this nutritious, delicious version.

Tip

If you prefer, you can substitute granulated sugar for the maple syrup.

Chocolate Nut Shake

- **Blender**

2 tsp	unsweetened cocoa powder	10 mL
1½ tbsp	natural almond butter, whole almonds or peanut butter	22 mL
⅓ cup	milk	75 mL
2 tsp	pure maple syrup (approx.)	10 mL
¼ cup	ice cubes	60 mL
2 tbsp	unflavored whey protein powder	30 mL

1. In blender, combine cocoa, almond butter, milk and maple syrup and blend until smooth. Add ice cubes and protein powder (if using) and blend until slushy. Sweeten with more syrup to taste, if desired. Serve immediately.

Nutritional Analysis per Serving

Calories...........254	Sodium........ 104 mg	Fiber .... 4 g
Fat .... 16 g	Carbohydrate ..... 17 g	Protein .... 16 g

Bananas are very appealing if you have mouth sores, thanks to their lack of acidity.

Banana Smoothie

- **Blender**

1	ripe banana	1
½ cup	probiotic plain yogurt	125 mL
½ cup	water	125 mL
½ cup	milk	125 mL
3	ice cubes	3

1. In blender, combine banana, yogurt, water, milk and ice and blend until smooth. Serve immediately.

This recipe courtesy of dietitian Jill Miller.

Nutritional Analysis per Serving

Calories...........120	Sodium........ 54 mg	Fiber .... 2 g
Fat .... 3 g	Carbohydrate ..... 19 g	Protein .... 5 g

Makes 4 servings

This smoothie, adapted from a recipe on the back of a tofu package, tastes sweet and rich, like dessert!

Tip

For extra frothiness, add 1 cup (250 mL) crushed ice when blending.

Pour into a chilled insulated cup or Thermos for a smoothie to go.

Survivor Wisdom

My kids would buy me milkshakes, and that was the only thing I could eat for a long time.

Decadent Fruit Smoothie

- **Blender**

1	ripe banana	1
10 oz	peach-mango-flavored or other fruit-flavored dessert tofu	300 g
1 cup	frozen peach or mango slices	250 mL
1 cup	orange juice	250 mL
	Liquid honey or granulated sugar (optional)	

1. In blender, combine banana, tofu, peach slices and orange juice and blend until smooth.
2. Sweeten with honey to taste, if desired. Serve cold.

This recipe courtesy of Eileen Campbell.

Nutritional Analysis per Serving

Calories..........149	Sodium........ 26 mg	Fiber .... 2 g
Fat............... 2 g	Carbohydrate..... 31 g	Protein .... 4 g

Makes 1 serving

You don't need an expensive juicer to make this über-healthy smoothie that will have you feeling empowered for the day.

Tip

Look for whey protein powder at health food and bulk food stores. Most come flavored as chocolate, strawberry or vanilla, although some are plain and some are sweetened. If you want the flavor of fresh fruit to be more dominant in your smoothie or shake, choose a plain protein powder. Read labels and buy the protein powder with the fewest ingredients — many have multiple unnecessary additives. Alternatively, old-fashioned and less expensive skim milk powder also gives an excellent protein boost.

Green Power Smoothie

- Blender

¼ cup	frozen chopped spinach (about 1 nugget)	60 mL
½	frozen banana, broken into chunks	½
¼	apple, chopped	¼
¼ cup	whey protein powder	60 mL
1 tbsp	ground flax seeds	15 mL
¼ cup	probiotic plain yogurt	60 mL
1 tbsp	liquid honey or agave nectar (approx.)	15 mL

1. In blender, combine spinach, banana, apple, protein powder, flax seeds, yogurt and honey and blend until smooth.

2. Sweeten with more honey to taste, if desired. Serve immediately.

Nutritional Analysis per Serving

Calories..........316	Sodium........ 98 mg	Fiber .... 5 g
Fat .... 7 g	Carbohydrate ..... 45 g	Protein .... 32 g

---

Makes 1 serving

Blueberries and green tea are two foods that should rank high on your cancer-fighting menu.

Tip

If you are nauseated or put off by food, try drinking from a cup with a lid and a straw.

Survivor Wisdom

The anxiety prior to chemo made it hard to eat.

Blueberry Green Tea Smoothie

- **Blender**

2 tsp	green tea leaves (or 1 bag)	10 mL
½ cup	boiling water	125 mL
1 tbsp	liquid honey or agave nectar	15 mL
½ cup	frozen blueberries	125 mL
½ cup	probiotic plain yogurt	125 mL

1. In a measuring cup or tea pot, combine green tea and boiling water; let steep for 8 minutes. Strain through a fine sieve (or discard tea bags), without squeezing leaves, into a bowl or container. Stir in honey until dissolved. Cover and refrigerate for at least 1 hour, until chilled, or for up to 1 day.

2. In blender, combine chilled tea, blueberries and yogurt and blend until smooth. Serve immediately.

Nutritional Analysis per Serving

Calories..........185	Sodium........ 57 mg	Fiber .... 2 g
Fat.............. 4 g	Carbohydrate..... 33 g	Protein .... 5 g

Makes 1 serving

Tropical fruit flavors get an even more exotic twist with a touch of coconut milk in this thick and decadent smoothie.

Tip

For a thinner texture, use a fresh banana rather than a frozen one.

Island Smoothie

- **Blender**

½	frozen ripe banana, broken in half	½
½ cup	frozen mango or pineapple cubes	250 mL
¼ cup	coconut milk	60 mL
¼ cup	probiotic plain yogurt	60 mL
1 tsp	vanilla extract	5 mL
	Agave nectar or liquid honey (optional)	

1. In blender, combine banana, mango, coconut milk, yogurt and vanilla and blend until smooth.
2. Sweeten with agave nectar to taste, if desired. Serve immediately.

Nutritional Analysis per Serving

Calories..........274	Sodium........ 37 mg	Fiber .... 4 g
Fat............. 14 g	Carbohydrate..... 35 g	Protein .... 5 g

Makes 2 servings

The idea for this refreshing cooler came from the beaches of southern Thailand. Carts line the beach, offering fruit concoctions to cool you down in the tropical heat. It's the perfect drink if you're feeling overheated.

Tropical Cooler

- **Blender**

1	ripe banana	1
1 cup	diced seedless watermelon	250 mL
1 cup	pineapple juice	250 mL
	Ice cubes (optional)	

1. In blender, combine banana, watermelon and pineapple juice until smooth and creamy. Serve over ice, if desired.

This recipe courtesy of Eileen Campbell.

Nutritional Analysis per Serving

Calories..........145	Sodium.........3 mg	Fiber .... 2 g
Fat............... 0 g	Carbohydrate..... 36 g	Protein .... 2 g

Makes 2 servings

This refreshing drink is a favorite at Indian restaurants. Now you can make it at home and taste why it's so popular.

Mango Lassi

- **Blender**

1	ripe mango, chopped (or 1 cup/250 mL frozen chopped mango)	1
½ cup	probiotic plain or vanilla-flavored yogurt	125 mL
½ cup	milk	125 mL
	Liquid honey	
½ cup	ice cubes	125 mL

1. In blender, combine mango, yogurt, milk, honey to taste and ice and blend until smooth. Serve immediately.

This recipe courtesy of Eileen Campbell.

Nutritional Analysis per Serving

Calories...........190	Sodium........ 72 mg	Fiber .... 3 g
Fat............... 3 g	Carbohydrate..... 39 g	Protein .... 6 g

---

Makes 1 serving

This beautiful beverage is like aromatherapy in a glass. The flavors of mint, melon, ginger and apple layer together effortlessly to create the ideal balance between refreshing and soothing.

Melon Mint Frosty

- **Blender**

4	fresh mint leaves	4
½ cup	frozen chopped melon (watermelon, cantaloupe or honeydew)	125 mL
½ cup	ginger ale	125 mL
¼ cup	unsweetened apple or cranberry juice	60 mL

1. In blender, combine mint, melon, ginger ale and apple juice and blend until smooth. Serve immediately.

Nutritional Analysis per Serving

Calories...........99	Sodium........ 29 mg	Fiber .... 1 g
Fat............... 0 g	Carbohydrate..... 25 g	Protein .... 1 g

This recipe from the World Health Organization is for those times when you find yourself dehydrated and without any store-bought oral electrolyte replacement on hand. It is meant to be sipped by the teaspoon (5 mL). Measure carefully.

Electrolyte Drink

2 tbsp	granulated sugar	30 mL
½ tsp	salt	2 mL
4 cups	water	1 L

1. In a container, combine sugar, salt and water, stirring well to dissolve sugar and salt. Drink small amounts frequently.

Nutritional Analysis per 2 tbsp (30 mL)

Calories............2	Sodium........ 36 mg	Fiber .... 0 g
Fat.............. 0 g	Carbohydrate...... 1 g	Protein .... 0 g

Ginger is soothing and, along with green tea, makes a refreshing iced tea. Adding the tea leaves to cold water and letting it steep slowly reduces bitterness from the tea.

Survivor Wisdom

I would cut limes into wedges and freeze them, then use them as my ice cubes.

Iced Ginger Green Tea

2 tbsp	chopped gingerroot	30 mL
4 cups	water, divided	1 L
¼ cup	honey	60 mL
2 tbsp	green tea leaves (or 4 tea bags)	30 mL
	Ice cubes	

1. In a small saucepan, combine ginger, ½ cup (125 mL) of the water and honey. Bring to a boil over medium heat. Reduce heat and simmer for about 10 minutes or until ginger is translucent and flavor is infused. Let cool.

2. Pour ginger syrup into a pitcher or other container; add remaining water and tea leaves. Cover and refrigerate for at least 8 hours, until tea is infused or overnight. Strain through a tea strainer or fine mesh sieve and discard ginger and tea leaves (do not squeeze). Serve immediately or store covered in refrigerator for up to 3 days. Serve cold over ice.

Nutritional Analysis per Serving

Calories...........70	Sodium..........0 mg	Fiber .... 0 g
Fat.............. 0 g	Carbohydrate..... 18 g	Protein .... 0 g

Makes 4 servings

This drink was served during a focus group with the cancer survivors who provided the "survivor wisdom" seen throughout this book. Everyone agreed it would be something they would drink during their treatment.

Grape Juice Sangria

1 cup	grape juice	250 mL
½ cup	orange juice	125 mL
3 cups	sparkling water	750 mL
1	orange, cut into wedges	1
	Ice cubes	

1. In a jug, combine grape juice, orange juice, sparkling water and orange wedges. (Store covered in refrigerator for up to 2 days). Serve over ice.

This recipe courtesy of dietitian Donna Bottrell.

Nutritional Analysis per Serving

Calories 58	Sodium . . . . 1 mg	Fiber . . . . 1 g
Fat . . . . 0 g	Carbohydrate . . . . . 14 g	Protein . . . . 1 g

Makes 1 serving

Cloves rank highest of all the spices in antioxidant content. Chai tea features cloves, as well as other beneficial spices, such as cinnamon, ginger, cardamom, nutmeg, black pepper and vanilla. Like the Mexican Hot Chocolate (page 303), this hot drink can be an appealing replacement for coffee.

Vanilla Chai Latte

1	chai tea bag	1
2 tsp	granulated sugar, agave nectar or liquid honey	10 mL
1 cup	milk	250 mL
1 tsp	vanilla extract	5 mL

1. In a saucepan, combine tea bag, sugar and milk. Bring to a simmer over medium-low heat, stirring occasionally (do not let boil). Remove from heat, cover and let steep for 5 to 8 minutes or until desired flavor is infused.

2. Discard tea bag, without squeezing tea bag (or strain through a fine-mesh sieve) and stir in vanilla. Pour into a mug and serve hot.

Nutritional Analysis per Serving

Calories 155	Sodium . . . . 100 mg	Fiber . . . . 0 g
Fat . . . . 5 g	Carbohydrate . . . . . 18 g	Protein . . . . 8 g

Recommended for:
- Constipation
- Dehydration
- Taste alterations

Bonus features:
- High protein
- Risk reduction

Makes 6 servings

Food aversions are very common during cancer treatment, and an aversion to coffee is one of the most common. Drinking a hot beverage can be beneficial for regular bowel movements, so if coffee no longer appeals to you, try this recipe.

Tip

If you have a manual milk frother, whirl the hot chocolate until very frothy before serving.

Survivor Wisdom

When it came to muscle strength, I had issues for a year post-treatment, despite the fact that I looked good.

Mexican Hot Chocolate

½ cup	granulated sugar	125 mL
½ cup	water	125 mL
⅓ cup	unsweetened cocoa powder	75 mL
½ tsp	ground cinnamon	2 mL
5 cups	milk	1.25 L
½ tsp	vanilla extract	2 mL
½ tsp	almond extract	2 mL

1. In a large saucepan, over medium heat, heat sugar, water, cocoa powder and cinnamon until sugar dissolves. Add milk; heat until steaming (do not boil). Remove from heat and stir in vanilla and almond extract. (Let any extra hot chocolate cool, then refrigerate in an airtight container for up to 2 days. Stir well and reheat individual portions in a saucepan or microwave.)

This recipe courtesy of Eileen Campbell.

Nutritional Analysis per Serving

Calories..........178	Sodium..........85 g	Fiber.............2 g
Fat..............5 g	Carbohydrate.....29 g	Protein..........8 g

Contributing Authors

Johanna Burkhard
500 Best Comfort Food Recipes
Recipes from this book are found on pages
161, 163, 167, 168, 173, 177, 178, 180,
183, 195, 204, 209, 210, 214, 215, 234,
241, 244, 245, 246, 255, 269, 278, 279, 286
and 288.

Dietitians of Canada
Cook Great Food
Recipes from this book are found on pages
148, 149, 153, 156, 162, 176, 179, 184,
185, 186, 187, 189, 191 (top), 193, 194,
198, 202, 203, 208, 213, 216, 219, 220,
221, 222, 223, 240, 264, 268, 270, 275,
276, 277, 281, 291 (top) and 294.

Dietitians of Canada
Simply Great Food
Recipes from this book are found on
pages 150, 152, 157, 160, 172, 175, 192,
199, 200, 201, 205, 211, 212, 218, 226,
228 (bottom), 238, 242, 243, 248, 250,
251, 252, 253, 260, 274, 287, 290, 292,
291 (bottom), 295 (bottom), 296, 299
(bottom), 300 (top), 302 (top) and 303.

Judith Finlayson
The Complete Whole Grains Cookbook
Recipes from this book are found on pages
174, 206, 236 and 239.

Judith Finlayson
The Convenience Cook
Recipes from this book are found on pages
169, 171, 181, 182, 188, 191, 237 and 262.

Judith Finlayson
The Healthy Slow Cooker
Recipes from this book are found on pages
151, 154, 155, 158, 159, 166, 257, 258, 282
and 283.

George Geary and Judith Finlayson
650 Best Food Processor Recipes
Recipes from this book are found on pages
170, 224, 225, 227, 228 (top), 230, 254,
261, 263, 265 and 284.

Jennifer MacKenzie
Recipes from this author are found on
pages 231, 235, 266, 280, 293, 295 (top),
297, 298, 299 (top), 300 (bottom), 301 and
302 (bottom).

Acknowledgments

I loved writing this book. I loved it because I enjoy researching, writing, and creating and because I strongly believe the book will make a difference for people with cancer. That belief kept me going, knowing there are people out there I can help. This book will allow me to reach them in a way private counseling never could. During this time, Monday became my favorite day of the week, because I got to sit at my computer and work on my book.

I am so grateful to have had a great team working with me, making the project such a joy. To the Robert Rose team — publisher Bob Dees; editors Bob Hilderley, Jennifer MacKenzie, and Sue Sumeraj; publicity manager Martine Quibell; and director of sales and marketing Marian Jarkovich — your expertise and guidance was exactly what this first-time writer needed, and I appreciate your nurturing. Thanks also to Kevin Cockburn of PageWave Graphics for the beautiful text design.

Writing a book is both an art and a science. When it comes to science, Serena Beber, Andrea Daley, Linda Kelemen, Anita McGowan, and Lucia Weiler set aside their own work to help me with research and keep the project moving forward, allowing me to produce an evidence-based work that professionals can trust.

I would also like to thank Sally Keefe Cohen, a most excellent literary consultant, and Daniela Fierini, who thought of me for this project and set the wheels in motion.

I appreciate all of the people who contributed recipes — the home economists, registered dietitians, and recipe developers who allowed me to select from their work recipes that would provide for the varied needs of these special readers. I am particularly grateful to Jennifer MacKenzie, the home economist who worked with me on the recipe section and whose experience, wisdom, and common sense provided much-needed direction and stability. Together, I believe we created a recipe section that cancer patients and their caregivers will find is tailored to their unique and specific needs — and I don't think that exists anywhere else.

Dr. Neil Berinstein literally saved my life in 1994, when I presented to him with Hodgkin's disease, which was filling my lungs with lymphatic fluids and drowning me in my own body. He saved me again, figuratively, when I so wanted to publish this book and he agreed to be my medical advisor on the project.

I want to acknowledge my focus group: the beautiful women of Wellspring who gave their time and wisdom. Until we met as a group, I don't think you realized how much your individual experiences with cancer could benefit others. Your goal of sharing your wisdom and sending it out into the universe can now be realized, and I know your survivor wisdom, scattered throughout the book, will resonate with readers.

Finally, this book would not have been possible without the unyielding support of my partner, Kathrin. You have always supported me, and that has kept me going through all the stages of this project. You remind regularly that "together we are strong."

Resources

Here's a sampling of some reliable cancer sites on the Internet.

Cancer Societies

American Cancer Society: www.cancer.org
Canadian Cancer Society: www.cancer.ca

Cancer Support

Cancer Support Community:
  www.cancersupportcommunity.org
Gilda's Club: www.gildasclub.org
Macmillan Cancer Support:
  www.macmillan.org.uk
Maggie's Cancer Caring Centres:
  www.maggiescentres.org
Paul D'Auria Cancer Centre:
  www.paulscancersupportcentre.org.uk
Virtual Hospice: www.virtualhospice.ca
Wellspring: www.wellspring.ca

Breast Cancer

American Breast Cancer Foundation:
  www.abcf.org
Breast Cancer: www.breastcancer.org
Canadian Breast Cancer Foundation:
  www.cbcf.org
National Breast Cancer Foundation:
  www.nationalbreastcancer.org

Colorectal Cancer

Bowel Cancer UK: www.bowelcanceruk.org.uk
Colon Cancer Foundation:
  www.coloncancerfoundation.org
Colorectal Cancer Association of Canada:
  www.colorectal-cancer.ca

Lung Cancer

Global Lung Cancer Coalition:
  www.lungcancercoalition.org
Lung Cancer Canada:
  www.lungcancercanada.ca
Lung Cancer Foundation of America:
  www.lcfamerica.org

Lymphoma

Lymphoma Foundation Canada:
  www.lymphoma.ca
Lymphoma Research Foundation:
  www.lymphoma.org

Prostate Cancer

Prostate Action: www.prostateaction.org.uk
Prostate Cancer Canada: www.prostatecancer.ca

Local Cancer Resources

BC Cancer Agency: www.bccancer.bc.ca
Memorial Sloan-Kettering Cancer Center:
  www.mskcc.org

Dietetic Associations

American Dietetic Association:
  www.eatright.org
British Dietetic Association: www.bda.uk.com
Dietitians of Canada: www.dietitians.ca

Nutrition and Health Information

American Institute of Cancer Research:
  www.aicr.org
Cancer Care Ontario: www.cancercare.on.ca.
Eat Right Ontario: www.eatrightontario.ca
Glycemic Index: www.glycemicindex.com
Health Canada: www.hc-sc.gc.ca/index-eng.php
HealthLink BC: www.healthlinkbc.ca
National Cancer Institute: www.cancer.gov
Office of Dietary Supplements, National
  Institutes of Health: www.ods.od.nih.gov

You Tube Channels

(go to www.youtube.com and type in these
organizations)
AICR (American Institute of Cancer Research;
  AICR also hosts video on Vimeo: www.vimeo.
  com/aicr)
American Cancer Society
Macmillan Cancer Support

References

Sources Used Throughout

American Cancer Society (www.cancer.org).
American Dietetic Association (www.eatright.org).
American Institute of Cancer Research (www.aicr.org).
BC Cancer Agency (www.bccancer.bc.ca).
British Dietetic Association (www.bda.uk.com).
Canadian Cancer Encyclopedia, Canadian Cancer Society (http://info.cancer.ca/cce-ecc/).
Canadian Cancer Society (www.cancer.ca).
Cancer Care Ontario (www.cancercare.on.ca).
Caring4Cancer (www.caring4cancer.com).
Eat Right Ontario (www.eatrightontario.ca).
Glycemic Index (www.glycemicindex.com).
Health Canada (www.hc-sc.gc.ca/index-eng.php).
HealthLink BC (www.healthlinkbc.ca).
National Academy of Sciences, The National Academies Press (www.nap.edu).
National Cancer Institute (www.cancer.gov).
Office of Dietary Supplements, National Institutes of Health (www.ods.od.nih.gov).
Practice-based Evidence in Nutrition (PEN), Dietitians of Canada (www.pennutrition.com).

Chapter 1: Conventional Cancer Therapies

McCallum PD, Grant B. *The Clinical Guide to Oncology Nutrition*, 2nd ed. New York: American Dietetic Association, 2006.

Chapter 2: Managing Side Effects and Concurrent Conditions

Fisher S, Bowman A, Mushins T, et al. *British Columbia Dietitians' and Nutritionists' Association Manual of Nutritional Care*. Vancouver: British Columbia Dietitians' and Nutritionists' Association, 1992:151–61.

Anemia

Pharmacist's Letter/Prescriber's Letter. 2008 Aug; 24(240811).

Appetite Loss, Anorexia and Cachexia

Choudry HA, Pan M, Karinch AM, Souba WW. Branched-chain amino acid-enriched nutritional support in surgical and cancer patients. *J Nutr*, 2006 Jan;136(1 Suppl):314S–18S.
Kumar NB, Kazi A, Smith T, et al. Cancer cachexia: Traditional therapies and novel molecular mechanism-based approaches to treatment. *Curr Treat Options Oncol*, 2010 Dec;11(3–4):107–17.
Liebman B. Under the influence: How external cues make us overeat. *Nutrition Action Health Letter* (Jacobson M, ed.), 2011 May;38(4):1–11.
Paccagnella A, Morassutti I, Rosti G. Nutritional intervention for improving treatment tolerance in cancer patients. *Curr Opin Oncol*, 2011 Jul;23(4): 322–30.
Tisdale MJ. Mechanisms of cancer cachexia. *Physiol Rev*, 2009 Apr;89(2):381–410.

Constipation

American Dietetic Association and Dietitians of Canada. *Manual of Clinical Dietetics*. Chicago: American Dietetic Association, 2000.
Tack J. Current and future therapies for chronic constipation. *Best Pract Res Clin Gastroenterol*, 2011 Feb;25(1):151–58.

Depression

Sánchez-Villegas A, Delgado-Rodríguez M, Alonso A, et al. Association of the Mediterranean dietary pattern with the incidence of depression: The Seguimiento Universidad de Navarra/University of Navarra follow-up (SUN) cohort. *Arch Gen Psychiatry*, 2009 Oct;66(10):1090–98.

Detox Diets

Detox Diets. *Mayo Clinic Women's HealthSource*, 2009 July;13(7):8. Available at: http://healthsource.mayoclinic.com/content/pdf.cfm?p=305/200907.PDF&d=OO8. Accessed June 13, 2011.

Diabetes

Canadian Diabetes Association. *Managing Your Blood Glucose*. Available at: http://www.diabetes.ca/diabetes-and-you/living/management/manage-glucose/. Accessed July 6, 2011.
Vigneri P, Frasca F, Sciacca L, et al. Diabetes and cancer. *Endocr Relat Cancer*, 2009 Dec;16(4): 1103–23.

Diarrhea

Brown AC, Valiere A. Probiotics and medical nutrition therapy. *Nutr Clin Care*, 2004 Apr–Jun;7(2):56–68.
Delia P, Sansotta G, Donato V, et al. Use of probiotics for prevention of radiation-induced diarrhea. *World J Gastroenterol*, 2007 Feb;13(6): 912–15.
Douglas LC, Sanders ME. Probiotics and prebiotics in dietetics practice. *J Am Diet Assoc*, 2008 Mar;108(3): 510–21.
Giralt J, Regadera JP, Verges R, et al. Effects of probiotic Lactobacillus casei DN-114 001 in prevention of radiation-induced diarrhea: Results from multicenter, randomized, placebo-controlled nutritional trial. *Int J Radiat Oncol Biol Phys*, 2008 Jul;71(4):1213–19.

Joneja J. Nutritional aspects of common food sensitivities: Celiac disease and lactose intolerance. *The Whitehall-Robins Report*, 2008 Sep;17(3).

McNeil Nutritionals. Lactose content list. Available at: http://www.lactaid.com/dairydigestion/dairy-digestion-test. Accessed June 30, 2011.

Visich KL, Yeo TP. The prophylactic use of probiotics in the prevention of radiation therapy-induced diarrhea. *Clin J Oncol Nurs*, 2010 Aug;14(4):467–73.

Dry Mouth

American Dietetic Association. Position of the American Dietetic Association: Ethical and legal issues in nutrition, hydration and feeding. *J Am Diet Assoc*, 2008 May;108:873–82.

GlaxoSmithKline. *Are You a Healthcare Professional Who Can Help with Symptoms of Dry Mouth?* Available at: http://www.biotene.com/Healthcare-professional/Symptoms.aspx. Accessed July 4, 2011.

National Institute of Dental and Craniofacial Research. *Oncology Pocket Guide to Oral Health.* Available at: http://www.nidcr.nih.gov/OralHealth/Topics/CancerTreatment/OncologyReferenceGuide. htm. Published March 25, 2011. Accessed July 4, 2011.

Oral Science. *X-PUR 100% Xylitol Gum/Mints.* Available at: http://www.oralscience.ca/en/products/gums_mints.html. Accessed July 4, 2011.

Pearce N. *Proper Dental Care for Cancer Patients.* Available at: http://blog.wellspring.ca/wp/2011/06/20/proper-dental-care-for-cancer-patients/. Published June 20, 2011. Accessed June 28, 2011.

Walsh L. Clinical assessment and management of the oral environment in the oncology patient. *Aust Dent J*, 2010;55(suppl 1):S66–S77.

Food Aversion

Hong JH, Omur-Ozbek P, Stanek BT, et al. Taste and odor abnormalities in cancer patients. *J Support Oncol*, 2009 Mar–Apr;7(2):58–65.

Heart Disease

Canadian Heart and Stroke Foundation website (www.heartandstroke.com).

Mayo Clinic Staff. *Mediterranean Diet: Choose This Heart-Healthy Diet Option.* Available at: http://www.mayoclinic.com/health/mediterranean-diet/CL00011. Published June 19, 2010. Accessed June 13, 2011.

Pauwels EK. The protective effect of the Mediterranean diet: Focus on cancer and cardiovascular risk. *Med Princ Pract*, 2011; 20(2):103–11.

Mouth Sores

Kuhn KS, Muscaritoli M, Wischmeyer P, Stehle P. Glutamine as indispensable nutrient in oncology: Experimental and clinical evidence. *Eur J Nutr*, 2010 Jun;49(4):197–210.

Mosel DD, Bauer RL, Lynch DP, Hwang ST. Oral complications in the treatment of cancer patients. *Oral Dis*, 2011 Sep;17(6):550–59.

National Institute of Dental and Craniofacial Research. *Oncology Pocket Guide to Oral Health.* Available at: http://www.nidcr.nih.gov/OralHealth/Topics/CancerTreatment/OncologyReferenceGuide. htm. Published March 25, 2011. Accessed July 4, 2011.

Pearce N. *Dental Care During Cancer Treatment.* Available at: http://blog.wellspring.ca/wp/2011/08/12/dental-care-during-cancer-treatment/. Published August 12, 2011. Accessed July 4, 2011.

Nausea

Dibble SL, Luce J, Cooper BA, et al. Acupressure for chemotherapy-induced nausea and vomiting: A randomized clinical trial. *Oncol Nurs Forum*, 2007 Jul;34(4):813–20.

Hickok JT, Roscoe JA, Morrow GR, Ryan JL. A phase II/III randomized, placebo-controlled, double-blind clinical trial of ginger (*Zingiber officinale*) for nausea caused by chemotherapy for cancer: A currently accruing URCC CCOP cancer control study. *Support Cancer Ther*, 2007 Sep 1;4(4):247–50.

Mandryk L. Ginger and chemo-induced nausea. *Oncology Network Infoletter*. Dietitians of Canada, 2010.

Morrow GR, Roscoe JA, Hickok JT, at al. Nausea and emesis: Evidence for a biobehavioral perspective. *Support Care Cancer*, 2002 Mar;10(2):96–105.

Murray M. *The Healing Power of Herbs: The Enlightened Person's Guide to the Wonders of Medicinal Plants*. Rocklin, CA: Prima Publishing, 1995.

Roscoe JA, Bushunow P, Morrow GR, et al. Patient expectation is a strong predictor of severe nausea after chemotherapy: A University of Rochester Community Clinical Oncology Program study of patients with breast carcinoma. *Cancer*, 2004 Dec 1; 101(11):2701–8.

Zick SM, Ruffin MT, Lee J, et al. Phase II trial of encapsulated ginger as a treatment for chemotherapy-induced nausea and vomiting. *Support Care Cancer*, 2009 May;17(5):563–72.

Taste Changes

Hong JH, Omur-Ozbek P, Stanek BT, et al. Taste and odor abnormalities in cancer patients. *J Support Oncol*, 2009 Mar–Apr;7(2):58–65.

Strasser F, Demmer R, Böhme C, et al. Prevention of docetaxel- or paclitaxel-associated taste alterations in cancer patients with oral glutamine: A randomized, placebo-controlled, double-blind study. *Oncologist*, 2008 Mar;13(3):337–46.

Vomiting

National Institute of Dental and Craniofacial Research. *Oncology Pocket Guide to Oral Health*. Available at: http://www.nidcr.nih.gov/OralHealth/Topics/CancerTreatment/OncologyReferenceGuide.htm. Published March 25, 2011. Accessed July 4, 2011.

Weight Gain and Obesity

McTiernan A. Obesity and cancer: the risks, science, and potential management strategies. *Oncology (Williston Park)*, 2005 Jun;19(7):871–81; discussion 881–82, 885–86.

Wound Healing

Guo S, Dipietro LA. Factors affecting wound healing. *J Dent Res*, 2010 Mar;89(3):219–29.

Chapter 3: Complementary Cancer Care

Barrett S. *Gastrointestinal Quackery: Colonics, Laxatives, and More*. Available at: http://www.quackwatch.org/01QuackeryRelatedTopics/gastro.html. Published August 4, 2010. Accessed August 17, 2011.

Courneya KS, Friedenreich CM. Physical activity and cancer: An introduction. *Recent Results Cancer Res*, 2011;186:1–10.

Faul LA, Jim HS, Minton S, et al. Relationship of exercise to quality of life in cancer patients beginning chemotherapy. *J Pain Symptom Manage*, 2011 May;41(5):859–69.

Gansler T, Kaw C, Crammer C, Smith T. A population-based study of prevalence of complementary methods use by cancer survivors: A report from the American Cancer Society's studies of cancer survivors. *Cancer*, 2008 Sep 1; 113(5):1048–57.

Hay L. *You Can Heal Your Life*. Carlsbad, CA: Hay House, Inc., 2004.

Ontario Breast Cancer Information Exchange Project. *A Guide to Unconventional Cancer Therapies*. 1994.

Chapter 4: Your Nutrition Toolbox

Inflammation

Béliveau R, Gingras D. *Foods That Fight Cancer: Preventing Cancer Through Diet*. Toronto: McClelland & Stewart, 2006.

Brasky TM, Lampe JW, Potter JD, et al. Specialty supplements and breast cancer risk in the VITamins And Lifestyle (VITAL) Cohort. *Cancer Epidemiol Biomarkers Prev*, 2010 Jul;19(7):1696–708.

Calder PC. n-3 polyunsaturated fatty acids, inflammation, and inflammatory diseases. *Am J Clin Nutr*, 2006 Jun;83(6 Suppl):1505S–19S.

Cavicchia PP, Steck SE, Hurley TG, et al. A new dietary inflammatory index predicts interval changes in serum high-sensitivity C-reactive protein. *J Nutr*, 2009 Dec;139(12):2365–72.

Daley CA, Abbott A, Doyle PS, et al. A review of fatty acid profiles and antioxidant content in grass-fed and grain-fed beef. *Nutr J*, 2010 Mar 10;9:10.

Field C. Workshop by Dr. Catherine J. Field, PhD, RD. April 26, 2010.

Gleissman H, Johnsen JI, Kogner P. Omega-3 fatty acids in cancer, the protectors of good and the killers of evil? *Exp Cell Res*, 2010 May 1;316(8):1365–73.

O'Sullivan A, O'Sullivan K, Galvin K, et al. Grass silage versus maize silage effects on retail packaged beef quality. *J Anim Sci*, 2002 Jun;80(6):1556–63.

Pierce BL, Ballard-Barbash R, Bernstein L, et al. Elevated biomarkers of inflammation are associated with reduced survival among breast cancer patients. *J Clin Oncol*, 2009 Jul 20;27(21):3437–44.

Prins RC, Rademacher BL, Mongoue-Tchokote S, et al. C-reactive protein as an adverse prognostic marker for men with castration-resistant prostate cancer (CRPC): Confirmatory results. *Urol Oncol*, 2012 Jan;30(1):33–37.

Fiber

Dong JY, He K, Wang P, Qin LQ. Dietary fiber intake and risk of breast cancer: A meta-analysis of prospective cohort studies. *Am J Clin Nutr*, 2011 Sep;94(3):900–905.

Finlayson J. *The Complete Whole Grains Cookbook: 150 Recipes for Healthy Living*. Toronto: Robert Rose Inc., 2008.

Schatzkin A, Mouw T, Park Y, et al. Dietary fiber and whole-grain consumption in relation to colorectal cancer in the NIH-AARP Diet and Health Study. *Am J Clin Nutr*, 2007 May;85(5):1353–60.

Villaseñor A, Ambs A, Ballard-Barbash R, et al. Dietary fiber is associated with circulating concentrations of C-reactive protein in breast cancer survivors: the HEAL study. *Breast Cancer Res Treat*, 2011 Sep;129(2):485–94.

Whole Grain Working Group. *UK Whole Grain Guidance*. Available at: http://www.igd.com/index.asp?id=1&fid=1&sid=4&tid=54&cid=169. Published November 21, 2007. Accessed July 2011.

Glycemic Index

Barclay AW, Petocz P, McMillan-Price J, et al. Glycemic index, glycemic load, and chronic disease risk — a meta-analysis of observational studies. *Am J Clin Nutr*, 2008 Mar;87(3):627–37.

Phytonutrients

Aune D, Lau R, Chan DS, et al. Nonlinear reduction in risk for colorectal cancer by fruit and vegetable intake based on meta-analysis of prospective studies. *Gastroenterology*, 2011 Jul;141(1):106–18.

Aravindaram K, Yang NS. Anti-inflammatory plant natural products for cancer therapy. *Planta Med*, 2010 Aug;76(11):1103–17.

Gupta SC, Kim JH, Prasad S, Aggarwal BB. Regulation of survival, proliferation, invasion, angiogenesis, and metastasis of tumor cells through modulation of inflammatory pathways by nutraceuticals. *Cancer Metastasis Rev*, 2010 Sep;29(3):405–34.

Kuhn KS, Muscaritoli M, Wischmeyer P, Stehle P. Glutamine as indispensable nutrient in oncology: Experimental and clinical evidence. *Eur J Nutr*, 2010 Jun;49(4):197–210.

Wayne SJ, Baumgartner K, Baumgartner RN, et al. Diet quality is directly associated with quality of life in breast cancer survivors. *Breast Cancer Res Treat*, 2006 Apr;96(3):227–32.

Soy and Breast Cancer

Caan BJ, Natarajan L, Parker B, et al. Soy food consumption and breast cancer prognosis. *Cancer Epidemiol Biomarkers Prev*, 2011 May;20(5):854–58.

Guha N, Kwan ML, Quesenberry CP Jr, et al. Soy isoflavones and risk of cancer recurrence in a cohort of breast cancer survivors: The Life After Cancer Epidemiology study. *Breast Cancer Res Treat*, 2009 Nov;118(2):395–405.

Kang X, Zhang Q, Wang S, et al. Effect of soy isoflavones on breast cancer recurrence and death for patients receiving adjuvant endocrine therapy. *CMAJ*, 2010 Nov 23;182(17):1857–62.

Shu XO, Zheng Y, Cai H, et al. Soy food intake and breast cancer survival. *JAMA*, 2009 Dec 9;302(22):2437–43.

Antioxidants

The Alpha-Tocopherol Beta Carotene Cancer Prevention Study Group. The effect of vitamin E and beta carotene on the incidence of lung cancer and other cancers in male smokers. *N Engl J Med*, 1994 Apr 14; 330(15):1029–35.

Doyle C, Kushi LH, Byers T, et al. Nutrition and physical activity during and after cancer treatment: An American Cancer Society guide for informed choices. *CA Cancer J Clin*, 2006 Nov–Dec;56(6):323–53.

Goodman M, Bostick RM, Kucuk O, Jones DP. Clinical trials of antioxidants as cancer prevention agents: Past, present, and future. *Free Radic Biol Med*, 2011 Sep 1; 51(5):1068–84.

Mocellin S. Vitamin D and cancer: Deciphering the truth. *Biochim Biophys Acta*, 2011 Dec;1816(2): 172–78.

Probiotics and Prebiotics

Bosscher D, Breynaert A, Pieters L, Hermans N. Food-based strategies to modulate the composition of the intestinal microbiota and their associated health effects. *J Physiol Pharmacol*, 2009 Dec;60 Suppl 6: 5–11.

Brown AC, Valiere A. Probiotics and medical nutrition therapy. *Nutr Clin Care*, 2004 Apr–Jun;7(2):56–68.

Choudry HA, Pan M, Karinch AM, Souba WW. Branched-chain amino acid-enriched nutritional support in surgical and cancer patients. *J. Nutr*, 2006 Jan;136(1 Suppl):314S–18S.

Douglas LC, Sanders ME. Probiotics and prebiotics in dietetics practice. *J Am Diet Assoc*, 2008 Mar;108(3): 510–21.

Paccagnella A, Morassutti I, Rosti G. Nutritional intervention for improving treatment tolerance in cancer patients. *Curr Opin Oncol*, 2011 Jul; 23(4):322–30.

Library and Archives Canada Cataloguing in Publication

LaMantia, Jean

The essential cancer treatment nutrition guide & cookbook : includes 150 healthy & delicious recipes / Jean LaMantia with Neil Berinstein.

Includes index.
ISBN 978-0-7788-0298-3

1. Cancer—Diet therapy—Recipes. 2. Cancer—Nutritional aspects. 3. Cookbooks I. Berinstein, Neil II. Title.

RC271.D52L36 2012   641.5'631   C2011-907460-5

Index